# Social Inequities and Contemporary Struggles for Collective Health in Latin America

This book explores the legacy of the Latin American Social Medicine and Collective Health (LASM-CH) movements and other key approaches—including human rights activism and popular opposition to neoliberal governance—that have each distinguished the struggle for collective health in Latin America during the twentieth and now into the twenty-first century.

At a time when global health has been pushed to adopt increasingly conservative agendas in the wake of global financial crisis and amidst the rise of radical-right populist politics, attention to the legacies of Latin America's epistemological innovations and social movement action are especially warranted. This collection addresses three crosscutting themes:

- First, how LASM-CH perspectives have taken root as an element of international cooperation and solidarity in the health arena in the region and beyond, into the twenty-first century.
- Second, how LASM-CH perspectives have been incorporated and restyled into major contemporary health system reforms in the region.
- Third, how elements of the LASM-CH legacy mark contemporary health social movements in the region, alongside additional key influences on collective action for health at present.

Working at the nexus of activism, policy, and health equity, this multidisciplinary collection offers new perspective on struggles for justice in twenty-first-century Latin America.

The chapters in this book were originally published as a special issue of the journal, *Global Public Health*.

**Emily E. Vasquez** is in the Department of Sociomedical Sciences at Columbia University, New York, NY, USA.

**Amaya Perez-Brumer** is at the Dalla Lana School of Public Health at the University of Toronto, Canada.

**Richard G. Parker** holds appointments at Columbia University, New York, NY, USA, the Federal University of Rio de Janeiro, Brazil, and the Brazilian Interdisciplinary AIDS Association.

T0175122

# Social Inequities and Contemporary Struggles for Collective Health in Latin America

*Edited by*
**Emily E. Vasquez, Amaya Perez-Brumer and Richard G. Parker**

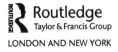

Routledge
Taylor & Francis Group
LONDON AND NEW YORK

First published 2020
by Routledge
2 Park Square, Milton Park, Abingdon, Oxon, OX14 4RN

and by Routledge
52 Vanderbilt Avenue, New York, NY 10017

*Routledge is an imprint of the Taylor & Francis Group, an informa business*

© 2020 Taylor & Francis

Chapter 1 © 2018 Eric D. Carter. Originally published as Open Access.
Chapter 9 © 2018 J. B. Spiegel, B. Ortiz Choukroun, A. Campaña, K. M. Boydell,
J. Breilh and A. Yassi. Originally published as Open Access.

*British Library Cataloguing in Publication Data*
A catalogue record for this book is available from the British Library

ISBN13: 978-0-367-90127-1

Typeset in Minion
by Newgen Publishing UK

**Publisher's Note**
The publisher accepts responsibility for any inconsistencies that may have arisen during
the conversion of this book from journal articles to book chapters, namely the inclusion
of journal terminology.

**Disclaimer**
Every effort has been made to contact copyright holders for their permission to reprint
material in this book. The publishers would be grateful to hear from any copyright holder
who is not here acknowledged and will undertake to rectify any errors or omissions in
future editions of this book.

# Contents

# Citation Information

The chapters in this book were originally published in the *Global Public Health*, volume 14, issue 6–7 (May 2019). When citing this material, please use the original page numbering for each article, as follows:

**Introduction**
*Social inequities and contemporary struggles for collective health in Latin America*
Emily E. Vasquez, Amaya Perez-Brumer and Richard G. Parker
*Global Public Health, volume 14, issue 6–7 (May 2019), pp. 777–790*

**Chapter 1**
*Social medicine and international expert networks in Latin America, 1930–1945*
Eric D. Carter
*Global Public Health, volume 14, issue 6–7 (May 2019), pp. 791–802*

**Chapter 2**
*Social medicine, feminism and the politics of population: From transnational knowledge networks to national social movements in Brazil and Mexico*
Rafael de la Dehesa
*Global Public Health, volume 14, issue 6–7 (May 2019), pp. 803–816*

**Chapter 3**
*Latin American social medicine across borders: South–South cooperation and the making of health solidarity*
Anne-Emanuelle Birn and Carles Muntaner
*Global Public Health, volume 14, issue 6–7 (May 2019), pp. 817–834*

**Chapter 4**
*Collective health and regional integration in Latin America: An opportunity for building a new international health agenda*
María Belén Herrero, Jorgelina Loza and Marcela Beatriz Belardo
*Global Public Health, volume 14, issue 6–7 (May 2019), pp. 835–846*

**Chapter 5**
*Revisiting the social determinants of health agenda from the global South*
Elis Borde and Mario Hernández
*Global Public Health, volume 14, issue 6–7 (May 2019), pp. 847–862*

For any permission-related enquiries please visit: www.tandfonline.com/page/help/permissions

# Notes on Contributors

**César Ernesto Abadía-Barrero** Department of Anthropology and Human Rights Institute, University of Connecticut, Storrs, CT, USA

**Martín Agrest** Proyecto Suma, Buenos Aires, Argentina

**Jana Villayzán Aguilar** Red Trans Perú, Lima, Peru

**Sara Ardila-Gómez** Facultad de Psicología, Instituto de Investigaciones, Consejo Nacional de Investigaciones Científicas y Técnicas (CONICET), Universidad de Buenos Aires, Buenos Aires, Argentina

**Eduardo Basz** Activist for the Human Rights of People with Disabilities, World Network of Users and Survivors of Psychiatry (WNUSP), Buenos Aires, Argentina

**Marcela Beatriz Belardo** Department of Public Law I, Faculty of Law, Universidad de Buenos Aires, Buenos Aires, Argentina

**Anne-Emanuelle Birn** Dalla Lana School of Public Health, University of Toronto, Toronto, Canada

**Elis Borde** Public Health, Universidad Nacional de Colombia, Bogotá, Colombia

**K. M. Boydell** Department of Psychiatry and Dalla Lana School of Public Health, University of Toronto, Toronto, Canada

**J. Breilh** Universidad Andina Simón Bolívar, Quito, Ecuador

**Brian J. Burke** Goodnight Family Sustainable Development Department, Appalachian State University, Boone, NC, USA

**Carlos F. Cáceres** Center for Interdisciplinary Studies in Sexuality, AIDS and Society, Universidad Peruana Cayetano Heredia, Lima, Peru

**A. Campaña** Universidad Andina Simón Bolívar, Quito, Ecuador

**Eric D. Carter** Geography Department, Macalester College, St. Paul, MN, USA

**H Daniel Castellanos** Hispanic AIDS Forum, New York, NY, USA

**B. Ortiz Choukroun** Universidad Andina Simón Bolívar, Quito, Ecuador

**Rafael de la Dehesa** Department of Sociology, City University of New York, New York, NY, USA

**Alberto Rodolfo Velzi Díaz** Facultad de Psicología, Universidad Nacional de Rosario, Santa Fe, Argentina

**Eduardo Faerstein** Department of Epidemiology, Institute of Social Medicine, State University of Rio de Janeiro, Rio de Janeiro, Brazil

**Ana Carolina Feldenheimer da Silva** Department of Nutrition in Public Health, University of State of Rio de Janeiro, Rio de Janeiro, Brazil

**Marina A. Fernández** Facultad de Psicología, Instituto de Investigaciones, Universidad de Buenos Aires, Buenos Aires, Argentina

**Mariana de Araújo Ferraz** School of Law, University of São Paulo, São Paulo, Brazil

**Karin Friederic** Department of Anthropology, Wake Forest University, Winston-Salem, NC, USA

**Fabio da Silva Gomes** Department of Noncommunicable Diseases and Mental Health, Pan-American Health Organization/World Health Organization, Washington, DC, USA

**Ignacio Méndez Gómez-Humaran** Centro de Investigación en Matemáticas - Sede Aguascalientes, Aguascalientes, Mexico

**Chris Hartmann** Department of Public Health, SUNY Old Westbury, New York, NY, USA

**Mario Hernández** Public Health, Universidad Nacional de Colombia, Bogotá, Colombia

**María Belén Herrero** Department of International Relations, Facultad Latinoamericana de Ciencias Sociales (FLACSO), Consejo Nacional de Investigaciones Científicas y Técnicas (CONICET), Buenos Aires, Argentina

**Paula Johns** ACT Health promotion, Rio de Janeiro, Brazil

**Deanna Kerrigan** Department of Sociology, Center on Health, Risk and Society, American University, Washington, DC, USA

**Guadalupe Ares Lavalle** Facultad de Psicología, Instituto de Investigaciones, Universidad de Buenos Aires, Buenos Aires, Argentina

**Lucila López** World Network of Users and Survivors of Psychiatry

**Jorgelina Loza** Instituto de Investigaciones Gino Germani, Universidad de Buenos Aires; Consejo Nacional de Investigaciones Científicas y Técnicas (CONICET), Buenos Aires, Argentina

**Jairo Ernesto Luna-García** Laboratorio de Ergonomía, Universidad Nacional de Colombia, Bogotá, Colombia

**Miluska Lusquiños** Movimiento Trans del Perú, Lima, Peru

**Qamar Mahmood** International Development Research Centre, Ottawa, Canada

**Oscar Javier Maldonado** Research group: Applied Ethics, Work and Social Responsibility, School of Human Sciences, Universidad del Rosario, Bogotá, Colombia

**Adriana Gisela Martinez-Parra** Doctorado en Ciencias en Salud Colectiva, Universidad Autónoma Metropolitana - Unidad Xochimilco, Mexico City, Mexico

**Hepzibah Muñoz Martínez** Department of History and Politics, University of New Brunswick, Saint John, Canada

**Amy Moran-Thomas** Anthropology, Massachusetts Institute of Technology, Cambridge, MA, USA

**Angélica Motta Ochoa** Center for Interdisciplinary Studies in Sexuality, AIDS and Society, Universidad Peruana Cayetano Heredia, Lima, Peru

**Carles Muntaner** Dalla Lana School of Public Health, University of Toronto, Toronto, Canada

**Chiharu Murata** Departamento de Metodología de la investigación, Instituto Nacional de Pediatría, Mexico City, Mexico

**Laura Rebecca Murray** Department of Health Policy, Planning, and Administration, Institute of Social Medicine, State University of Rio de Janeiro, Rio de Janeiro, Brazil

**Arón Núñez-Curto** Center for Interdisciplinary Studies in Sexuality, AIDS and Society, Universidad Peruana Cayetano Heredia, Lima, Peru

**Vera Silvia Paiva** Department of Social Psychology, Institute of Social Psychology – University of São Paulo, São Paulo, Brazil

**Richard G. Parker** Institute for the Study of Collective Health (IESC), Federal University of Rio de Janeiro, Rio de Janeiro, Brazil

**Ann Pederson** Population Health Promotion, BC Women's Hospital andHealth Centre, Vancouver, Canada

**Amaya Perez-Brumer** Dalla Lana School of Public Health, University of Toronto, Toronto, Canada.

**Ignacio Méndez Ramírez** Instituto de Investigaciones en Matemáticas Aplicadas y Sistemas, Universidad Nacional Autónoma de México, Mexico City, Mexico

**Elisabetta Recine** Observatory of Food and Nutrition Security Policies, Department of Nutrition, University of Brasilia, Brasília, Brazil

**Melina Rosales** Facultad de Psicología, Instituto de Investigaciones, Universidad de Buenos Aires, Buenos Aires, Argentina

**Ximena Salazar** Center for Interdisciplinary Studies in Sexuality, AIDS and Society, Universidad Peruana Cayetano Heredia, Lima, Peru

**Pamela Scorza** Department of Psychiatry, Columbia University, New York, NY, USA

**J. B. Spiegel** Department of English and Department of Theatre, Concordia University, Montreal, Canada

**Alicia Stolkiner** Facultad de Psicología, Instituto de Investigaciones, Universidad de Buenos Aires, Buenos Aires, Argentina

**Mauricio Torres-Tovar** Departamento de Salud Pública, Universidad Nacional de Colombia, Bogotá, Colombia

**Emily E. Vasquez** Department of Sociomedical Sciences, Columbia University, New York, NY, USA

**Santiago Javier Vivas** Facultad de Psicología, Universidad de Buenos Aires, Buenos Aires, Argentina

**A. Yassi** Global Health Research Program, School of Population and Public Health, University of British Columbia, Vancouver, Canada

# Introduction: Social inequities and contemporary struggles for collective health in Latin America

Emily E. Vasquez, Amaya Perez-Brumer and Richard G. Parker

**ABSTRACT**

As part of a planned series from *Global Public Health* aimed at exploring both the epistemological and political differences in diverse public health approaches across different geographic and cultural regions, this special issue assembles papers that consider the legacy of the Latin American Social Medicine and Collective Health (LASM-CH) movements, as well as additional examples of contemporary social action for collective health from the region. In this introduction, we review the historical roots of LASM-CH and the movement's primary contributions to research, activism and policy-making over the latter-half of the twentieth century. We also introduce the special issue's contents. Spanning 19 papers, the articles in this special issue offer critical insight into efforts to create more equitable, participatory health regimes in the context of significant social and political change that many of the countries in the region have experienced in recent decades. We argue that as global health worldwide has been pushed to adopt increasingly conservative agendas, recognition of and attention to the legacies of Latin America's epistemological innovations and social movement action in the domain of public health are especially warranted.

## Introduction

The field of global health has evolved significantly since the beginning of the twenty-first century with the rebranding of 'international health' to 'global health' (Birn, Pillay, & Holtz, 2017; Cueto, 2015). While this shift recognised and aimed to create new flows of health-related knowledge, resources and interconnected platforms for health governance (Brown, Cueto, & Fee, 2006), its impact has also had a homogenising effect on understandings of varied approaches to health. Paralleling criticism of globalisation more broadly (Labonte, Schrecker, Packer, & Runnels, 2009; Navarro, 1998), the field of global health has been leveraged primarily by actors from the global North (Beaglehole & Bonita, 2010; Macfarlane, Jacobs, & Kaaya, 2008), prioritising understandings of health problems and solutions from a northern perspective (Adams, Behague, Caduff, Löwy, & Ortega, 2019; Birn, 2011; Brown & Bell, 2008; Lakoff, 2010; Ollila, 2005; Ottersen et al., 2014). Indeed, roughly two decades after the rebranding to 'global health', little attention is paid to country or regional diversity regarding frameworks of public health and how these approaches fit under the umbrella of 'global health'. Certainly, frequent failure to recognise, teach, and meaningfully incorporate southern perspectives is not a condition in which the field arbitrarily finds itself. Instead, this reflects fundamental distributive injustices inherent to late global capitalism that have led to the political and financial empowerment of particular actors within the apparatus of global health, including the World Bank, International Monetary Fund, influential philanthropists, and corporations, in addition to multilaterals and state actors (Birn, 2014; Laurell, 2008; Mitchell & Sparke, 2016; Waitzkin & Jasso-Aguilar, 2015b). In response, this special issue is part of a planned series from *Global Public Health* aimed at encouraging recognition of epistemological and political alternatives reflected in public health approaches outside the global North. While *Global Public Health* itself is situated within flows of global North and English language scholarship, this series is committed to thinking broadly and deeply about public health traditions and approaches often unrecognised.

To contribute to greater recognition of epistemological diversity in how public health is understood and practiced, this collection of articles emphasises the legacy and applications of a distinct approach to public health that falls under the rubric of what we are designating as LASM-CH – Latin American Social Medicine and Collective Health (the latter an alternative terminology used especially [though not exclusively] in Brazil). LASM-CH is best understood as a rich and diverse intellectual current, shaped by both academics and activists and driven by key research centres, graduate programmes, and academic networks established in the region (Birman, 2005; Breilh, 2013; Granda Ugalde, 2008; Laurell, 1989; Paim & Almeida Filho, 1998; Tajer, 2003; Waitzkin, Iriart, Estrada, & Lamadrid, 2001). In particular moments, the LASM-CH movement has significantly influenced health policy reforms in Latin America, especially through the ascendance of actors who ascribe to the tradition to policymaking positions at the level of municipal, state, and regional governance (Briggs & Mantini-Briggs, 2009; Laurell, 2003; Tajer, 2003; Waitzkin, 2005). Broadly speaking, however, the LASM-CH movement has remained counter-hegemonic in the arenas of health policy and research alike (Almeida Filho, 1989, 2000; Breilh, 2003, 2008). Although it is not the only approach to public health in the region, and it co-exists in different ways with more conservative and technocratic perspectives in many countries, the LASM-CH movement has been the source of critical, innovative scholarship and policy alternatives from which the broader field of global health has and should continue to benefit (see also Adams et al., 2019; Holmes, Greene, & Stonington, 2014). Below we highlight the LASM-CH movement, as well as additional key approaches from the region at the nexus of activism, policy and health equity that have been influenced by or expanded on the LASM-CH legacy – particularly in the areas of human rights activism and recent popular opposition to neoliberal governance – in order to advance understanding of twenty-first century health politics in the region and the lessons they offer.

## The LASM-CH approach

Many accounts of the LASM-CH movement's history tie its intellectual roots to nineteenth century European social medicine and, in particular, to the scholarship of German pathologist and social scientist Rudolph Virchow, who viewed the material conditions of everyday life – especially those linked to class structure – as key causes of illness and early death and the state as having a key role in the protection of health (Tajer, 2003; Waitzkin, 2006; Waitzkin et al., 2001). Students and followers of Virchow's vision immigrated to Latin America, where social medicine perspectives increasingly gained footing, interacting with the importance of Marxist perspectives in Latin American social theory, and shaping a unique intellectual trajectory in response to the region's particular political conditions (Waitzkin et al., 2001).

By the 1930s social medicine had a stronghold in Chile and significantly influenced medical student Salvador Allende, who first as Minister of Health, later as Senator and ultimately as President would oversee the founding of Chile's first national health service – the first in the Americas to guarantee universal access to health services (Waitzkin, 2005). Over the course of his political career, Allende would also promote a range of additional reforms to achieve a more equitable income distribution and improve social conditions broadly, efforts that eventually inspired to a violent coup d'état in which he was killed in 1973 (Waitzkin et al., 2001). Other early key figures whose politics either reflected or resonated deeply with social medicine perspectives include (but are by no means limited to) anarchist physician Juan Lazarte who was active in the 1930s–1950s as a leader of one of

Argentina's medical unions; Peruvian hygiene expert Carlos Paz Soldán; Josúe De Castro of Brazil, who wrote 'The Geography of Hunger' (1952), analyzing of the structural roots of malnutrition and hunger; Ernesto ('Che') Guevara who would help lead the Cuban revolution in 1959; and physician and sociologist Juan César García who would serve as research coordinator within the Pan American Health Organization (PAHO) from 1966 to 1984 (Cueto & Palmer, 2015; Waitzkin et al., 2001).

Social medicine perspectives coalesced most visibly as a social movement in Latin America in reaction to authoritarian regimes that held power in the region through the 1970s and into the 1980s. Drawing on Marxist perspectives – the hegemonic theoretical current in Latin American social sciences at the time (Laurell, 1989) – and also particularly Engels' report on the condition of the working class in England, which was widely circulated among them, scholars, student activists, and political dissidents came together in nodes to critique of the prevailing capitalist social order fortified under these regimes and the associated decline in living and health conditions. Their organising and attempts to promote reform were at times met with violent consequences, as Allende and his followers earlier experienced in Chile (Tajer, 2003; Waitzkin et al., 2001). But despite instances of repression, this period spurred the founding of key organisations that united social medicine proponents in the region – particularly under the umbrellas of the Centro Brasileiro de Estudos de Saúde (CEBES) in 1976, the Associação Brasileira de Saúde Coletiva (ABRASCO) formed in 1979 (both in Rio de Janeiro), and the Latin American Social Medicine Association (ALAMES) founded in Ouro Preto, Brazil, in 1984. As re-democratisation swept the region understanding of health as a social right and one intimately connected to the full exercise of democracy was well-established across these groups (Cueto & Palmer, 2015). In Brazil, for example, activists in the sanitary reform movement and proponents of Collective Health in many ways spearheaded this moment of re-democratisation and the articulation of a new social contract broadly. They also developed a comprehensive plan for participatory health reform that would be written into the 1988 constitution and provide the architecture for the Brazilian Unified Health System or *Sistema Único de Saúde* (de Camargo, 2009; Paim, Travassos, Almeida, Bahia, & Macinko, 2011; Vieira-da-Silva & Pinell, 2014; Weyland, 1995).

Moreover, across these networks and centres – as well as key graduate programmes in social medicine and collective health being consolidated across the region – an anti-hegemonic approach to epidemiology itself emerged. This approach stood (and remains) in contrast to more conservative or mainstream public health approaches throughout the region and beyond and in opposition the principles underpinning decades of initiatives spearheaded by actors like the Rockefeller Foundation – initiatives that often involved vertical programming focused, especially, on enhancing the productivity of labour linked to US-based multinational corporations with presence in the region (Birn & Solórzano, 1999; Cueto, 1994). In this sense, early on, LASM-CH proponents recognised the science of epidemiology as an epistemological battleground and a direct expression of relations of power in society (Barreto, 2004; Breilh, 2003, 2008; Breilh & Granda, 1989). As Elis Borde and Mario Hernández have detailed in this issue, LASM-CH proponents have produced extensive critiques of mainstream epidemiological approaches, in particular regarding limitations to mainstream conceptualizations of causality and validity (Almeida Filho, 1989, 2000) and to risk-factor logic (Ayres, 1997; Breilh, 2003; Castiel, 1999; Castiel, Rodrigues Guilam, & Ferreira, 2010). Accordingly, Tajer (2003) has written, 'thus began a new and distinctive methodological tradition in the field: the critical and ideological analysis of what is usually presented as purely technical knowledge' (p. 2023).

Beyond these critiques, the LASM-CH movement has offered numerous proposals for re-approaching both epidemiology and public health practice more broadly. Classic tenets of the movement include: the integration of social science theory into health analyses (in particular Marxist perspectives, but also contributions from Foucault, Gramsci, Bourdieu, Althusser, Giddens, and Habermas, among others) and special attention to the impact of capitalist development on health; epidemiological analysis conducted through the lens of collectives (e.g. social class) rather than on groups of individuals; a commitment to *praxis* or the union of theory and practice so that academic analysis is also, at once, a political intervention; and an analytic focus on the dialectic relationship between health, disease, and care, rather than on static health outcomes (Franco, Nunes, Breilh, &

Laurell, 1991; Granados Cosme & Delgado Sánchez, 2006; Granda Ugalde, 2008; Irwin & Scali, 2007; Tajer, 2003; Waitzkin et al., 2001).

## Latin America as a laboratory for neoliberal reform

The LASM-CH movement's consolidation in the 1970s and 80s coincided with – and, in important ways, directly contributed to – an upwelling of support for health equity as a broad social goal and access to primary care services as articulated in the 1978 Alma-Ata declaration issued at the World Health Organization's International Conference on Primary Health Care. There now exists a well-developed historical literature on medicine and public health in Latin America that helps to situate the LASM-CH movement's contributions from this watershed moment in international health politics to the present (Birn et al., 2017; Birn & Necochea López, 2011; Cueto & Palmer, 2015; Palmer, 2010; Waitzkin & Jasso-Aguilar, 2015a). This begins with the resistance that arose almost immediately to Alma-Ata's articulation of its progressive (if not radical) Primary Health Care goals (Thomas & Weber, 2004). The Alma-Ata declaration contained three central themes cross-cutting its focus on comprehensive preventive services – it opposed expensive technology irrelevant to the needs of the poor, in favour of 'appropriate technology'; it opposed overspecialisation and medical elitism, in favour of community participation and intersectoral institutional engagement in meeting health goals; and, finally, it positioned health as an instrument for development, rather than its outcome (Cueto & Palmer, 2015). In opposition to these goals, a more conservative approach under the label of 'selective primary health care' was rapidly articulated under the purview of institutions including the World Bank, the Rockefeller Foundation, and UNICEF, as well as the influence of the for-profit sector. Proponents of 'selective primary health care' would advocate for a more limited understanding of primary health care centred, especially, on preventing childhood diseases through growth monitoring, oral rehydration techniques, breast-feeding, and immunisation (or GOBI).

As Cueto and Palmer (2015) have noted, 'though it did not provide the main impetus for the official push codified at Alma Ata, Latin America would become one of the great battlegrounds of its implementation' (p. 209). Indeed, although early progress toward establishing holistic primary health in settings like Costa Rica and Cuba had fuelled Alma-Ata's goals and values, over the course of the 1980s the conservative 'selective' approach to primary health care would become far more amenable to health policy makers in Latin America. This, as economic crisis swept the region in the wake of the Latin American debt crisis and given the clear preference at the time among international agencies like UNICEF for more focused, short-term, and technical interventions. The repression of comprehensive primary health care, however, was just a start.

Through the 1980s and into the 1990s, the World Bank (with the International Monetary Fund, the Interamerican Development Bank, and the U.S. Government) would increasingly assume the reins of international health policy making, promoting the Washington Consensus throughout the region and converting Latin America into a living laboratory of neoliberal macroeconomic reform (Laurell, 2000). This era of structural adjustment would entail the reduction and privatisation of state social services and safety-nets, the expansive opening of national economies to foreign trade and investment, the deregulation of finance capital, and the overall promotion of the market and its logic over a state-based social contract. In the domain of health this would mean the contraction and decentralisation of health care services and programmes, increasing precariousness of health professionals' terms of labour, emphasis on management efficiency, and growing prominence of private insurance and other forms of public-private partnerships in the sector (Cueto & Palmer, 2015; Pfeiffer & Chapman, 2010; Schrecker, 2016).

## Pushing beyond neoliberal public health

In response, LASM-CH proponents have taken as a central task the 'demystification of the processes of neoliberal health system reform' (Tajer, 2003, p. 2025) through the production of systematic evidence about its deleterious impact on the right to health. This work counts important points of intersection with research on the social determinants of health that fuelled WHO-level interest in this area as of the early 2000s. However, LASM-CH approaches to the social determinants of health should not be equated with discourse linked solely to the WHO Commission on the Social Determinants of Health launched in 2005. LASM-CH scholarship stands to offer more, particularly with regard to identifying and radically addressing the fundamental relations of power that drive social determinants of health, as various scholars from the region have articulated (Borde, Hernández-Álvarez, & Porto, 2015; Buss & Pellegrini Filho, 2007; CEBES, 2010; Eibenschutz, Tamez González, & González Guzmán, 2011; Gonzalez Guzman, 2009; Spiegel, Breilh, & Yassi, 2015). We return to this point further below.

Offering a further framework through which to oppose neoliberalism's impact on health, the LASM-CH central tenet of health as a universal, human right increasingly has taken a central role in state-level and regional health policy through the 1990s and into the twenty-first century (Meier & Ayala, 2014). This is perhaps not surprising in light of the important role that Latin American thinkers and activists have historically had in advocating for human rights considerations in international relations (Sikkink, 2015). But this was reinforced in significant ways over the course of the 1990s in relation to the emerging field of health and human rights (Stolkiner, 2010; Yamin & Frisancho, 2015). During this period, several Latin American countries were key sites for the development of participatory, rights-based approaches to reproductive health, playing key roles in and around the 1994 International Conference on Population and Development in Cairo (Shepard, 2006) and the Fourth World Conference on Women in Beijing in 1995 (Alvarez, 1999). Heavily influenced by LASM-CH approaches, policy-making in the region related to HIV and AIDS was also at the forefront of pioneering rights-based approaches to the global epidemic (Berkman, Garcia, Muñoz-Laboy, Paiva, & Parker, 2005; Cueto, 2001, 2019; Parker, 2009; Smallman, 2007). Rights-based policy-making related to mental health also underpinned a restructuring of psychiatric care throughout the Americas (Meier & Ayala, 2014). In addition, Latin American policymakers and activists have played an especially important role in questioning intellectual property rights and trade regimes that have limited access to medicines (Loyola, 2008; Vieira & Di Giano, 2019), and in promoting flexibilities such as the Doha Declaration on TRIPS and Public Health (Amorim, 2017a, 2017b).

Broad opposition to neoliberal governance culminated in the region over the early 2000s with the rise of leftist governments and constitutional reforms, comprising Latin America's populist 'pink tide'. These shifts ushered in a wave of health sector reforms across the region – most prominently in Venezuela, Uruguay, Bolivia, Ecuador, and Nicaragua. Such reforms were also visible in Mexico City, where LASM leader, physician, and sociologist Asa Cristina Laurell put LASM-CH principals into action as the city's Secretary of Health between 2000 and 2006 and in 2019 ascended to national leadership in the public health sector with the election of president Andrés Manuel López Obrador. Around the region, these reforms have explicitly recognised health as a socio-political endeavour, involved efforts to democratise health policymaking, and most importantly included steps to re-centre health as a state-guaranteed social right (Hartmann, 2016; Laurell, 2008). In Ecuador, Bolivia and Nicaragua, specifically, these 'post-neoliberal' strategies have been marked by fragile but hopeful attempts to redistribute capital surplus to social policies, to institute interculturality, to strengthen civil-society relations, and to articulate health-related objectives through the concept of 'living well' (i.e. Buen Vivir), even as states have struggled to overcome economic continuities from their neoliberal pasts and largely remained mired by market-oriented extractivism and varying degrees of fiscal restraint (Grugel & Riggirozzi, 2012; Hartmann, 2016; Rojas, 2017).

As we discuss below, during this period – and now especially as the region's 'pink tide' recedes and more conservative forces return to power in many countries across the region – LASM-CH researchers have taken up the work of evaluating these reforms to understand what lessons we might draw from them (Birn, Nervi, & Siqueira, 2016; Breilh, 2011). On the international stage as the field of global health has struggled to recover from the 2007/2008 global financial crisis (Navarro

& Muntaner, 2014), interest in the social determinants of health and human rights has similarly experienced a retreat in favour of 'cost-effectiveness', continued reliance on public-private partnerships, and public health interventions evermore narrowly targeting groups deemed to be at highest risk. Indeed, investments and political momentum in the field of global health are now moving away from action on the fundamental social processes that determine health, wellbeing and disease (Bekker et al., 2018; Benatar, Gill, & Bakker, 2011; Marmot & Bell, 2009; Schrecker, 2012; Schrecker & Bambra, 2015). In this context, Latin America and in particular the LASM-CH movement offers not only rich epistemological alternatives, but also systematic evidence and lessons drawn from attempts to move beyond neoliberal health policymaking and establish more just, equitable, and inclusive approaches.

## Into the twenty-first century: LASM-CH legacies and contemporary health social movements

What is the on-going legacy LASM-CH in the twenty-first century? This special issue brings together a collection of papers that respond to this question by addressing three cross-cutting themes: First, articles in this special issue examine the ways in which LASM-CH perspectives have remained an element of international cooperation and solidarity in the health arena in the region, and beyond, into the twenty-first century. Second, articles examine recent efforts toward major health system reforms carried out during what some scholars have termed the region's 'post-neoliberal era' (Hartmann, 2016). These articles foreground how LASM-CH perspectives have been incorporated and restyled in the midst of these reforms. Third, we include articles that examine cases of contemporary health social movements in the region, pointing to elements of the LASM-CH legacy within them and also to a range of other factors more broadly structuring collective action for health at present. These case studies bring forth aspects of the landscape of health politics in twenty-first century Latin America that have posed both opportunities for and challenges to struggles for improved health equity.

### Networks of international cooperation, solidarity, and knowledge

Although the influence of the LASM-CH tradition is often overlooked on the international stage, its impact on transnational circuits of intellectual and political exchange – within and beyond the region – is longstanding (Birn, 2006). Indeed, scholars in this issue, tracing the historic and contemporary trajectories of the LASM-CH approach, offer new understanding of the multidirectional and multi-level exchanges through which this tradition developed and disseminated.

In the first article included in this special issue, Eric Carter (2018) addresses the origins of social medicine's unique articulation in Latin America. While, as noted above, the ideals of social medicine are frequently believed to have migrated to Latin America from Europe – originating first among pioneers like Virchow, then travelling through academic circles, and later gaining institutional ground via the interwar efforts of international organisations – Carter argues that these were not simply one-way channels through which the ideals of social medicine were imported into the region. Instead, he shows that formal meetings sponsored by organisations including the League of Nations (LN) and the International Labour Organization (ILO) were 'sites of contestation over the causes of health inequalities, the universality of liberal welfare state policy models, and the role of science in policy' (p. 2). Carter writes that in the context of such venues 'Latin American experts seldom took their cues from European social medicine, and offered their own integrative and politically sophisticated analysis of social and structural causes of local public health crises' (p. 4). Indeed, he argues, in the 1930s and 1940s LASM perspectives avidly coalescing in the region clearly transcended the technocratic recommendations and less politically radical approaches to social medicine promoted by the Geneva-based institutions, in such policy domains as nutrition and social security.

In decades following those on which Carter focuses in this issue, repression of left-leaning health activists in the region would take place at the hands of the authoritarian regimes that came to power across Latin America during the Cold War era. In response, networks of cross-border solidarity and intellectual exchange would paradoxically increasingly solidify. Indeed, LASM-CH proponents not only built strong networks of solidarity across national borders through academic and civil society alliances, but they also formed key partnerships across and between activist networks. As Rafael de la Dehesa (2018) describes in his contribution to this issue, by the early 1970s LASM-CH and feminist groups in Brazil (and to a more limited extent in Mexico) formed key alliances through which to confront the global reproductive regime. Given the 'inscription of family planning within larger projects of economic development and geopolitical oppositions' (p. 3) the issue served as a 'bridge' between social medicine advocates and feminist collectives.

Networks of solidarity and knowledge exchange in which LASM perspectives were disseminated through the region also formed beyond the level of civil society, marking official foreign policy, as well, as Anne-Emanuelle Birn and Carles Muntaner (2018) clarify in their contribution to the issue. Focusing especially on Cuba as a key champion of official regional cooperation in the health sector, Birn and Muntaner note that this example of inter-state cooperation is often 'deliberately overlooked by most mainstream (Northern) observers' (p. 8), but has represented an important alternative to U.S.-dominated and conservative international cooperative efforts like the Pan-American Sanitary Bureau and initiatives of the International Health Division (IHD) of the Rockefeller Foundation.

Tracing the legacy of this south-south cooperation into the twenty-first century, María Belén Herrero, Jorgelina Loza, and Marcela Beatriz Belardo (2019), in their contribution to the special issue, describe the on-going impact of LASM-CH perspectives in the context of the Union of South American Countries (UNASUR). Founded in 2008 with the rise of leftist and progressive governments in many countries of the region (which vowed to restore the role of the state and counteract the effects of neoliberal policies on social welfare), this new project of regional integration has focused on health, its political determinants, and its implications for human rights. Drawing significantly on the intellectual resources available through the region's ALAMES network, the UNASUR Health Council has promoted 'movement toward horizontal cooperation and technical support, away from what its leaders view as an out-dated vertical model of donor and recipients' (p. 8–9). Although currently threatened with the rise of conservative leaders in the region, UNASUR member countries over the last decade have negotiated as a block to defend their interests 'in multilateral spaces, in front of the market and other international and transnational organizations' (p.8).

On the global stage of international cooperation in the context of WHO policy and programming, although the social determinants of health (SDH) approach has gained important ground, in this issue Elis Borde and Mario Hernández (2019) clarify that it is critical to recognise that the LASM-CH perspectives remain peripheral to these international efforts. Specifically, they argue the work and advances of the WHO's Commission on Social Determinants of Health (SDH) should not be understood to fully encompass or subsume more the radical and potentially more transformative LASM-CH perspectives. Indeed, they argue, the SDH approach falls far short of LASM-CH perspectives especially with regard to a 'comprehensive analysis of society, of power relations in society and the processes in which these determinants develop and are reproduced' (p. 6). Absent, as well, is 'discussion on political struggle, oppression and exploitation, that is, social processes that generate and substantiate unequal power relations in capitalist development models, let alone alternatives to capitalist development' (p. 6). In this sense, Borde and Hernández argue, LASM-CH perspectives remain a source of under-recognised alternative and notably progressive vision for how we may move forward globally toward a systematic reduction of health inequities, even as LASM-CH perspectives and concepts are continually being revised, advanced, and strengthened by researchers in the region (see Martinez-Parra, Abadía-Barrero, Murata, Méndez Ramírez, & Méndez Gómez-Humaran, 2018).

### National health system reforms

At the national level, Brazil represents a particularly notable stage on which the perspectives shared by the LASM and CH movements coalesced and gained broad recognition in the context of political transformation and associated health system reform. In the 1970s, amid collective action for democratisation in the face of military dictatorship and an upwelling of protest against the deteriorating social conditions brought about with Brazil's neoliberal 'economic miracle', the collective health or *saúde coletiva* movement emerged as an ideological approach to health as a social right (Cueto & Palmer, 2015). As noted above, by the late 1980s, the movement's representatives or *sanitaristas* had gained sufficient political strength to incorporate into Brazil's new constitution the framing for a universal, decentralised and participatory Unified Health System (SUS), a national project that continues to evolve today. In their contribution to this issue, Mahmood & Muntaner (2018) analyse the *sanitaristas'* efforts to integrate into the architecture of the SUS institutional spaces that would permit community participation and control over public policy – spaces that *sanitaristas* viewed as key to fostering an alternative social order to economic neoliberalism, under which private interests most often monopolised the ear of government. As Mahmood & Muntaner describe, this was achieved through the SUS, most notably, with the creation of Health Councils, where civil society would have the opportunity to formally engage in health policymaking at national, state, and municipal levels. In parallel with the construction of the SUS, in this issue Feldenheimer da Silva et al. (2018) detail the extraordinary achievements made toward integrating civil society into food and nutrition security (FNS) policy-making in Brazil. However, in parallel with challenges faced by the SUS, these authors note that with time it has become clear that 'while Brazil stands out as a reference in social participation and control in relation to FNS actions, the established participatory bodies have not been sufficient to avoid the deleterious political influence of agribusiness and big food companies' (p. 7).

Mahmood & Muntaner (2018), in their contribution to the issue, also describe similar attempts to democratise decision-making in health in Venezuela's *Barrio Adentro* programme established in 2003. Here they offer important insight into the health reform efforts initiated under the wave of leftist, anti-neoliberal governments that began to take power in Latin America at the turn of the millennium. Other contributors to this issue examine more recent examples of the region's 'pink tide' – most notably Ecuador, Bolivia, and Nicaragua – and efforts through state-led initiatives to engineer progressive, anti-neoliberal health sector reforms. These reforms to an extent incorporate LASM-CH values, even while maintaining ties to previous neoliberal models of health governance (see also Hartmann, 2016). Authors analysing these reforms in this issue point to the complexities involved under these 'post-neoliberal' regimes in establishing a new social contract that would account for broader dimensions of well-being in development goals, better address the social production of disease and strengthen state-society relations through civil society engagement.

For example, in this issue Friederic and Burke (2018) write that 'under President Rafael Correa's administration (2007–2017), the Ecuadorean Ministry of Health has established a state-centred, populist health care regime that incorporates elements of Latin American social medicine into a post-neoliberal platform' in a 'backlash against nearly two decades of neoliberal policies that aimed to radically marketise society, minimise the welfare and regulatory arms of the state, and convert basic social services into commodities' (p. 2) in Ecuador. However, through analysis focused on the particular community of Las Colinas in rural northwest Ecuador, the authors argue that Correa's National Plan for Good Living (*Buen Vivir*) and its state-centred healthcare reforms, have in this case paradoxically weakened existing community organising for collective health. In another of the issue's articles, Spiegel et al. (2018) examine a community-arts based intervention carried out in Ecuador under Rafael Correa's National Plan for Good Living (*Buen Vivir*), critically assessing its potential to support collective well-being in marginalised communities of urban Ecuador. Finally, Hartmann (2018) analyses in this issue the comparable 'Live Beautiful, Live Well' ('*Vivir Bonito, Vivir Bien*') initiative implemented in Nicaragua beginning in 2013 under President Daniel Ortega. Hartmann points to the ways in which environmental public health messaging disseminated through this government programme, only narrowly, if at all, escapes classic neoliberal invocations of individual responsibility for health and well-being, even while the campaign is veiled in rhetoric championing solidarity, shared responsibility, and recognition of cultural plurality. For these authors, contemporary efforts that engage social medicine in Latin America invoke LASM-CH perspectives, but do not constitute their broad adoption in the context of national reforms. Instead, LASM-CH ideals remain aspirational, indeed often radical, especially in comparison to more mainstream approaches to public health.

## Case studies in contemporary social action for health

The final group of articles in this special issue is dedicated to case studies of contemporary social action for health taking place across the region. Here we open the issue to scholars analysing action beyond the lens of LASM-CH perspectives. As a counter-hegemonic intellectual current in the region, proponents of LASM-CH perspectives have in many contexts and moments joined forces, worked parallel to or been complemented by other approaches to mobilisation for health as a social right. Here we draw out themes that emerge across these cases in order to contextualise the legacy of LASM-CH perspectives within a broader field of health politics in the region.

First, while LASM-CH proponents in some contexts historically subordinated identity-based struggles to a broader class-based or general social struggle (as noted by de la Dehesa, 2018), the entanglement of identity, citizenship and health has powerfully propelled key social movements in Latin America as elsewhere, particularly in the context of the struggle against HIV, as several contributions to the collection demonstrate. In this issue Laura Murray, Deanna Kerrigan, and Vera Silva Paiva (2018), for example, track the mobilisation of sex workers in Brazil who time and again have provocatively affirmed their rights as *'putas'*, defending prostitution both as work and as a sexual right. Sex workers in this context have fought for HIV policy and programming that explicitly acknowledges the link between HIV vulnerability and key structural factors including stigma, gender inequalities, and the criminalisation of sex work. In their contribution to the issue, Salazar et al. (2019) argue that the HIV-research industry in Peru has provided a context in which emergent transgender women's activism has taken shape. But this contribution to the issue and that of Castellanos (2019), which analyses LGBT activism in the Dominican Republic taking place amidst international funding for HIV prevention, both foreground an important cautionary: social action agendas carried out under the heavy shadow of international aid and research dollars has, in some cases, succumbed to a narrower public-health focus rather than assiduously pursing demands for political recognition and broader social rights.

Identity-linked struggles for health citizenship of course have not been limited to the domain of HIV. In their contribution to the issue, addressing a classic domain of LASM research and political action, Mauricio Torres-Tovar and Jairo Ernesto Luna-García (2019) describe the formation of associations of sick and disabled workers in Colombia. These have coalesced as a consequence of changes related to neoliberal labour, health and social security reforms of the early 1990s, which contributed to the erosion of working conditions and occupational health protections. Arising in response to a distinct set of political conditions, in this issue Ardila-Gómez et al. (2018) analyse the similar expansion of users' participation in the arena of mental health policymaking with the proliferation of user's associations in Argentina. These associations – though not to be confused with a social movement in and of themselves – have multiplied in the wake of national legislation mandating that psychiatric reform in Argentina follow a rights-based approach and engage users in participatory decision-making, which in turn took its cue from the United Nations Convention on the Rights of People with Disabilities.

Indeed, as several contributions to the special issue indicate, in Latin America, as elsewhere, leaders of contemporary social action initiatives for health are successfully leveraging international human rights treaties to advance their agendas. Most prominently in our collection, Hepzibah Muñoz Martínez and Ann Pederson (2018) offer insight into how civil society organisations in Argentina creatively mobilised the United Nations Convention on the Elimination of all Forms of Discrimination Against Women in order to win tobacco control legislation in the late 2000s. Arguing that marketing practices of tobacco predatorily targeted women, especially economically marginalised women, activists were able to leverage gender-based anti-discrimination protections to garner a public health win.

Another trend evident in the region in the context of social action over issues from violence to obesity, our collection points to activist coalitions' increasing reliance on health metrics and indicators as instruments to support struggles for health equity. Oscar Maldonado (2018), in his contribution, offers a cautionary narrative with regard to the use of 'scientized', quantitative data as the basis for health equity claims. He describes how feminist scholars and women's organisations mobilising in Colombia for the decriminalisation of abortion came to rely heavily on arguments grounded in global health logic and metrics (accounting for the burden of unsafe abortion in terms or women's mortality and morbidity) in order to re-frame debate away from issues of morality or gender-based rights. Although this move was key to the Colombian Constitutional Court's decision to decriminalise abortion, Maldonado explains that anti-abortion groups are now in turn mobilising quantitative evidence. Where statistics regarding the public health burden of unsafe abortion at first seemed to carry an illusion of 'objectivity', opponents have successfully cast doubt around the production and validity of these epidemiological facts, imperilling the infrastructure on which abortion decriminalisation was established.

Finally, our collection concludes with observations from Amy Moran-Thomas (2019) on Belize – an often-overlooked part of the region where, she writes, basic healthcare access has not historically been framed as a right of citizens. Moran-Thomas reminds us that while the legacy of health social movements may be exceptionally strong in Latin America, there are many patients whose experiences remain at the margins and who are still struggling to gain a collective voice in contexts of persistent neglect, if not abandonment. Describing the first rights-based patient activism in the history of Belizean national medicine, which emerged among patients seeking access to dialysis, Moran-Thomas points to measured, tenuous, but nonetheless hopeful signs that 'future visions of rights' could find footing even in where their legacies are absent.

## Conclusion

In the process of editing this special issue, we sought to bring together a wide array of scholars, working within the LASM-CH movement or studying advances in social action for collective health across multidisciplinary perspectives – history, epidemiology, anthropology, geography, and health policy. We were pleased by the response from Latin American authors, who constitute the majority of contributors to this collection. Indeed, contributing scholars are located across top institutions in the region, including the Universidad Andina Simón Bolívar, Universidad Nacional de Colombia, the Universidad Autónoma Metropolitana-Unidad Xochimilco, the Universidade do Estado do Rio de Janeiro, and FLASCO Argentina, to name a few. While this collection advances scholarship exploring the often under-recognised epistemological and political differences in public health across global regions, here we only brush the surface of the dynamic currents of LASM-CH-influenced research and other strands of health activism on-going in the region. We encourage readers to look to core LASM-CH institutions for additional resources, including ALAMES (alames.org), CEBES (cebes.org.br) and ABRASCO (abrasco.org.br). At a time when global health worldwide has been pushed to adopt increasingly conservative agendas in the wake of an extended global financial crisis, the rise of radical right populist politics, and the rupture of liberal democratic regimes, attention to legacies of Latin America's epistemological innovations and social movement action are especially warranted.

## Acknowledgements

This special issue has benefitted enormously from the involvement of contributing authors, many of whom also served as peer-reviewers on multiple papers for this issue. We are particularly grateful to Marcos Cueto and Anne-Emanuelle

Birn for their support in helping us shape the vision for this special issue and for supporting us in the dissemination of the call for papers. Additionally, we owe Eric Carter, Kenneth Camargo Jr., and César Torres Cruz a very special thank you for their close review of the introduction and their important suggestions for improvement which led us to, again, acknowledge the importance of collective health mobilisation in Latin America, not only historically but its contemporary application and re-articulations.

## Disclosure statement

No potential conflict of interest was reported by the authors.

## References

Adams, V., Behague, D., Caduff, C., Löwy, I., & Ortega, F. (2019). Re-imagining global health through social medicine. *Global Public Health*, 1–18. doi:10.1080/17441692.2019.1587639

Almeida Filho, N. d. (1989). *Epidemiologia sem números*. Rio de Janeiro: Editora Campus.

Almeida Filho, N. d. (2000). *La ciencia tímida. Ensayos de desconstrución de la epidemiología*. Buenos Aires: Lugar Editorial.

Alvarez, S. E. (1999). Advocating feminism: The Latin American feminist NGO 'boom'. *International Feminist Journal of Politics*, 1(2), 181–209. doi:10.1080/146167499359880

Amorim, C. (2017a). *Acting globally: Memoirs of Brazil's assertive foreign policy*. Lanham, Maryland: Hamilton Books.

Amorim, C. (2017b). Antecedentes internacionais da nova lei de patentes brasileira. In ABIA (Ed.), *As políticas de acesso a medicamentos e os direitos humanos no Brasil e no mundo* (pp. 7–10). Rio de Janeiro: ABIA.

Ardila-Gómez, S., Agrest, M., Fernández, M. A., Rosales, M., López, L., Velzi Díaz, A. R., … Stolkiner, A. (2018). The mental health users' movement in Argentina from the perspective of Latin American collective health. *Global Public Health*, 14(6–7), 1008–1019. doi:10.1080/17441692.2018.1514063

Ayres, J. R. (1997). *Sobre o risco*. São Paulo: Hucitec.

Barreto, M. L. (2004). The globalization of epidemiology: Critical thoughts from Latin America. *International Journal of Epidemiology*, 33(5), 1132–1137. doi:10.1093/ije/dyh113

Beaglehole, R., & Bonita, R. (2010). What is global health? *Global Health Action*, 3, 10.3402/gha.v3403i3400.5142. doi:10.3402/gha.v3i0.5142

Bekker, L.-G., Alleyne, G., Baral, S., Cepeda, J., Daskalakis, D., Dowdy, D., … Beyrer, C. (2018). Advancing global health and strengthening the HIV response in the era of the Sustainable development goals: The international AIDS society— *Lancet* commission. *The Lancet*, 392(10144), 312–358. doi:10.1016/S0140-6736(18)31070-5

Benatar, S. R., Gill, S., & Bakker, I. (2011). Global health and the global economic crisis. *American Journal of Public Health*, 101(4), 646–653. doi:10.2105/AJPH.2009.188458

Berkman, A., Garcia, J., Muñoz-Laboy, M., Paiva, V., & Parker, R. (2005). A critical analysis of the Brazilian response to HIV/AIDS: Lessons learned for controlling and mitigating the epidemic in developing countries. *American Journal of Public Health*, 95(7), 1162–1172. doi:10.2105/AJPH.2004.054593

Birman, J. (2005). A physis da saúde coletiva. *Physis: Revista de Saúde Coletiva*, 15, 11–16.

Birn, A.-E. (2006). O nexo nacional-internacional na saúde pública: O Uruguai e a circulação das políticas e ideologias de saúde infantil, 1890-1940. *História, Ciências, Saúde-Manguinhos*, 13, 675–708.

Birn, A.-E. (2011). Remaking international health: Refreshing perspectives from Latin America. *Revista Panamericana de Salud Publica*, 30, 106+.

Birn, A.-E. (2014). Philanthrocapitalism, past and present: The Rockefeller Foundation, the Gates Foundation, and the setting(s) of the international/global health agenda. *Hypothesis*, 12(1), e8. doi:10.5779/hypothesis.v12i1.229

Birn, A.-E., & Muntaner, C. (2018). Latin American social medicine across borders: South–South cooperation and the making of health solidarity. *Global Public Health*, 14(6–7), 817–834. doi:10.1080/17441692.2018.1439517

Birn, A.-E., & Necochea López, R. (2011). Footprints on the future: Looking forward to the history of health and medicine in Latin America in the twenty-first century. *Hispanic American Historical Review*, 91(3), 503–527. doi:10.1215/00182168-1300164

Birn, A.-E., Nervi, L., & Siqueira, E. (2016). Neoliberalism redux: The global health policy agenda and the politics of cooptation in Latin America and beyond. *Development and Change*, 47(4), 734–759. doi:10.1111/dech.12247

Birn, A.-E., Pillay, Y., & Holtz, T. H. (2017). *Textbook of global health* (4th ed.). New York: Oxford University Press.

Birn, A.-E., & Solórzano, A. (1999). Public health policy paradoxes: Science and politics in the Rockefeller Foundation's hookworm campaign in Mexico in the 1920s. *Social Science & Medicine*, 49(9), 1197–1213. doi:10.1016/S0277-9536(99)00160-4

Borde, E., & Hernández, M. (2019). Revisiting the social determinants of health agenda from the global south. *Global Public Health*, 14(6–7), 847–862. doi:10.1080/17441692.2018.1551913

Borde, E., Hernández-Álvarez, M., & Porto, M. F. d. S. (2015). Uma análise crítica da abordagem dos determinantes sociais da saúde a partir da medicina social e saúde coletiva latino-americana. *Saúde em Debate, 39*, 841–854.

Breilh, J. (2003). *Epidemiología crítica. Ciencia emancipadora e intercultural*. Buenos Aires: Universidad Nacional de Lanus, Lugar Editorial.

Breilh, J. (2008). Latin American critical ('social') epidemiology: New settings for an old dream. *International Journal of Epidemiology, 37*(4), 745–750. doi:10.1093/ije/dyn135

Breilh, J. (2011). La subversión del buen vivir (rebeldía esclarecida para el siglo XXI: Una perspectiva crítica de la obra de Bolívar Echeverría). *Salud Colectiva, 7*(3), 389–397.

Breilh, J. (2013). La determinación social de la salud como herramienta de transformación hacia una nueva salud pública (salud colectiva). *Revista Facultad Nacional de Salud Pública, 31*, 13–27.

Breilh, J., & Granda, E. (1989). [Epidemiology and heterogeny]. *Social Science & Medicine (1982), 28*(11), 1121-1127. doi:10.1016/0277-9536(89)90004-x

Briggs, C. L., & Mantini-Briggs, C. (2009). Confronting health disparities: Latin American social medicine in Venezuela. *American Journal of Public Health, 99*(3), 549–555. doi:10.2105/AJPH.2007.129130

Brown, T., & Bell, M. (2008). Imperial or postcolonial governance? Dissecting the genealogy of a global public health strategy. *Social Science & Medicine, 67*(10), 1571–1579. doi:10.1016/j.socscimed.2008.07.027

Brown, T. M., Cueto, M., & Fee, E. (2006). The World Health Organization and the transition from "international" to "global" public health. *American Journal of Public Health, 96*(1), 62–72. doi:10.2105/AJPH.2004.050831

Buss, P. M., & Pellegrini Filho, A. (2007). A saúde e seus determinantes sociais. *Physis: Revista de Saúde Coletiva, 17*, 77–93.

Carter, E. D. (2018). Social medicine and international expert networks in Latin America, 1930–1945. *Global Public Health, 14*(6–7), 791–802. doi:10.1080/17441692.2017.1418902

Castellanos, H. D. (2019). Santo Domingo's LGBT social movement: At the crossroads of HIV and LGBT activism. *Global Public Health, 14*(6–7), 963–976. doi:10.1080/17441692.2019.1585467

Castiel, L. D. (1999). *A medida do possível ... saúde, risco e tecnobiociências*. Rio de Janeiro: Editora Fiocruz.

Castiel, L. D., Rodrigues Guilam, M. C., & Ferreira, M. S. (2010). *Correndo o risco: Uma introdução aos riscos em saúde*. Rio de Janeiro: Editora Fiocruz.

CEBES. (2010). *Determinação social da saúde e reforma sanitária* Retrieved from http://cebes.org.br/biblioteca/determinacao-social-da-saude-e-reforma-sanitaria/.

Cueto, M. (1994). *Missionaries of science: The Rockefeller Foundation and Latin America*. Bloomington: Indiana University Press.

Cueto, M. (2001). *Culpa y coraje: Historia de las políticas sobre el VIH/Sida en el Perú*. Lima: Consorcio de Investigación Económica y Social / Universidad Peruana Cayetano Heredia.

Cueto, M. (2015). *Saúde global: Uma breve história*. Rio de Janeiro: Editora FIOCRUZ.

Cueto, M. (2019). Brazil and the changing meanings of 'universal access' to antiretrovirals during the early 21st century. In R. G. Parker, & J. García (Eds.), *Routledge Handbook on the politics of global health* (pp. 266–275). London and New York: Routledge.

Cueto, M., & Palmer, S. (2015). *Medicine and public health in Latin America: A history*. New York, NY: Cambridge University Press.

de Camargo, K. R. (2009). Celebrating the 20th anniversary of Ulysses Guimaraes' rebirth of Brazilian democracy and the creation of Brazil's national health care system. 2008. *American Journal of Public Health, 99*(1), 30–31. doi:10.2105/AJPH.2008.147868

de Castro, J. (1952). *The geography of hunger*. Boston: Little Brown.

de la Dehesa, R. (2018). Social medicine, feminism and the politics of population: From transnational knowledge networks to national social movements in Brazil and Mexico. *Global Public Health, 14*(6–7), 803–816. doi:10.1080/17441692.2018.1443486

Eibenschutz, C., Tamez González, S., González Guzmán, R., & Asociación Latinoamericana de Medicina Social, Universidad Autónoma Metropolitana, & Taller Latinoamericano sobre Determinantes Sociales de la Salud (2011). *Determinación social o determinantes sociales de la salud?: Memoria del Taller Latinoamericanos sobre Determinantes Sociales de la Salud*. Mexico, D.F.: Universidad Autónoma Metropolitana.

Feldenheimer da Silva, A. C., Recine, E., Johns, P., Gomes, F. d. S., Ferraz, M. d. A., & Faerstein, E. (2018). History and challenges of Brazilian social movements for the achievement of the right to adequate food. *Global Public Health, 14*(6–7), 875–883. doi:10.1080/17441692.2018.1439516

Franco, S., Nunes, E. D., Breilh, J., & Laurell, A. C. (1991). *Debates en medicina social. Organización Panamericana de la Salud—ALAMES*. Quito, Ecuador: Imprenta Non Plus Ultra.

Friederic, K., & Burke, B. J. (2018). La revolución ciudadana and social medicine: Undermining community in the state provision of health care in Ecuador. *Global Public Health, 14*(6–7), 884–898. doi:10.1080/17441692.2018.1481219

Gonzalez Guzman, R. (2009). Latin American social medicine and the report of the WHO commission on social determinants of health. *Social Medicine, 4*(2), 113–120.

Granados Cosme, J. A., & Delgado Sánchez, G. (2006). Temas médico-sociales en México: La maestría en Medicina Social y la revista Salud Problema. *Perfiles Educativos, 28*, 129–141.

Granda Ugalde, E. H. (2008). Alames turns 24. *Social Medicine, 3*(2), 165–172.

Grugel, J., & Riggirozzi, P. (2012). Post-neoliberalism in Latin America: Rebuilding and reclaiming the state after crisis. *Development and Change, 43*(1), 1–21. doi:10.1111/j.1467-7660.2011.01746.x

Hartmann, C. (2016). Postneoliberal public health care reforms: Neoliberalism, social medicine, and persistent health inequalities in Latin America. *American Journal of Public Health, 106*(12), 2145–2151. doi:10.2105/ajph.2016. 303470

Hartmann, C. (2018). 'Live beautiful, live well' ('Vivir Bonito, Vivir Bien') in Nicaragua: Environmental health citizenship in a post-neoliberal context. *Global Public Health, 14*(6–7), 923–938. doi:10.1080/17441692.2018.1506812

Herrero, M. B., Loza, J., & Belardo, M. B. (2019). Collective health and regional integration in Latin America: An opportunity for building a new international health agenda. *Global Public Health, 14*(6–7), 835–846. doi:10. 1080/17441692.2019.1572207

Holmes, S. M., Greene, J. A., & Stonington, S. D. (2014). Locating global health in social medicine. *Global Public Health, 9*(5), 475–480. doi:10.1080/17441692.2014.897361

Irwin, A., & Scali, E. (2007). Action on the social determinants of health: A historical perspective. *Global Public Health, 2*(3), 235–256. doi:10.1080/17441690601106304

Labonte, R. N., Schrecker, T., Packer, C., & Runnels, V. (eds.). (2009). *Globalization and health: Pathways, evidence and policy.* New York: Routledge.

Lakoff, A. (2010). Two regimes of global health. *Humanity: An International Journal of Human Rights, Humanitarianism, and Development, 1*(1), 59–79. doi:10.1353/hum.2010.0001

Laurell, A. C. (1989). Social analysis of collective health in Latin America. *Social Science & Medicine, 28*(11), 1183–1191. doi:10.1016/0277-9536(89)90011-7

Laurell, A. C. (2000). Structural adjustment and the globalization of social policy in Latin America. *International Sociology, 15*(2), 306–325. doi:10.1177/0268580900015002010

Laurell, A. C. (2003). What does Latin American social medicine do when it governs? The case of the Mexico city government. *American Journal of Public Health, 93*(12), 2028–2031. doi:10.2105/AJPH.93.12.2028

Laurell, A. C. (2008). Bringing Latin America's progressive health reforms out of the closet. *Social Medicine, 3*(2), 56–56.

Loyola, M. A. (2008). Medicamentos e saúde pública em tempos de AIDS: Metamorfoses de uma política dependente [Drugs, health policy and AIDS: Changes in a dependent policy]. *Ciência & Saúde Coletiva, 13*(1), 763–778. doi:10. 1590/S1413-81232008000700027

Macfarlane, S. B., Jacobs, M., & Kaaya, E. E. (2008). In the name of global health: Trends in academic institutions. *Journal of Public Health Policy, 29*(4), 383–401. doi:10.1057/jphp.2008.25

Mahmood, Q., & Muntaner, C. (2018). Theoretical underpinnings of state institutionalisation of inclusion and struggles in collective health in Latin America. *Global Public Health, 14*(6–7), 863–874. doi:10.1080/17441692. 2018.1455886

Maldonado, O. J. (2018). The decriminalisation of abortion in Colombia as cautionary tale. Social movements, numbers and socio-technical struggles in the promotion of health as a right. *Global Public Health, 14*(6–7), 1031–1043. doi:10.1080/17441692.2018.1504101

Marmot, M., & Bell, R. (2009). How will the financial crisis affect health? *BMJ: British Medical Journal, 338*(7699), 858–860.

Martinez-Parra, A. G., Abadía-Barrero, C. E., Murata, C., Méndez Ramírez, I., & Méndez Gómez-Humaran, I. (2018). Social class for collective health research: A conceptual and empirical challenge. *Global Public Health, 14*(6–7), 977–995. doi:10.1080/17441692.2018.1541098

Meier, B. M., & Ayala, A. S. (2014). The Pan American Health Organization and the mainstreaming of human rights in regional health governance. *The Journal of Law, Medicine & Ethics, 42*(3), 356–374. doi:10.1111/jlme.12152

Mitchell, K., & Sparke, M. (2016). The New Washington consensus: Millennial philanthropy and the making of global market subjects. *Antipode, 48*(3), 724–749. doi:10.1111/anti.12203

Moran-Thomas, A. (2019). Struggles for maintenance: Patient activism and dialysis dilemmas amidst a global diabetes epidemic. *Global Public Health, 14*(6–7), 1044–1057. doi:10.1080/17441692.2019.1596292

Muñoz Martínez, H., & Pederson, A. (2018). Global frameworks, local strategies: Women's rights, health, and the tobacco control movement in Argentina. *Global Public Health, 14*(6–7), 1020–1030. doi:10.1080/17441692.2018. 1442488

Murray, L. R., Kerrigan, D., & Paiva, V. S. (2018). Rites of resistance: Sex workers' fight to maintain rights and pleasure in the centre of the response to HIV in Brazil. *Global Public Health, 14*(6–7), 939–953. doi:10.1080/17441692.2018. 1510020

Navarro, V. (1998). Comment: Whose globalization? *American Journal of Public Health, 88*(5), 742–743.

Navarro, V., & Muntaner, C. (eds.). (2014). *Financial and economic crises and their impact on health and social well.* Amityville, NY: Baywood Publishing Co, Inc.

Ollila, E. (2005). Global health priorities – priorities of the wealthy? *Globalization and Health, 1*(1), 6. doi:10.1186/ 1744-8603-1-6

Ottersen, O. P., Dasgupta, J., Blouin, C., Buss, P., Chongsuvivatwong, V., Frenk, J., ... Scheel, I. B. (2014). The political origins of health inequity: Prospects for change. *The Lancet, 383*(9917), 630–667. doi:10.1016/S0140-6736(13)62407-1

Paim, J., & Almeida Filho, N. d. (1998). Saúde coletiva: Uma "nova saúde pública" ou campo aberto a novos paradigmas? *Revista de Saúde Pública, 32,* 299–316.

Paim, J., Travassos, C., Almeida, C., Bahia, L., & Macinko, J. (2011). The Brazilian health system: History, advances, and challenges. *The Lancet, 377*(9779), 1778–1797. doi:10.1016/S0140-6736(11)60054-8

Palmer, S. P. (2010). *Launching global health: The Caribbean odyssey of the Rockefeller Foundation.* Ann Arbor: University of Michigan Press.

Parker, R. G. (2009). Civil society, political mobilization, and the impact of HIV scale-up on health systems in Brazil. *Journal of Acquired Immune Deficiency Syndromes (1999), 52*(1), S49–S51. doi:10.1097/QAI.0b013e3181bbcb56

Pfeiffer, J., & Chapman, R. (2010). Anthropological perspectives on structural adjustment and public health. *Annual Review of Anthropology, 39*(1), 149–165. doi:10.1146/annurev.anthro.012809.105101

Rojas, R. (2017). The ebbing "pink tide": An autopsy of left-wing regimes in Latin America. *New Labor Forum, 26*(2), 70–82. doi:10.1177/1095796017700136

Salazar, X., Núnez-Curto, A., Villayzán Aguilar, J., Lusquiños, M., Motta Ochoa, A., & Cáceres, C. F. (2019). Confluent paths: Research and community participation to protect the right to health among transgender women in Peru. *Global Public Health, 14*(6–7), 954–962. doi:10.1080/17441692.2019.1599982

Schrecker, T. (2012). Multiple crises and global health: New and necessary frontiers of health politics. *Global Public Health, 7*(6), 557–573. doi:10.1080/17441692.2012.691524

Schrecker, T. (2016). Neoliberalism and health: The llinkages and the dangers. *Sociology Compass, 10*(10), 952–971. doi:10.1111/soc4.12408

Schrecker, T., & Bambra, C. (2015). *How politics makes us sick: Neoliberal epidemics.* New York, NY: Palgrave Macmillan.

Shepard, B. (2006). *Running the obstacle course to sexual and reproductive health: Lessons from Latin America.* Westport, Conn: Praeger Publishers.

Sikkink, K. (2015). Latin America's protagonist role in human rights. *Sur International Journal on Human Rights, 12* (22), 207–219.

Smallman, S. C. (2007). *The AIDS pandemic in Latin America.* Chapel Hill: University of North Carolina Press.

Spiegel, J. B., Ortiz Choukroun, B., Campaña, A., Boydell, K. M., Breilh, J., & Yassi, A. (2018). Social transformation, collective health and community-based arts: 'Buen Vivir' and Ecuador's social circus programme. *Global Public Health, 14*(6–7), 899–922. doi:10.1080/17441692.2018.1504102

Spiegel, J. M., Breilh, J., & Yassi, A. (2015). Why language matters: Insights and challenges in applying a social determination of health approach in a North-South collaborative research program. *Globalization and Health, 11*(1), 9. doi:10.1186/s12992-015-0091-2

Stolkiner, A. I. (2010). Human rights and the right to health in Latin America: The two faces of one powerful idea. *Social Medicine, 5*(1), 58–63.

Tajer, D. (2003). Latin American social medicine: Roots, development during the 1990s, and current challenges. *American Journal of Public Health, 93*(12), 2023–2027. doi:10.2105/AJPH.93.12.2023

Thomas, C., & Weber, M. (2004). The politics of global health governance: Whatever happened to "health for all by the year 2000"? *Global Governance, 10*(2), 187–205.

Torres-Tovar, M., & Luna-García, J. E. (2019). Struggles for the right to health at work in Colombia: The case of associations of workers with work-related illnesses. *Global Public Health, 14*(6–7), 996–1007. doi:10.1080/17441692.2018. 1552982

Vieira, M. F., & Di Giano, L. (2019). Taking on the challenge of implementing public health safeguards on the ground: The experience of Argentina and Brazil from a civil society perspective. In R. G. Parker, & J. García (Eds.), *Routledge Handbook on the politics of global health* (pp. 332–345). London and New York: Routledge.

Vieira-da-Silva, L. M., & Pinell, P. (2014). The genesis of collective health in Brazil. *Sociology of Health & Illness, 36*(3), 432–446. doi:10.1111/1467-9566.12069

Waitzkin, H. (2005). Commentary: Salvador Allende and the birth of Latin American social medicine. *International Journal of Epidemiology, 34*(4), 739–741. doi:10.1093/ije/dyh176

Waitzkin, H. (2006). One and a half centuries of forgetting and rediscovering: Virchow's lasting contributions to social medicine. *Social Medicine, 1*(1), 5–10.

Waitzkin, H., Iriart, C., Estrada, A., & Lamadrid, S. (2001). Social medicine then and now: Lessons from Latin America. *American Journal of Public Health, 91*(10), 1592–1601. doi:10.2105/AJPH.91.10.1592

Waitzkin, H., & Jasso-Aguilar, R. (2015a). Empire, health, and health care: Perspectives at the end of empire as we have known it. *Annual Review of Sociology, 41*(1), 271–290. doi:10.1146/annurev-soc-071913-043243

Waitzkin, H., & Jasso-Aguilar, R. (2015b). Imperialism's health component. *Monthly Review, 67,* 114–129.

Weyland, K. (1995). Social movements and the state: The politics of health reform in Brazil. *World Development, 23* (10), 1699–1712. doi:10.1016/0305-750X(95)00079-R

Yamin, A. E., & Frisancho, A. (2015). Human-rights-based approaches to health in Latin America. *The Lancet, 385* (9975), e26–e29. doi:10.1016/S0140-6736(14)61280-0

# Social medicine and international expert networks in Latin America, 1930–1945

Eric D. Carter

**ABSTRACT**
This paper examines the international networks that influenced ideas and policy in social medicine in the 1930s and 1940s in Latin America, focusing on institutional networks organised by the League of Nations Health Organization, the International Labour Organization, and the Pan-American Sanitary Bureau. After examining the architecture of these networks, this paper traces their influence on social and health policy in two policy domains: social security and nutrition. Closer scrutiny of a series of international conferences and local media accounts of them reveals that international networks were not just 'conveyor belts' for policy ideas from the industrialised countries of the US and Europe into Latin America; rather, there was often contentious debate over the relevance and appropriateness of health and social policy models in the Latin American context. Recognition of difference between Latin America and the global economic core regions was a key impetus for seeking 'national solutions to national problems' in countries like Argentina and Chile, even as integration into these networks provided progressive doctors, scientists, and other intellectuals important international support for local political reforms.

## Introduction

In recent years there has been rising interest in the history of social medicine in Latin America (Birn & Nervi, 2015; Galeano, Trotta, & Spinelli, 2011; Krieger, 2003; Porter, 2006; Waitzkin, 2011). Meanwhile, there have been calls in the history of public health in Latin America to go beyond national case studies (and even comparative studies) to more fully understand the dynamics of international and/or transnational institutions and networks (Birn, 2006; Birn & Necochea López, 2011; Borowy, 2009). This paper examines the international networks that influenced ideas and policy in social medicine in the 1930s and 1940s in Latin America. While the character, functions, and influence of international networks in Latin American social medicine since the 1970s are relatively well understood, as a result of living participants, better documentation, and the existence of key coordinating institutions, such as ALAMES (Galeano et al., 2011), for the 'first wave' of Latin American social medicine, rising in the interwar period and continuing into the 1940s, the contours of such international networks are less well understood.

Nevertheless, there are many assumptions about how ideas travelled internationally in social medicine. One commonplace notion is that the idea of social medicine migrated to Latin America from Europe, passed down from pioneers like Rudolph Virchow, in the mid-1800s, via his intellectual progeny, through academic networks, into Latin American countries, starting with 'early adopters' like Uruguay, Argentina, and Chile (Cueto & Palmer, 2015; Waitzkin, 2011). Another school of thought points to the efforts of progressive international institutions, such as the League of Nations (LN) and the International Labour Organization (ILO), which helped foster more integrative analyses of population health problems in line with social medicine (Dubin, 1995; Weindling, 1995, 2006).

Such narratives demand further scrutiny. One problem is that the influence of international networks is often inferred from the mere existence of associations or relationships (such as membership in organisations or attendance at conferences). Relatedly, ideas are often seen to flow, in a top-down or centre–periphery pattern, without due consideration of the give-and-take between Latin Americans and their counterparts abroad. We actually know little about how ideas in international health and social policy were received by the Latin American social medicine milieu.

This paper focuses primarily on the role of Latin American scientists and experts in formal institutional networks organised by the LN and the International Labour Organization during the 1930s, in two major policy domains, social security and nutrition. I argue that international networks were not just 'conveyor belts' (Plata-Stenger, 2015, p. 108) for policy ideas in these domains from the industrialised countries of the US and Europe into Latin America. Rather, international meetings were sites of contestation over the causes of health inequalities, the universality of liberal welfare-state policy models, and the role of science in policy. Latin Americans' participation in these networks tended to reinforce perceptions of difference between Latin America and the global geopolitical core regions; prompted the search for 'national solutions to national problems' in some Latin American countries; and fostered stronger intra-regional ties among progressive doctors, scientists, and other intellectuals interested in social medicine.

Thus, this paper embraces the newer historiographic tendency to 'fully reconsider so-called centre–periphery and imperial-colonial relations, emphasising how each party shapes and is shaped by others through multidirectional influences' (Birn & Necochea López, 2011, p. 519). To understand these relations, I build upon the work of historians who have pored over the Geneva archives for evidence of Latin American participation in the international health and welfare organisations of the interwar period. I extend this important research by emphasising the local reception of proposals from the international health and social policy episteme in two Latin American countries, Chile and Argentina, as conveyed in published and unpublished local materials, such as medical journals and conference proceedings.

Analysis of formally structured networks around social medicine is complicated by the fact that there were no prominent international organisations for the promotion and advancement of social medicine *per se*, despite the fact that the interwar period is understood as a period of florescence for social medicine. Generally rising usage of the term in noun (*medicina social*) or compound adjective (*médico-social*) forms during the 1930s – in journal, book, and article titles; academic departments; conferences and conference sections; and government programmes in Latin American countries – is a cue that the concept was gaining relevance. While no international meetings on social medicine, as such, were organised in the region during this time, it was a cross-cutting approach employed to analyze an array of health and social problems.

Although defining the field of social medicine is a challenge, two features made social medicine distinctive for its proponents and recognisable as an approach in health science and policy in the interwar period. First and foremost, social medicine advocated for an *integrative causal framework* that stressed the social, economic, and political causes of health problems, in tension with reductionist and increasingly prominent 'biomedical' frameworks (Löwy, 2011; Packard, 2016). Second, social medicine questioned the model of *liberal medicine* and called for the state to take a strong role in developing and regulating health systems to serve the collective needs of national populations. With faith in classically liberal, free-market principles at perhaps a low ebb during the economic crisis of the 1930s, such proposals were aligned with the ideological tendencies of the era.

In this paper, after examining the architecture of formal international networks I trace their influence on social and health policy in two areas: social security and nutrition. These were key issue domains that were both shaped by international networks and testing grounds for the relevance of social medicine ideas.

## Institutional panorama

Major Geneva institutions of the interwar period, the LN and the ILO, were idealistic experiments to sustain an international liberal political order. Due mainly to its failure to prevent the catastrophe of World War II, the LN particularly has long been dismissed as a failure in international governance, but a revisionist history emphasises the Geneva institutions' roles as pioneer in humanitarian internationalism and as a laboratory for social policy (Borowy, 2009; Kott & Droux, 2013; McPherson & Wehrli, 2015). The Geneva institutions developed a technocratic approach to governance, an ostensibly non-ideological style of policy innovation and transfer, which made them a forerunner to postwar international institutions such as the World Health Organization (WHO), United Nations, and the World Bank (Guthrie, 2013).

The League of Nations Health Organization (LNHO) played a key role in international health governance during the interwar period. The economic dislocations of the Great Depression moved the LNHO towards a 'social medicine' orientation in the research it sponsored and policies it supported (Packard, 2016). Ludwik W. Rajchman, a Polish bacteriologist who served in the key role of medical director of the LNHO from 1921 to 1939, was known for promoting a 'conception of a social medicine serving humanity' and the LNHO paid 'growing attention to social medicine in the 1930s, when [member] governments turned toward social welfare policies' (Dubin, 1995, pp. 59–63). The LNHO's activities shifted, from a focus on technical assistance in programmes to combat specific diseases and epidemiological surveillance, to a 'broader inquiry into disease etiology that encompassed the roles of nutrition, housing, working conditions, agricultural production, and the economy' (Packard, 2016, p. 57). In Europe, this new orientation was especially evident in rural hygiene and malaria policies (Packard, 2007, 2016; Weindling, 1995). But institutional weaknesses and concerns over political neutrality tempered the LNHO's leftward tilt (Dubin, 1995).

Similar to the LN, the ILO – generally known in Latin America as the OIT, Organización Internacional del Trabajo – had a high-minded purpose: that 'lasting peace can be established only if it is based on social justice,' and social justice – often used interchangeably with the concept of 'social peace' – could be achieved only through agreements between labour, capital, and the state, meeting together on equal footing (Guthrie, 2013; International Labour Office, 1944, p. 16). Intrinsic to the ILO's governance practices was the 'tripartite' format, whereby representatives of three parties (labour, employers, and the state) were supposed to negotiate and hammer out resolutions, which initially dealt with regulating industrial working conditions, at regular meetings in Geneva. Though the ILO was not conceived as a public health organisation, its policy models integrated labour and health issues in a variety of ways, first by seeking to address workplace safety, such as a ban on the manufacture of 'white lead' (basic lead carbonate), one of the first examples of international regulation of a chemical occupational hazard. In the 1930s, the ILO increasingly looked beyond questions of occupational safety, workplace conditions, and fair labour contracts towards broader questions of worker health and security.

The Geneva institutions, especially the LNHO, were notoriously 'Eurocentric,' and relations with Latin America were sporadic and slow to develop. Partly due to the costly and time-consuming travel to Geneva, Latin American presence in the LNHO was weak, although notables such as Carlos Chagas of Brazil and Gregorio Aráoz Alfaro of Argentina represented their countries at the LNHO (Dubin, 1995; Weindling, 2006). In dialogue with a French school of 'puericulture,' this Latin American contingent pushed for LN involvement in child and maternal health issues. The LN sponsored a conference on this topic in Montevideo in 1927, leading to the creation of the Instituto Internacional Americano de Protección de la Infancia (IIPI), also based in Uruguay. The IIPI served as a 'bridge' between the LN and American states, including the US though mainly Latin American countries, but at the same time it had considerable autonomy, both in financial terms and in setting an agenda on child health (Birn, 2006; Scarzanella, 2003). Meanwhile, ILO involvement in Latin America began in 1925 when Albert Thomas, the organisation's director, visited Chile to recognise the progressive labour and social laws its government had enacted in 1924. These included the creation of the

Caja del Seguro Obrero (CSO), a large social insurance fund that offered medical services, and Chile's prompt ratification of several ILO declarations (Wehrli, 2012).

During the tumultuous 1930s, in a push for legitimacy and to ensure their survival, the Geneva institutions increased their activities outside of Europe (Packard, 2016). The ILO intensified its engagements with the region in the 1930s, not least because the ILO leadership 'was aware that the organisation was in dire need of Latin American support if it wanted to survive the looming European crisis' (Plata-Stenger, 2015, p. 97). The ILO also recognised that, in comparison to Europe, Latin American countries were relatively peaceful and politically stable, and already showing demonstrable advances in welfare state policies (Herrera González, 2012). With much of the world's territory still colonised by European powers, Geneva found it hard to ignore Latin America's independent states, who were already involved with closely allied US-led health institutions, the Pan-American Sanitary Bureau (PASB) and the International Health Division (IHD) of the Rockefeller Foundation (RF). Such engagements, argue Cueto and Palmer (2015, p. 106), 'would provide the principal blueprint for the fully "international" health apparatus that emerged in the post-World War II era, when the nation-state became the global norm.'

Relations between the US- and Geneva-based institutions were complicated and inconsistent. While the US remained outside of the LN system, some Americans were well-placed within the LNHO's advisory body, and the RF enjoyed a 'symbiotic relationship' with the LNHO, supplying about 30 percent of its budget (Dubin, 1995). And while the ILO's relocation to Montreal, Canada during the war facilitated its work in the Americas, its leadership had to be mindful of Washington's desires and 'the competitive force of Pan-Americanism' (Singleton, 2012, p. 241). Meanwhile the United States reasserted its hemispheric hegemony with the soft diplomacy of initiatives like the Good Neighbor Policy of 1933 and an attempt to create a Pan-American Labor Organization to supplant the ILO in the Americas. As a result, the planning of meetings to discuss seemingly innocuous and technical policy matters often entailed fraught diplomatic negotiations behind the scenes (Herrera González, 2012; Singleton, 2012).

Ultimately, friction with the US kept Geneva's health institutions from developing strong and sustainable ties with Latin America. For example, the PASB was initially indifferent to child health initiatives, so it did not block the LN's sponsorship of the IIPI. However, just a few years later, PASB director Hugh Cumming (of the US) influenced the composition of the expert team conducting the LNHO-sponsored nutritional survey of Chile in 1935 and intervened to block LNHO sponsorship of a rural hygiene conference in Mexico the same year (Birn, 2006). The IHD's heavy involvement in the control of infectious and vector-borne diseases in Latin America deterred all LNHO efforts in this domain, except for a leprosy research centre in Rio de Janeiro (Birn, 2006).

Thus, during this period Latin American social policy experts, bureaucrats, and sympathetic politicians were often required to gauge and triangulate their interests against those of Europe and the United States. However, the root of these tensions did not necessarily lie in philosophical differences about health and social policy. Packard (2016), among others, has suggested that the Geneva institutions championed social medicine's programme of broader, systemic social and economic reforms, in sharp contrast with the outlook of the PASB and the IHD, which tended to support laboratory research and narrow, technical public health interventions, especially against infectious and vector-borne disease. Yet during the 1930s and 1940s the US supported the expansion of welfare states in Latin America, by promoting its own model of social security developed during Roosevelt's New Deal (Cohen, 1942; Jensen, 2011; Singleton, 2012). No doubt, the US exercised outsized influence in the PASB, but at the regular Pan-American Sanitary Conferences, US representatives exercised only loose control over the meeting agendas, and these meetings became a forum for discussion of a wide range of policy approaches, including some inspired in social medicine. As I discuss below, at international conferences on social security and nutrition, Latin American experts seldom took their cues from European social medicine, and offered their own integrative and politically sophisticated analyses of social and structural causes of local public health crises.

## Social security

The ILO was pivotal in disseminating social insurance, a product of Western European liberal state-craft, as a policy model around the world. ILO leaders viewed social insurance as one means to adjust the social contract between labour, capital, and the state, and thus to promote social peace. For some Latin American governments, social insurance was attractive since it offered a practical way to fund the expansion of healthcare services to reach a greater share of national populations. Indeed, one reason for governments to be involved with the ILO was to avail themselves of the technical expertise necessary to launch, finance, and administer these complex social insurance systems (Singleton, 2012).

Not surprisingly, the Latin American governments most involved with the ILO already had some semblance of a social insurance system, and Chile stands out in this respect (Cueto & Palmer, 2015; Labra, 2004). The official publications of Chile's CSO, *Acción Social* and *Boletín Médico-Social*, closely followed ILO meetings and conferences, the travels of its functionaries, and the fate of its many resolutions during the 1930s. In Chile, sustained involvement with the ILO depended on the entrepreneurial energy of people such as Francisco Walker Linares, who served as a 'correspondent' to the LN, and Moisés Poblete Troncoso, a lawyer and one of the few Latin Americans to actually hold a position in the central office of the ILO in Geneva (Wehrli, 2012). Poblete Troncoso was recommended as a candidate for this position because of his immersion in social and labour policy in Chile, along with his avoidance of partisan politics, and would go on to serve as advisor to other Latin American countries on social insurance issues (Martínez Franzoni & Sánchez-Ancochea, 2016; Pernet, 2013; Yáñez Andrade, 2012). Poblete Troncoso and Walker Linares also created a Chilean association in support of the LN; it was a small group, but one composed of influential members of a progressive Chilean political-intellectual elite (Wehrli, 2012).

Given Chile's already high level of participation in the ILO, Santiago was a natural choice for the first ILO Regional Labor Conference in Latin America, in January 1936 (Singleton, 2012). Unlike other networks around social medicine – such as eugenics, puericulture, hygiene, and nutrition, which were largely dominated by members of the medical profession and allied sciences – the ILO meetings brought together a wider range of professions, interests, and outlooks. Lawyers, economists, accountants, actuaries, and an increasingly professionalised labour union sector convened to discuss the intricacies of social insurance and industrial labour conditions, while medical professionals, who were protagonists in other expert networks, were mostly at the margins. Labour leaders, for their part, used the occasion of the 1936 Santiago conference to collaborate, strategize, and organise their own networks while adopting a cautious stance toward the ILO governance process (Herrera González, 2013). Coincidentally, the first Chilean National Medical Convention, a landmark in the history of the development of social medicine in the country, was held at the very same time, in Valparaíso, which might also explain the low turnout of physicians at the ILO meeting.

Despite several months of planning for the conference, led by Poblete Troncoso, the deliberations of the meeting largely departed from the narrow agenda set by the ILO. Adrien Tixier, the head of the ILO social security office, wanted to focus on moving Latin American countries toward ratification of declarations on just two issues: 'social insurance and the working conditions of women and children' (Plata-Stenger, 2015, p. 106), but in their speeches delegates covered a wide range of subjects, including immigration, monopolies, international trade, minimum salaries, the special problems of indigenous groups, and housing conditions. Labour union representatives made use of conversations outside of sessions to discuss the common interests of labour across the hemisphere and signed a pact to form a Latin American labour confederation, eventually realised in the formation of the CTAL, the Confederación de Trabajadores de América Latina (Herrera González, 2015). A lengthy discussion of *alimentación popular* (popular or public nutrition, roughly), discussed in more detail further on, was also a surprising departure from the conference agenda.

The discussion of social insurance policy was marked by a general affirmation of the ILO's objectives, but there were also intriguing silences, divergences, and skepticism, particularly from organised labour. The ILO's social insurance model centred on adjusting the labour contract to include 'sickness insurance' that encompassed, first, 'compensation' for lost wages, and second, 'restoration' of 'health and working capacity' (International Labour Office, 1935, pp. 50–51). The Latin American delegates at the Santiago conference offered a more expansive concept of social insurance, in line with social medicine, 'especially the need to link social insurance to other policies such as medical services' and 'to prevention, worker education on hygiene, and nutrition' (Plata-Stenger, 2015, p. 107). Voicing the concerns of the conference's social insurance committee, Edgardo Rebagliati, the governmental delegate from Peru, pointed to the special circumstances of Latin American countries, 'still in the critical stages of their organization,' which called for integrating social insurance into 'the fight against diseases, [which are] the eternal source of poverty, desperation, and decrepitude of nations' (O.I.T., 1936, p. 245). Some labour delegates viewed social insurance programmes with skepticism. Luis Solís Solís, the Chilean labour representative, rather than praising his country's social security system argued that the CSO was underfunded (due mainly to the meagre contribution required from employers), ineffectual (the country continued to suffer from rampant infectious diseases and high infant mortality, giving Chile 'one of the lowest life expectancies in the world'), and did nothing to address the underlying structural problem for Chilean labour, the gap between low wages and the extremely high cost of living (O.I.T., 1936, pp. 64, 255–256).

In the following decade, the ILO continued to strengthen its ties to Latin American states, by holding two more regional conferences in Havana in 1939 and Mexico in 1946, establishing several branch offices in the region, and working to develop a cadre of technical experts in social security (Jensen, 2011; Plata-Stenger, 2015). Meanwhile, social security was integrated into the hemispheric public health agenda: the Tenth Pan-American Sanitary Conference in Bogotá in 1938, sponsored by the PASB, offered express support for social security as a 'means to defend collective health' (Oficina Sanitaria Panamericana, 1938, p. 4). Unfortunately, the ideological and material commitments of the US to promoting social security systems and labour rights more generally in the region, through its influence on the ILO, diminished rapidly after World War II, while the PASB (reborn as PAHO) largely neglected social insurance as it concentrated efforts on the control of infectious and vector-borne diseases (Cueto, 2007; Jensen, 2011).

## Nutrition

During the 1930s, the Geneva Institutions became increasingly focused on the problem of adequate nutrition. Because of its 'clear connections with broader social and economic processes related to the production and consumption of food,' nutritional research was often caught between the integrative approach of social medicine and the reductionist tendencies of physiology and cell biology (Packard, 2016). Corinne Pernet (2013) contends that, compared to the ILO's broad social vision, the LNHO supported 'pure science' research in nutrition, with priority placed on defining international nutrition standards and tracing the health impacts of malnutrition, while largely neglecting how underlying social and economic conditions contributed to malnutrition. Even with this integrative approach, the ILO valued scientific research on nutrition to establish baseline standards for nutritional needs of workers and their families, a key component for calculating a 'living wage' (Pernet, 2013).

Both the LNHO and ILO supported expert missions to Latin America and sponsored conferences on nutrition. Absent a coherent policy agenda from Geneva, discussions of nutrition in Latin American circles were open, fluid, and wide-ranging. However, the same tensions between 'integrative approaches' and 'reductionist tendencies' played out among Latin American experts in nutrition, particularly with the region-wide leadership of Pedro Escudero of Argentina, who sought to elevate nutrition to a science and, quixotically, to isolate the realm of food and agriculture from everyday politics.

In one well-studied event in this larger process, in 1935 the LN sponsored a survey of nutritional conditions in Chile, led by Carlo Dragoni, of the University of Rome and the International Institute of Agriculture, and Etienne Burnet, formerly of the LNHO and then-director of the Pasteur Institute in Tunisia (Pernet, 2013; Scarzanella, 2003; Weindling, 2006; Yáñez Andrade, 2017). The Dragoni-Burnet survey 'bewildered European nutritionists' who found it hard to believe that many Chileans could survive on fewer than 900 calories per day, believed to be less than the minimum for survival (Borowy, 2009, p. 390; Wehrli, 2012). The report was 'not limited to information about food consumption, but also covered spending on housing, electricity, [and] fuel, offering a complete picture of the living conditions of the Chilean working class' (Scarzanella, 2003, p. 10).

Some Chilean commentators used the Dragoni-Burnet survey to expose the macro-structural causes of the country's nutrition crisis. One left-leaning medical journal asserted:

> Two technical experts of the League of Nations have reaffirmed what we have so often said about our country. Our people are dying of hunger, live in pigsties, and the level of abandonment and misery can be compared only with the most backwards countries on earth. The figures from Dragoni-Burnet completely confirm our tragedy, which is the same as all the Indo-American countries; a semi-feudal economy, overpowering influence of foreign imperialists and the creole oligarchy of bankers and landowners at their service. (*Boletín Médico de Chile*, 27 March 1937, p. 4.)

Here, as was so often the case, the pronouncements of respected international experts were used by local actors to support their insistent claims against recalcitrant governments and powerful social sectors (Weindling, 2006). The prestige of LN scientists validated what were becoming widespread calls for reform of the agricultural sector in Chile and attention to the social causes of malnutrition (Mardones Restat & Cox, 1942).

At the same time, however, the substance of Dragoni and Burnet's report was distorted to support certain political arguments. For example, while these European nutrition experts did collect social and economic data, they did not actually go so far as to ascribe the malnutrition crisis to imperialism and latifundia. The fact that the entire report was published only in French in Chile, and not until 1938, probably encouraged wide-ranging and competing interpretations of its findings (Dragoni & Burnet, 1938).

Nutrition dominated an entire day of discussion at the 1936 Labor Conference in Santiago, organised by the ILO, under the rubric of *alimentación popular*. Many delegates called for governments to intervene more directly in the production, distribution, and commercialisation of food, ranging from strict control of food advertising, subsidies and price-setting to reduce the cost of food, adjustments to wages in response to the high cost of living, and the reorganisation of national economies to improve markets for domestic food products, which involved road building and other infrastructure.

More radical perspectives on nutrition came from the labour sector. Vocal Chilean labour delegate Luis Solís Solís said, 'we are not interested' in participating in national partisan politics, because 'we are the opposition to a regime, to a system of exploitation' (O.I.T., 1936, p. 192). He went on to say, 'men will eat when food production and trade are in the service of the collective, and not for profit; that is, in a socialist society' (O.I.T., 1936, p. 192). 'In the meantime,' though, he proposed a more practical set of resolutions, calling for the ILO to support conducting more detailed surveys of salaries, diets, and the cost of living in member countries. Solís apparently understood the power of appealing to such numbers to establish the factual basis for policy discussions, even while dismissing the general reformist approach in social policy.

The ILO leadership was caught off-guard by the interest in *alimentación popular* at the 1936 Santiago Conference, and the resolutions related to nutrition approved at the meeting received little attention back in Geneva (Pernet, 2013). But persistent Latin American interest in the issue, along with political uncertainties in Europe, compelled the LN to hold its Third International Nutrition Conference in Buenos Aires in 1939. While the first two of these conferences, held in Geneva in 1937 and 1938, had almost exclusively European representation, in Buenos Aires the situation was reversed. With the exception of the LN's own representative, Louis Rasminsky, and the U.S. delegate Hazel K. Stiebeling, all of the attendees were from Latin America and the Caribbean. And in contrast to the 1936 ILO-sponsored Santiago conference, where medical and scientific professionals were largely absent, the 1939 Buenos Aires meeting was dominated by those with a medical background, led by Pedro Escudero, whose Argentine National Institute of Nutrition was widely admired by nutritionists across Latin America (Buschini, 2016). Notably, only one person attended both the 1936 Santiago labour conference and the 1939 Buenos Aires nutrition conference: Alejandro Unsain, Argentina's representative to the ILO (Ramacciotti, 2015).

There was scant consensus at the conference on the best approach to addressing persistent nutritional problems. Escudero and the other Argentine delegates tended to emphasise the high quality of their research on nutrition, including the advanced state of data collection on working class consumption habits. Juan Collazo explained how Uruguay's government had, for at least a decade, given priority to managing and regulating all aspects of the food economy, making the country almost self-sufficient in food, available at reasonable prices, with high nutritional standards that were largely being met. José J. Rada of Peru promoted 'comedores populares' (also called 'restaurantes populares'), which were large government-run cafeterias that offered standardised, balanced menus at subsidised prices, aimed especially at urban industrial workers (Drinot, 2005). Peruvian delegates had also showcased this programme at the 1936 Santiago labour conference, and similar strategies had recently been attempted in Chile, as part of an effort spearheaded by Minister of Health Eduardo Cruz-Coke to improve 'alimentación popular' (Zárate Campos, 2012). Yet Escudero, for his part, worried that restaurantes populares were mainly a tool of political patronage, with the potential to 'break apart the family' at meal time, which should be 'the family hour, serving to gather the family together for its spiritual integration.' By contrast, restaurantes populares, absent any 'social and technical control' from nutritional experts, would lead to comunización, an allusion to socialist collectives of the time in the Soviet Union (Escudero, 1940b, p. 333; 1940c, p. 246).

Despite these differences, by sharing their national experiences, delegates discovered a common set of development problems across the region that tended to make food more expensive and less healthful: lack of good roads, monopolies in the food industry, export agriculture, imported foods, deficient salaries, regional diets, ignorance of the science of nutrition, and economic policy priorities. Summarising the proceedings, Escudero stated that the conference 'had demonstrated the reality of a spiritual union of the Latin countries: the same problem concerns them, the same malady burdens them. All [delegates] felt united to seek out the path towards liberation' (Escudero, 1940b, p. 335). Distinctive socioeconomic conditions and shared cultural roots meant that 'South America should take on the problem of nutrition with an American approach.'

The notion of a culturally distinctive Latin America faced with common social and public health problems was typical of the time, and evidence of a rising class of regional scientific experts resistant to longstanding European hegemony in their fields (Cueto & Palmer, 2015). But this project of Latin American identity formation took on new texture in a pair of articles Escudero wrote in 1940 for the Argentine magazine *Viva Cien Años*, which served as a popular forum for advice on healthy living. Drawing on some of the national cases presented at the 1939 conferences, Escudero adopted an idiom familiar to eugenicists, explaining that, 400 years after the Conquest, indigenous and mestizo peoples of the continent continued in a state of biological 'slavery,' holding on to diets that made them 'obedient, lacking in rebelliousness, without a spirit of improvement' (Escudero, 1940a, pp. 140–145). In line with the prevailing spirit of eugenics, a movement that he was not formally affiliated with, Escudero perceived that social discord and political tensions had biological roots, specifically in the degenerative effects of malnutrition concentrated and passed down, over time, in distinct ethnic groups. In this way, the nutritional studies of Escudero and others fit with the central tendency of so-called 'Latin' eugenics, that genetic endowment was not determinative of health or life chances, which could be shaped by medical and social interventions, guided by science, in nutrition, hygiene, sanitation, and education (Reggiani, 2010).

Despite Escudero's interpretations for a general Argentine audience, the discourse on race was muted during the 1939 conference. Possibly, delegates perceived that it was impolitic to speak in highly racialized terms in international scientific forums. In late 1939, when the conference took place, Europe was already at war and the LN was seen as a failure in international governance.

But the LN was also anti-fascist and its agenda aimed, albeit unsuccessfully, to limit the excesses of virulent nationalisms underwritten, in part, by the science of eugenics. In a way, the LNHO and its sponsorship of nutrition studies anticipated the 'anti-racist' rationale of international research in biomedicine of the post-war period (Wade, 2017, pp. 28–29). Thus, international networks fostered by the prestigious Geneva institutions may have tamed or moderated racialized explanations of social problems.

## Discussion: Latin America and international social medicine

In contrast to core–periphery or imperial-colonial models, Anne-Emanuelle Birn's model of 'circulation' helps us make sense of how ideas in social medicine flowed through international networks. By circulation, Birn means that 'health and scientific ideologies, policies, and practices undergo an intricate process of give and take among multiple actors who are linked in particular professional, political, and practical circles' (Birn, 2006, p. 57). Using this lens, we can see that there was no purposeful diffusion and slavish emulation of a school of social medicine thought from Europe. Ultimately, the Geneva-led initiatives in Latin America added little to advance an already vibrant 'social medicine' movement. If anything, Latin Americans presented a more politically radical and epistemologically integrative view of social medicine and the welfare state that exceeded the modest and technocratic recommendations of the Geneva institutions.

Engagement with broader international networks brought another tension into sharp relief for Latin American experts, between internationalism and universalism (Wehrli, 2012). The ILO, in particular, tried to diffuse social policy models it saw as viable everywhere. Latin Americans at the regional labour conferences were not convinced, instead contending that many ILO resolutions were not relevant for Latin American countries, where industrial development was incipient. At these meetings, Latin American delegates had the eye-opening experience of finding some common interests and even a common frame around the experience of international economic depression from a dependent, semi-colonial position. These core–periphery tensions were subtle at the ILO meetings, but they reflect a larger intellectual project of Latin American identity construction of the 1930s, and anticipate the appeal of geopolitically attuned structuralist and dependency theories in Latin American development during the Cold War era.

The activities of the Geneva institutions may have helped to temper the influence of the Latin American eugenics movement. While ideas about racial degeneration of national populations permeated social policy discourse in the interwar period, at the Latin American conferences sponsored by the ILO and the LN, calls for eugenicist measures to raise the quality of the population were infrequent. Experts in social security and nutrition apparently saw little explanatory power in eugenics, which privileged constitutional-biological or genetic mechanisms to explain population health conditions. In a study of José Francisco Socarrás, a Colombian doctor, Stefan Pohl-Valero persuasively demonstrates that there was no inherent contradiction between reductionist nutrional science and the key eugenicist project of preventing 'racial degeneration' (Pohl-Valero, 2016). Yet as the case of Pedro Escudero shows, by the late 1930s Latin American experts were perhaps mindful that the rhetoric of race science and eugenics was inappropriate on the international stage but still acceptable and even persuasive for national audiences. Quite possibly, as the 1930s progressed, the Latin American eugenicists' network became tighter but also more isolated, cut off from more important currents in health and social policy, and out of step with the movement towards more expansive welfare states, a key legacy of social medicine.

Overall, formal international networks influenced the development of social medicine in Latin America in the 1930s, but probably in a limited way. Latin American experts' awareness of international health and social policy trends probably resulted more from a lettered culture of scientific publication and diffusion, while interpersonal contacts in professional networks at specific events like conferences may have been secondary in importance. Journals such as *Acción Social* or *Boletín Médico-Social* in Chile reported constantly on health and social policy innovations elsewhere in the region, the US, the Soviet Union, Western Europe, and even Asia. The news of the 1939 Buenos Aires conference reverberated widely and quickly, thanks to widely disseminated publications like the *Boletín de la Oficina Sanitaria Panamericana*. For example, within months of the conference, the young doctor José Maria Bengoa – apparently disconnected from these formal networks – incorporated Escudero's recommendations into his treatise on social medicine in the Venezuelan countryside (Bengoa, 1992 [1940], pp. 82–84).

The Geneva institutions were able to conduct studies and convene conferences on important issues like nutrition and social security, but hardly established the deep and integrated networks that led to the building of strong and lasting institutions in Latin America. Unlike international development institutions of the Cold War era, the Geneva institutions had almost no financial or geopolitical leverage, such as development aid, to promote their agenda in the region. The ILO and LN worked most effectively in countries with existing pro-Geneva associations and energetic policy entrepreneurs, like Chile and Argentina. Moreover, it is fair to say that the 'circulation' of ideas was not complete, as Latin America's influence on European social medicine appears to have been minimal. However, it may be the case that their impact was delayed, given the key role played by Latin American states in forming the WHO, based on principles of universal social and health rights (Cueto & Palmer, 2015).

## Conclusions

Tracing these international networks is valuable for understanding the development of social medicine and the expansion of welfare states in Latin America. One little-recognized role of these networks is that they did a lot of epistemological 'work,' i.e. defining problems, delineating boundaries between fields of study, propelling the development of new fields, and exploring explanations that crossed between disciplinary domains. Social medicine's tendencies were always centrifugal, integrative, and anti-reductionist, expanding the boundaries of the study and practice of medicine to include the study of the political-economic and social structures that shaped life chances. If the ILO and the LN offered something like a 'social medicine' perspective and advanced the development of strong welfare states, they did so in a Latin American context where such proposals were already gaining acceptance. And while the US stance towards Geneva institutions was often aloof, it is important not to exaggerate philosophical and policy differences between them. At least into the late 1940s, the US lent support to welfare state initiatives in Latin America, through the example of its own progressive social security legislation and the wide-ranging agendas of the Pan-American Sanitary Conferences.

One limitation of this paper is the necessarily partial analysis of international networks, focused on Geneva- and US-based multilateral institutions. More analysis is needed of less obvious, even dissident networks in social medicine, outside the boundaries of international scientific technocracy. As Weindling (2006) and Pernet (2013) point out, most of the Latin Americans involved in Geneva-sponsored policy networks were well-established public health officials, who valued stability and order, and thus looked for ways to manage and reform society scientifically, or technocratically, while staying above the fray of ordinary politics. Yet more politically radical groups of medical professionals, which are often recognised in national histories of social medicine (e.g. anarcho-syndicalist doctors such as Juan Lazarte in Argentina or the socialist-leaning 'Vanguardia Médica' group in Chile that included a young Salvador Allende), were not integrated at all into the networks analyzed in this paper. Tracing these networks would be challenging but rewarding, as their influence shows in the radical, collectivist strands of thought that characterise Latin American social medicine.

## Disclosure statement

No potential conflict of interest was reported by the authors.

## Funding

This work was supported by American Council of Learned Societies (ACLS).

## References

Bengoa, J. M. (1992 [1940]). *Sanare–hace 50 años: medicina social en el medio rural venezolano*. Caracas.

Birn, A.-E. (2006). The national-international nexus in public health: Uruguay and the circulation of child health and welfare policies, 1890–1940. *História, Ciências, Saúde-Manguinhos, 13*(3), 675–708.

Birn, A.-E., & Necochea López, R. (2011). Footprints on the future: Looking forward to the history of health and medicine in Latin America in the twenty-first century. *Hispanic American Historical Review, 91*(3), 503–527.

Birn, A.-E., & Nervi, L. (2015). Political roots of the struggle for health justice in Latin America. *The Lancet, 385*(9974), 1174–1175. doi:10.1016/s0140-6736(14)61844-4.

Borowy, I. (2009). *Coming to terms with world health: The League of Nations Health Organisation 1921–1946.* Frankfurt am Main: Peter Lang.

Buschini, J. D. (2016). La alimentación como problema científico y objeto de políticas públicas en la Argentina: Pedro Escudero y el Instituto Nacional de la Nutrición, 1928–1946. *Apuntes: Revista de Ciencias Sociales, 43* (79), 129–156.

Cohen, W. J. (1942). The first Inter-American Conference on Social Security. *Social Security, 5*(10), 4–7.

Cueto, M. (2007). *The value of health: A history of the Pan American Health Organization.* Rochester, NY: University of Rochester Press.

Cueto, M., & Palmer, S. (2015). *Medicine and public health in Latin America: A history.* New York, NY: Cambridge University Press.

Dragoni, C., & Burnet, E. (1938). L'alimentation populaire au Chili. *Revista Chilena de Higiene y Medicina Preventiva, 1*(10-12), 407–611.

Drinot, P. (2005). Food, race and working-class identity: Restaurantes populares and populism in 1930s Peru. *The Americas, 62*(2), 245–270.

Dubin, M. D. (1995). The League of Nations Health Organisation. In P. Weindling (Ed.), *International health organisations and movements, 1918–1939* (pp. 56–80). Cambridge: Cambridge University Press.

Escudero, P. (1940a). El problema de la alimentación en América Latina. *Viva Cien Años, 9*(3), 140–145.

Escudero, P. (1940b). La Tercera Conferencia Internacional de la Alimentación. *Oficina Sanitaria Panamericana, 19*, 330–336.

Escudero, P. (1940c). Mejoremos la alimentación en América. *Viva Cien Años, 9*(4), 232–236, 244–246.

Galeano, D., Trotta, L., & Spinelli, H. (2011). Juan César García and the Latin American social medicine movement: Notes on a life trajectory. *Salud Colectiva, 7*(3), 285–315.

Guthrie, J. (2013). The ILO and the international technocratic class, 1944–1966. In S. Kott & J. Droux (Eds.), *Globalizing social rights* (pp. 115–134). New York, NY: Palgrave Macmillan.

Herrera González, P. (2012). La primera conferencia regional del trabajo en América: su influencia en el movimiento obrero (1936). In F. Herrera León & P. Herrera González (Eds.), *América Latina y la OIT: Redes, cooperación técnica e institucionalidad social (1919-1950)* (pp. 175-213). Morelia: Instituto de Investigaciones Históricas, Universidad Michoacana de San Nicolás de Hidalgo.

Herrera González, P. (2013). El pacto por la unidad obrera continental: sus antecedentes en Chile y México, 1936. *Estudios de Historia Moderna y Contemporánea de México, 46,* 87–119.

Herrera González, P. (2015). Beyond social legislation: Worker unity in Latin America and its links to the International Labour Organization, 1936–1938. In A. McPherson & Y. Wehrli (Eds.), *Beyond geopolitics: New histories of Latin America at the League of Nations* (pp. 115–134). Albuquerque: UNM Press.

International Labour Office. (1935). *Report on social insurance. First item on the agenda, Conference of American States Members of the International Labour Organisation, Santiago de Chile, December 1935–January 1936.* Geneva: International Labour Office.

International Labour Office. (1944). 'Declaration of Havana,' adopted 30 Nov 1939 at Second Labor Conference of the American States, Havana. *International Labour Office Official Bulletin, 25*(1), 16–17.

Jensen, J. (2011). From Geneva to the Americas: The International Labor Organization and inter-American social security standards, 1936–1948. *International Labor and Working-Class History, 80,* 215–240.

Kott, S., & Droux, J. (2013). *Globalizing social rights: The International Labor Organization and beyond.* New York, NY: Palgrave Macmillan.

Krieger, N. (2003). Latin American social medicine: The quest for social justice and public health. *American Journal of Public Health, 93*(12), 1989–1991.

Labra, M. E. (2004). Medicina Social en Chile: propuestas y debates (1920–1950). *Cuad Méd Soc, 44*(4), 207–219.

Löwy, I. (2011). Historiography of biomedicine: "Bio," "medicine," and in between. *Isis, 102*(1), 116–122. doi:10.1086/658661.

Mardones Restat, J., & Cox, R. (1942). *La alimentación en Chile. Estudios del Consejo Nacional de Alimentación.* Santiago: Imprenta Universitaria.

Martínez Franzoni, J., & Sánchez-Ancochea, D. (2016). *The quest for universal social policy in the south: Actors, ideas and architectures.* Cambridge: Cambridge University Press.

McPherson, A., & Wehrli, Y. (2015). *Beyond geopolitics: New histories of Latin America at the League of Nations.* Albuquerque: UNM Press.

O.I.T. (1936). *Conferencia del Trabajo de los Estados de América miembros de la Organización Internacional del Trabajo: Santiago de Chile 2 al 14 de enero de 1936, actas de las Sesiones.* Ginebra: O.I.T.

Oficina Sanitaria Panamericana. (1938). Acta final, Décima Conferencia Sanitaria Panamericana (celebrada en Bogotá, Colombia, septiembre 4–14, 1938). *Boletín de la Oficina Sanitaria Panamericana, 126,* 1–14.

Packard, R. M. (2007). *The making of a tropical disease: A short history of malaria.* Baltimore, MD: Johns Hopkins University Press.

Packard, R. M. (2016). *A history of global health: Interventions into the lives of other peoples.* Baltimore, MD: Johns Hopkins.

Pernet, C. A. (2013). Developing nutritional standards and food policy: Latin American reformers between the ILO, the League of Nations Health Organization, and the Pan-American Sanitary Bureau. In S. Kott & J. Droux (Eds.), *Globalizing social rights: The international labour organization and beyond* (pp. 249–261). New York, NY: Palgrave Macmillan.

Plata-Stenger, V. (2015). 'To raise awareness of difficulties and to assert their opinion': The international labour office and the regionalization of international cooperation in the 1930s. In A. McPherson & Y. Wehrli (Eds.), *Beyond geopolitics: New histories of Latin America at the League of Nations* (pp. 97–113). Albuquerque: UNM Press.

Pohl-Valero, S. (2016). Alimentación, raza, productividad y desarrollo. Entre problemas sociales nacionales y políticas nutricionales internacionales (Colombia, 1890–1940). In G. Mateos & E. Suárez-Díaz (Eds.), *Aproximaciones a lo local y lo global: América Latina en la historia de la ciencia contemporánea* (pp. 115–154). México: Centro de Estudios Filosóficos, Políticos y Sociales Vicente Lombardo Toledano.

Porter, D. (2006). How did social medicine evolve, and where is it heading? *PLoS Medicine, 3*(10), e399.

Ramacciotti, K. I. (2015). Transnational dialogues between specialist and institutional knowledge in occupational accident legislation, first half of the twentieth century. *História, Ciências, Saúde-Manguinhos, 22,* 201–219.

Reggiani, A. H. (2010). Depopulation, fascism, and eugenics in 1930s Argentina. *Hispanic American Historical Review, 90*(2), 283–318.

Scarzanella, E. (2003). Los pibes en el Palacio de Ginebra: Las investigaciones de la Sociedad de las Naciones sobre la infancia latinoamericana (1925–1939). *Estudios interdisciplinarios de América Latina y el Caribe, 14*(2), 5–30.

Singleton, L. (2012). The ILO and social security in Latin America, 1930–1950. In F. Herrera León & P. Herrera González (Eds.), *América Latina y la OIT: Redes, cooperación técnica e institucionalidad social (1919–1950)* (pp. 215-243). Morelia: Instituto de Investigaciones Históricas, Universidad Michoacana de San Nicolás de Hidalgo.

Wade, P. (2017). *Degrees of mixture, degrees of freedom: Genomics, multiculturalism, and race in Latin America.* Durham: Duke University Press.

Waitzkin, H. (2011). *Medicine and public health at the end of empire.* Boulder, CO: Paradigm Publishers.

Wehrli, Y. (2012). Francisco Walker Linares: un actor del internacionalismo ginebrino en Chile (1927–1946). In F. Herrera León & P. Herrera González (Eds.), *América Latina y la OIT: Redes, cooperación técnica e institucionalidad social (1919–1950)* (pp. 56–85). Morelia: Instituto de Investigaciones Históricas, Universidad Michoacana de San Nicolás de Hidalgo.

Weindling, P. (1995). Social medicine at the League of Nations Health Organisation and the International Labour Office compared. In P. Weindling (Ed.), *International health organisations and movements, 1918–1939* (pp. 134–153). Cambridge: Cambridge University Press.

Weindling, P. (2006). The League of Nations Health Organisation and the rise of Latin American participation, 1920–40. *História, Ciências, Saúde – Manguinhos, 13*(3), 1–14.

Yáñez Andrade, J. C. (2012). La OIT y la red sudamericana de corresponsales. El caso de Moisés Poblete, 1922–1946. In F. Herrera León & P. Herrera González (Eds.), *América Latina y la OIT: Redes, cooperación técnica e institucionalidad social (1919–1950)* (pp. 22–55). Morelia: Instituto de Investigaciones Históricas, Universidad Michoacana de San Nicolás de Hidalgo.

Yáñez Andrade, J. C. (2017). El problema de la alimentación: un enfoque desde las encuestas de nutrición. Chile, 1928–1938. *América Latina en la Historia Económica, 24*(1), 66–97.

Zárate Campos, M. S. (2012). Alimentación y previsión biológica: La política médico-asistencial de Eduardo Cruz-Coke. In E. Cruz-Coke (Ed.), *Medicina Preventiva y Medicina Dirigida* (pp. ix–lxv). Santiago: Cámara Chilena de la Construcción, Pontífica Universidad Católica de Chile, Dibam.

# Social medicine, feminism and the politics of population: From transnational knowledge networks to national social movements in Brazil and Mexico

Rafael de la Dehesa

**ABSTRACT**
This article examines the role of national actors articulated with an explicitly counter-hegemonic transnational knowledge network (TKN) mobilising around social medicine in policy debates on population control and family planning. It focuses primarily on Brazil, using Mexico as a shadow case to highlight salient points of contrast. In doing so, it makes two contributions to larger debates about TKNs. First, it highlights the plural and contested nature of the knowledge production they enact, underscoring contestation around a global reproductive regime that consolidated around family planning. Second, it underscores how the position and relative influence of actors articulated with TKNs is shaped by political and institutional contexts at the national level, producing variable opportunities for the mobilisation of applied knowledge. Reflecting its advocates' embeddedness in larger opposition movements to authoritarian states, social medicine had a greater influence on these debates in Brazil, where synergies with a resurgent feminist movement reinforced a shared insistence on comprehensive women's healthcare and increased the salience of sterilisation abuse on the political agenda.

Scholars have called attention to the growing importance of transnational knowledge networks (TKNs) in global governance in public health and other areas of development.[1] Such networks can articulate, with varying degrees of formalisation, public and private actors at the local, national and supranational levels, potentially including government agencies, international organisations, foundations, research institutes, professional associations, corporations and nongovernmental organisations (NGOs). TKNs link 'the production, collection and movement of knowledge to technologies of government' through the coordination of research, intellectual exchange and 'capacity-building' activities such as academic scholarships and professional trainings (Stone, 2013, p. 44). Through the Foucauldian lens of governmentality, one can understand them as 'assemblages of forms of practical knowledge, with practices of calculation and types of authority and judgments' (Ilcan & Phillips, 2008, p. 713). Scholars have hailed TKNs for encouraging horizontality, flexibility and innovation; placing overlooked issues on the policy agenda and incorporating local actors and knowledge into the policymaking process (Kothari et al., 2016). More critical assessments have underscored their embeddedness in cartographies of knowledge production long shaped by geopolitical imbalances and their reliance on technocratic rather than democratic forms of legitimation (Bang & Esmark, 2009; Natividad, Fiereck, & Parker, 2012).

This article examines the role of TKNs in the politics of population control and family planning as they played out in Latin America's two most populous countries, Mexico and Brazil. The Cold War politics of population policy is noteworthy as a site deeply marked by north–south tensions in which TKNs played an early, central and strategic role. Through the funding and coordination of demographic research centres, fellowships, trainings and fertility and attitudinal surveys, a global network of international agencies and foundations, bilateral aid organisations and NGOs fostered the production and dissemination of applied knowledge to promote the creation of national population programmes and ultimately changes in gender norms and reproductive practices in the global south. This reliance on networks of state and non-state actors and capacity-building activities to promote knowledge production in the global south responded in part to (geo)political sensitivities surrounding this project, to avoid the appearance of neocolonial imposition while building a consensus on population dynamics (Barrett, Kurzman, & Shanahan, 2010; Connelly, 2008). But as the historian Matthew Connelly (2003) reminds us, it is easy to misread the history of population control and family planning through a top-down focus on the discourses and policy prescriptions of global elites and institutions. Such an approach ignores the national actors that selectively embraced, rejected or adapted global prescriptions. Indeed, the field mobilised an array of diverse, if overlapping globalised constituencies – feminists, neo-Malthusians, development planners, environmentalists, demographers and healthcare professionals, among others – in ways that played out differently in different national contexts.

The article seeks to contribute to this literature in two ways. First, it highlights the plural and contested nature of knowledge production enacted by TKNs around a global reproductive regime constructed around family planning. Second, it underscores how national political and institutional contexts shape the position and influence of national actors articulated with TKNs, producing different opportunities for the mobilisation of knowledge. To be clear, my intention here is not to posit a unidirectional flow of ideas and political energy from transnational networks to national movements, nor to suggest that transnational networks necessarily have a declining influence over time. The framing in the title, 'From (TKNs) to national social movements,' rather, is intended to denote an analytic move, focusing attention on how actors' embeddedness in national polities conditions the selective deployment and the salience of the knowledge circulated by TKNs. Knowledge-production is understood here, in the Gramscian sense, not as the activity of individual intellectuals but as encompassing internally differentiated institutionalised fields of social relations within which various forms of collective knowledge are produced and distributed. It thus encompasses activities not just in the academy or research laboratories but in other institutions such as state bureaucracies and NGOs (Crehan, 2017).

To develop these arguments, I examine national instantiations of an explicitly counter-hegemonic TKN mobilising around the banner of 'social medicine' or 'collective health.' Since the late 1960s, social scientists and healthcare specialists in Latin America mobilised, initially through informal networks and regional conferences and eventually through university-based research centres and academic programmes (Duarte, 1991). The movement posed an epistemological challenge to the biologizing, medicalizing and individualising tendencies of mainstream epidemiology and public health, calling for the incorporation of social scientific methodologies and approaches, particularly historical materialism, into health research. In ways that echoed the contemporaneous Latin American project of dependency theory, researchers focused critically on questions like the social determination of health and illness, the production of medical knowledge and the formation of human resources in healthcare, with the goal of producing applied knowledge to confront persistent health disparities specific to Latin American conditions of dependent development (Laurell, 1982; Waitzkin, Iriart, Estrada, & Lamadrid, 2001). The movement gained an important institutional foothold in the Pan-American Health Organization (PAHO), with the arrival of the Argentine physician and sociologist Juan César García in 1966, who worked initially in its Human Resources Development Department and subsequently as Director of Research, until his death in 1984, a position from which he and his colleagues promoted regional seminars, research, scholarships and publications

(Nunes, 2015). Since 1984, its principal transnational expression has been the Latin American Association of Social Medicine (ALAMES) founded that year, consolidating as a TKN that produces counter-hegemonic knowledge and policy alternatives to the dominant healthcare prescriptions of the World Bank and other international agencies (Almeida, 2006).

The inscription of family planning within larger projects of economic development and geopolitical oppositions made it a potential bridge between advocates of social medicine and Latin American feminist movements, which experienced a contemporaneous resurgence in the 1970s. In both Brazil and Mexico, this resurgence occurred against the backdrop of authoritarian governments confronting opposition movements demanding democratic and sometimes revolutionary change. Synergies between feminists and advocates of social medicine found much greater expression in Brazil, in part reflecting the latter's institutional location within these larger polities. This influence contributed to the course of women's health activism and policy by reinforcing the salience of sterilisation abuse and an insistence on women's comprehensive healthcare, ultimately delaying the passage of a National Family Planning Law until 1996, over two decades after Mexico's. This article focuses primarily on Brazil, given the much greater influence of social medicine on feminist politics there, with particular attention to debates on female sterilisation, around which (geo)political contestation often crystalised. Mexico is discussed primarily as a shadow case to highlight salient political contrasts. The article draws on a larger research project on sexual and reproductive rights movements' engagement with healthcare. This project has involved extensive research in archives belonging to social movement organisations, public health institutes, state agencies and international foundations as well as 81 interviews in Mexico and 100 in Brazil with sexual and reproductive rights activists, health officials and other relevant political actors.

## The politics of population

Until the 1970s, the prevailing view among Mexican and Brazilian political elites regarding population policy might be summarised by the famous phrase first uttered by the nineteenth-century Argentine liberal Juan Carlos Alberdi, 'To govern is to populate' (*Gobernar es poblar*). In both countries, this essentially pronatalist view had deep historical roots, linked to geopolitical concerns that territorial security and social progress required the occupation of vast empty tracts of land by national populations (Fonseca Sobrinho, 1993; Welti-Chanes, 2011). Pronatalist understandings informed public policies in various areas, from the criminalisation of abortion to early protections for maternal-child health. Mexico's General Population Laws of 1934 and 1947, for example, established the state's obligation to increase population size through immigration and 'natural growth,' involving the promotion of marriage and social protections for mothers and children. Brazil's 1934 constitution introduced stipulations that called for protecting mothers and children and supporting families with numerous offspring. Mexico's Sanitary Code of 1949 and Brazil's Criminal Infractions Law of 1941 banned advertisements for birth control, remaining on the books until 1973 and 1979 respectively. While enforcement of these laws was lax – contraceptives, for instance, came to be advertised and freely dispensed by pharmacies for the purposes of menstrual regulation – they nonetheless shaped the public face of a double discourse that powerfully influenced the political landscape (Márquez, 1984; Mora Bravo, 2017; Werneck Vianna, 1977).

The 1974 World Population Conference at Bucharest framed the geopolitical backdrop against which changes in official government positions in both countries began to take shape. Deep divisions emerged leading up to that conference between global south countries, organised as the Group of 77, and countries of the global north. Against the premise advanced by the latter that overpopulation impeded economic development and must be contained, the G-77 inverted the causal arrow, countering that if economic development happened, fertility declines would follow. Mobilising around the banner, 'Development is the best contraceptive,' the G-77 pushed back against the single-minded focus on population growth as the cause of all ills. Conflict also centred on particular tactics, including quantitative targets for population growth and 'acceptors' of contraceptives and the use of incentives and disincentives to promote them. At stake in these debates were competing biopolitical framings that inscribed family planning as either a tool to achieve aggregate goals or an individual human right, demanding state protection. This debate found echo among advocates of family planning in Mexico and Brazil, who routinely distinguished it from demographic control.

Brazilian and Mexican officials at the Conference echoed the G-77 position. The Brazilian military government (1964–1985) officially broke with pronatalism, spelling out what came to be called the 'Brazilian Demographic Policy,' stipulating that population policy is a matter of national sovereignty; that birth control is a family decision, not the government's; but that the state must provide contraceptives and information to ensure access across class lines (Rodrigues, 1983). Despite this discursive shift and inclusion of family planning in the II National Development Plan of 1974, the government took little action, reflecting the contentious political dynamics surrounding the issue. In 1977, its attempt to include family planning for the first time in a public health programme for high-risk pregnancies met such broad resistance that the project was never implemented (Costa, 1999). In 1983, the regime's efforts took a surprising turn, with the announcement of the Program of Integral Attention to Women's Health (PAISM). PAISM was widely hailed as a victory by feminist activists and bore the strong imprint of social medicine, as I elaborate below, though again, implementation fell short. While the right to family planning was incorporated in the 1988 Constitution, a National Family Planning Law regulating services, including sterilisation, was only passed in 1996 after protracted, heated contestation.

The case of Mexico was quite different. As the presidential candidate (and heir apparent) of the ruling Institutional Revolutionary Party (PRI), Luis Echeverría responded to World Bank president Robert McNamara's call to make family planning a conditionality for lending by reiterating Alberdi's famous expression, 'To govern is to populate' (Mora Bravo, 1986). During his presidency (1970–76), however, Echeverría oversaw a dramatic reversal that would eventually lead to adoption of some of the most problematic tactics in the global repertoire. In 1974, prior to the Bucharest Conference, the government promulgated a new National Population Law that created a National Population Council (CONAPO) to coordinate policy. Though Mexico's statement at Bucharest echoed the G-77 position and excluded any reference to quantitative targets, its first National Family Planning Program, launched in 1977 under Echeverría's successor José López Portillo, called for reducing population growth from 3.2% in 1976 to 2.5% by 1982 and 1% by 2000 (Mora Bravo, 1986). It also set targets for the number of new acceptors and active users and subsequently for consultations and acceptance of specific methods, which were applied from the federal, state and municipal levels to individual health centres (Navarro & Manautou, 1986).

The Program for Surgical Contraceptives was also launched in 1977 and by 1982 had performed 122,888 cases of female sterilisation, almost entirely postnatal. These were initially conducted in public hospitals, requiring patients to be at least 30, with at least 4 children, and 'the husband's consent,' though these requirements were subsequently dropped to increase numbers. An internal assessment of the programme identified a 'lack of motivation among medical and paramedical personnel, which made it difficult to convince patients.' To resolve it, specialised family planning services and personnel were incorporated into hospitals and health centres, including mobile health services for rural areas, verticalising services (SSA, n.d., pp. 2–3). Three-day site visits were also instituted for all health centres entering the programme and surgical units showing 'low output.' Of the 249 surgeons evaluated in 242 site visits in 1982, 92 had not received any training and 13 were considered inadequately trained (p. 4). Recalling his visit in 1984 to villages with fewer than 2,500 residents as part of a team sent by the Mexican Social Security Institute to evaluate its family planning programme, Joseph Potter (1999) recalled that the practitioners interviewed gave 'nearly uniform answers' in terms of the number of children they thought women should have, the methods they recommended and the suitability of sterilisation as a postpartum method. Reflecting both socialisation within the public health system and 'guidelines and priorities transmitted down the chain of supervision,' the result, he concluded, was a highly interventionist approach (pp. 717–18). Though changes were subsequently implemented, particularly after the International Conference on Population and Development at

Cairo in 1994, a 1996 survey conducted by CONAPO of clinics, hospitals and practitioners providing family planning services in rural areas of nine states found that normative guidelines were not well-known but that virtually all doctors knew their institutions had quantitative targets and over half had targets for their personal performance (cited in Potter, 1999, pp. 721–722). While the Mexican government has taken steps to institute improvements, charges of forced sterilisation and other forms of 'obstetric violence,' particularly in indigenous communities, have periodically been brought to national and international human rights bodies (Menéndez, 2009).

The table below shows the percentage of women of reproductive age, married or in unions, using any contraceptive method in both countries over time, and the percentage of this group using selected methods. The growing reliance on female sterilisation is striking, used by over half of this population in Brazil by the mid-1990s and in Mexico by 2009. Also worth noting is the reversal of this trend in Brazil in the 1990s. While not entirely attributable to the passage of the Family Planning Law in 1996, this reversal is particularly noteworthy, given that the growing practice of sterilisation in the earlier period occurred in semi-clandestine ways, its cost not covered by the public health system or private insurance plans, generally performed in conjunction with cesarean sections or other procedures (Caetano, 2010; Potter, 1999) (Table 1).[2]

A final point might be made to situate this story in political context. While both governments officially abandoned pronatalist stances in the 1970s, with Mexico going further to institute national family planning policies, these changes grew out of an earlier history of mobilisation around the issue by nongovernmental actors. Population growth in Latin America, I should note, received growing attention from international organisations during the 1960s, due partly to a greater focus on the region by established actors and partly to new actors' entry into the field. Most notably, USAID established a population office in 1965 and soon became the largest donor to family planning efforts in the region (Bertrand, Ward, & Santiso-Gálvez, 2015). The role of three national actors engaged in the debate is worth underscoring, all of which were heavily articulated with TKNs.

First, university-based demographic research centres became key sites for the production of demographic knowledge about national population dynamics, and indeed, global actors extensively promoted demographic research as a first step toward the adoption of national family planning programmes (Connelly, 2008). In 1957, the United Nations established the Latin American Demography Center (CELADE) in Chile. It was the second of seven UN regional and interregional demographic research and training centres created by 1982 to train demographers, produce and standardise statistical knowledge and offer governments technical assistance. In the early 1960s, CELADE launched its Program of Comparative Fertility Surveys in Latin America (PECFAL). Grounding the so-called KAP (Knowledge-Attitudes-Practices) surveys in the region, the programme coordinated pioneering research on reproductive practices, initially in seven metropolitan areas, including Mexico City and Rio de Janeiro, and subsequently in rural areas (Berquó & Baltar da Rocha, 2005; Zarate Campos & González Moya, 2013). In Mexico, the Center for Economic and Demographic Research (CEED) founded at the Colegio de México in 1964, was particularly influential. Its Masters Program in Demography, the first in Latin America, trained experts throughout the region, and its researchers produced studies that laid the groundwork for policy and consulted with

Table 1. Percentage of married or in-union women of reproductive age* using any contraceptive method; and those using selected methods as a percentage of all married or in-union women of reproductive age using contraceptives.

| | Brazil | | | Mexico | | | |
|---|---|---|---|---|---|---|---|
| | 1986 | 1996 | 2006–7 | 1976–77 | 1987 | 1995 | 2009 |
| Any method | 66.2 | 76.7 | 80.3 | 30.3 | 52.7 | 66.5 | 72.5 |
| Female sterilisation | 40.5 | 52.3 | 36.2 | 8.9 | 35.3 | 41.1 | 50.1 |
| IUD | 1.5 | 1.4 | 2.4 | 18.8 | 19.4 | 22.0 | – |
| Pill | 38.1 | 27.0 | 30.8 | 35.6 | 18.4 | 12.6 | – |

Source: Calculated from, United Nations Population Division, http://www.un.org/en/development/desa/population/publications/dataset/contraception/wcu2015.shtml.
*The 1986 Brazil survey includes women ages 15–44; the others include women ages 15–49.

government agencies working with population policy and statistics-keeping. On the eve of the government's embrace of family planning, for instance, the Mexican interior minister called on then CEED director Gustavo Cabrera – the first director of the Masters Program and among the first Mexican demographers trained at CELADE – and demographer Susana Lerner to draft the proposal for the country's Family Planning Law of 1974.[3]

Second, private-sector family planning organisations also entered the public sphere in the 1960s. While not the first or only such organisations, the most important were the Brazilian Civil Society for Family Welfare (BEMFAM) in Brazil and the Foundation for Population Studies (FEPAC) in Mexico (rebaptised the Mexican Family Planning Foundation, MEXFAM, in 1983). Both were founded in 1965 and became affiliates of the International Planned Parenthood Federation (IPPF) two years later. IPPF had had a limited Latin American presence in its Western Hemisphere Region, with only one affiliate in 1961 (Puerto Rico, alongside six others from Anglophone countries). As the first such event in the region, its VIII International Conference, held in 1967 in Santiago at the invitation of Chilean President Eduardo Frei, gave a 'seal of legitimacy to family planning,' and within five years, virtually all Latin American countries had affiliated organisations.[4] In addition to building national networks of family planning clinics, BEMFAM and FEPAC also engaged in biomedical and social research and extensive education efforts, organising seminars targeting doctors and other professionals. They also spearheaded efforts to press national governments to adopt national family planning programmes, efforts that to some extent aligned these organisations with an authoritarian political status quo.

Finally, the Catholic Church also became a key player in global and national debates on population policy. Key encyclicals issued at the Second Vatican Council sanctioned the use of 'natural' birth control methods within a paradigm of 'responsible parenthood' (*Humanae Vitae*, 1967) and recognised a government role in addressing problems derived from 'accelerated population growth' (*Popularum Progressio*, 1968) While the Church undoubtedly influenced reproductive politics in Mexico as well, particularly sustaining restrictions on abortion, the Brazilian Church gained a more direct role shaping the course of women's health policy. For example, it negotiated directly with the Health Ministry team that designed PAISM, resulting in its incorporation of 'natural methods' and the exclusion of others, like IUDs, which it considered abortifacient (Fonseca Sobrinho, 1993). While retaining some leverage in official circles, the Brazilian Church also occupied a unique institutional position that extended its influence across the ideological spectrum. A Latin American movement of liberation theology found among its strongest expressions in Brazil, where the Church became a leading voice in the democratic opposition to the military regime and a key agent fostering progressive social mobilisation via grassroots Christian base communities.

In Mexico, FEPAC, CONAPO and the CEED constituted an arena of knowledge production that was institutionally positioned to undergird early family planning policy, selectively grounding the work of TKNs in the national polity. To be clear, this is not to suggest that demography was inextricably bound to a global project of population control. There were counter-hegemonic voices within Latin American and Mexican demography, and indeed, within the CEED. As Felitti (2012) observes, the fact that many Latin American countries under pressure to institute family planning programmes in fact had relatively low population densities, though often concentrated in rapidly growing cities, heightened a critical awareness that the problems cited were really about distribution, not scarcity. A historical-structural school developed within Latin American demography – like social medicine influenced by dependency theory – which articulated this critique, finding expression, for instance, in the Population Commission of the Latin American Social Science Council (CLACSO). The institutional constellation of CONAPO-CEED-FEPAC, however, strengthened positions within the national polity that were generally supportive of the government's policy directions and echoed global concerns over population growth. In Brazil, advocates mobilising around the banner of collective health – participants in an explicitly counterhegemonic TKN – became as significant, in part because of synergies with a resurgent feminist movement. I turn now to that story.

## Transnational knowledge networks and counter-hegemonies

Again, a transnational movement advancing social medicine found different institutional expressions and levels of influence at the national level, conditioned by advocates' embeddedness in national polities, with implications for debates on family planning and women's health. In Mexico, its primary institutional expression is the Masters Program in Social Medicine, established in 1975 at the Autonomous University of Mexico (UAM)-Xochimilco, with the idea of creating a Latin American research and training centre that would attract scholars and students from throughout the region.[5] The UAM-Xochimilco had itself been founded only the previous year. Its rector Ramón Villarreal had worked with Juan César García at PAHO, and PAHO worked closely with the Program's architects 'to develop [its] curriculum, look for staff and finance scholarships.'[6] While the programme remains an important research centre nationally and regionally, its influence on national policy has been circumscribed by larger dynamics associated with the country's democratic transition, particularly by the marginalisation of the partisan left, which coalesced around the Party of the Democratic Revolution (PRD) in the late 1980s. The PRD has yet to capture the presidency but maintains a stronghold in Mexico City, holding the executive there since 1997. Social medicine's most direct policy influence, notably, occurred in the capital, with the appointment of Asa Cristina Laurell, one of the founders of the Masters Program and a leading figure in the regional movement, as health secretary (2000–2006) (Laurell, 2003; Pêgo & Almeida, 2004).

In Brazil, on the other hand, the larger and more politically influential *movimento sanitario* erupted in the 1970s, finding institutional expression in numerous graduate and undergraduate programmes around the country, professional associations and independent organisations (Nunes, 2016). Key among these was the Brazilian Center for Health Research (CEBES), founded in 1976, which published the journal *Saúde em Debate*. CEBES occupied a unique institutional position within a changing public sphere, as a social movement organisation that bridged the academy and other institutions. Reflecting many of its members' participation in clandestine leftist organisations, particularly the Brazilian Communist Party (PCB), CEBES replicated the left's model of party cells, creating 'nuclei,' or discussion groups, throughout the country. CEBES activists had ongoing discussions about its institutional role in the context of *abertura*, the gradual democratic opening announced by the military government in the late 1970s. By 1978, *abertura* had restored alternative spaces for critical debate in universities and health sector unions, precipitating a 'crisis' in CEBES's second oldest and largest nucleus, in Rio de Janeiro, by drawing mobilisation elsewhere. Responding to the crisis, the CEBES National Assembly of Delegates rejected the functional segmentation of opposition across unions, parties and universities. Instead, it called for a 'synergistic' relationship and approved a programme defining its nuclei's essential role as unifying struggles by articulating networks across popular movements, unions, women's groups and other organisations.[7] An editorial appearing in *Saúde em Debate* in 1980 explicitly linked this institutional position to knowledge production in Gramscian terms. Against the constraints of the individualising and proprietary intellectual work performed in universities and of the intellectual work of organising and applying existing knowledge that occurred in healthcare bureaucracies, bound by a political project, CEBES was in a unique position to move from 'specialist' to 'leader' by collaboratively developing 'counter-policies … and new models of actions.'[8] The synergies created by this institutional position would mark CEBES's relationship with feminism.

*Sanitaristas'* knowledge-production and medical practice reflected their embeddedness in larger movements opposing rightwing authoritarianism at both the national and regional levels. For example, Albertina Takiuti Duarte, a gynecologist and early activist with CEBES and the PCB, recalled organising a sort of 'red cross group' in the mid-1970s that provided medical attention to relatives of political prisoners and leftist exiles living clandestinely in the city. This experience, she recalled, fostered exchanges within clandestine networks that contributed to a pioneering study on women's health: 'We would invite a woman from Chile, for instance, to tell us about healthcare organisations in Chile – in Uruguay, in Argentina – about women's movements. This created the basis for us to conduct the study.' Obtaining letters of support from the United Nations Office in Brazil and the progressive São Paulo Archdiocese, activists coordinated a study in 49 maternity hospitals, presenting their results at the First Diagnostic of the Paulista Woman. That conference, held in City Hall in October 1975 to mark the UN International Women's Year, in turn prompted the establishment of the Brazilian Women's Development Center, among the first organisations of a resurgent feminist movement.[9]

The related epistemological and political stakes of *sanitaristas'* work was suggested by a dispatch that Health Minister Paulo de Almeida Machado sent to President General Ernesto Geisel in 1977. The report regarded with suspicion a draft document presented at the Fourth Special Meeting of Health Ministers at PAHO, which recommended that health centres 'raise community awareness to promote the institutional changes needed to improve income distribution and social justice.' Noting 'the same tone used by the groups of social medicine and community medicine in Brazil, with roots in Allende's Chile,' it celebrated the effective coordination by health officials from Argentina, Brazil, Chile, Uruguay and Paraguay at the meeting to achieve a 'more discrete tone,' transposing the right-wing military alliance Operation Condor to the field of public health. The dispatch also reported on a recent *sanitarista* conference in São Paulo, warning of the 'infiltration of CEBES' and the outsized role of departments of social, preventive or collective medicine in medical education. 'Previously,' it lamented, 'Every professor methodically taught the appropriate preventive measures in analyzing each sickness and even, among the most skilled, each sick person.' Now that these departments were attracting 'students with a greater vocation for social problems,' it recommended that the government maintain 'an attitude of reserve' toward these departments, 'looking into their gradual emptying' while promoting undergraduate public health courses 'with a focused curriculum, [that left students] little time for fun in the area of "social" sciences'.[10]

Over the course of democratisation, the *movimento sanitario* eventually established a hegemonic position in defining the direction of healthcare reform, in part facilitated by its position within the public sphere. In contrast to the political marginalisation of the partisan left in Mexico, the Brazilian Democratic Movement (MDB), as the only officially recognised opposition party under military rule, united a broad-based opposition movement that ranged from centrist liberals to sectors of the revolutionary left. Within this broad coalition, the *sanitaristas* were well-positioned to influence national healthcare debates, no less so because of the number of activists affiliated with the Brazilian Communist Party, which at the time operated clandestinely within the MDB. The political scientist Sonia Fleury, an important leader of the movement who participated in both CEBES and the PCB, refers to an oppositional strategy of occupying state healthcare bureaucracies that began in municipalities and states won by the opposition and proceeded to the national level when the healthcare system operated by the National Social Security and Healthcare Institute (INAMPS) fell into crisis in the 1980s: 'The dictatorship lacked competent technical specialists who could rationalise the system, so they called this group on the left which had already gained prominence and whose ideas already appeared with the idea of rationalisation.'[11] In 1985, the movement leader Hésio Cordeiro was appointed to head INAMPS. The following year, *sanitaristas* dominated VIII National Healthcare Conference, where the proposal to create the country's Unified Healthcare System (SUS) was hammered out. The inclusion of SUS, along with the right to healthcare, in the 1988 constitution marked the movement's most important victory, though its subsequent implementation was sharply constrained by neoliberal austerity.

In addition to being better positioned to influence national health policy than their counterparts in Mexico, *sanitaristas* also demonstrated somewhat greater openness to the women's health concerns being introduced into national public spheres by feminist movements, which experienced a contemporaneous resurgence in the 1970s. Unlike the case in Mexico, an important Foucauldian current emerged among *sanitaristas* relatively early in Brazil. In 1974, Foucault gave a series of lectures at the Institute of Social Medicine (IMS) at the State University of Rio de Janeiro. The Institute created the first Masters Program in social medicine in the country that same year, like the UAM-

Xochimilco, with strong collaboration from PAHO. This Foucauldian current heightened critical attention to bodily discipline, sexuality and the family among *sanitaristas*.

In neither country was the relationship between advocates of social medicine and feminists free of tensions. To some extent, the former shared the left's tendency to subordinate identity-based 'specific struggles' to the larger class-based 'general struggle.' In the case of social medicine, this translated into an emphasis on class-based inequities and universal healthcare over sector-specific demands and a tendency to dismiss feminist demands as secondary, if not outright conservative. Catalina Eibenschutz, one of the founders of the Masters Program at the UAM-Xochimilco, recalled that these topics had only entered the research agenda very recently and in a limited way:

> There is very little on gender and sexuality in social medicine [in Mexico]. There is a space in psychology and another with questions of gender, but these have arisen primarily in the last 10 or 15 years ... The first discussions did not admit anything besides class interests between the state and society; no mediations.[12]

Ana Maria Costa, an early activist with the Brazilian feminist movement and CEBES who worked in the Health Ministry where she became the principal architect of PAISM, recalled her position as one of the few dual militants participating in both movements and 'a certain mocking assessment of feminism [among *sanitaristas*], as if feminism were a petit bourgeois struggle that brought individual, not collective, issues onto the stage.' Population control and family planning, however, bridged the concerns of feminists and *sanitaristas*:

> There was not much communication at first [between the movements]. There were a few instances. For instance, the *movimento sanitario* constructed a formal political plank on family planning ... The argument for demographic control was very strong in the 1970s. The feminist movement was very inspired by the thinking of the Boston Feminist Collective, and also French feminists, for whom the question of autonomy over the body and autonomy of choice were central. The *movimento sanitario* critiqued that line of thought although not based on autonomy over the body but of autonomy of the population against demographic control ... for national sovereignty.[13]

Because of its inscription in larger debates on economic development and geopolitics, very much bound with social medicine's attention to the social determination of health in contexts of dependent development, population control thus became an important early bridge between both movements. In 1977, the CEBES nucleus in Rio de Janeiro and the feminist Brazilian Women's Center organised a panel discussion decrying the government's announced intention to incorporate family planning into its programme for 'high-risk pregnancy,' an initiative, again, that never got off the ground.[14] At its National Assembly of Delegates in 1980, CEBES defined demographic policy (along with environmental and workplace health and national healthcare policy) as three key priorities in the upcoming years, calling on its nuclei to engage in research, denunciations and mobilisation around the issue.[15] Several nuclei created family planning commissions. Feminists in the CEBES nucleus in São Paulo created a Women's Health Group, which published a short-lived bulletin *Mulher e Saúde*. One issue included translations of several articles on women's health by Giovanni Berlinguer, the Italian professor of social medicine, brother of then General Secretary of the Italian Communist Party Enrico Berlinguer and a frequent interlocutor of Latin American activists.

The synergy created between feminism and the *movimento sanitario* in Brazil played out in several ways in relation to women's health policy. Most importantly, it reinforced a shared insistence on attention to women's comprehensive healthcare, as opposed to vertical family planning programmes, and a critical attention to the structural conditioning of health and healthcare. With regard to the growing rates of female sterilisation, for instance, this extended to a problematization of structural conditions shaping what would come to be understood as 'informed consent.' In an article appearing in *Saúde em Debate*, Ana Maria Canesqui (1981), a professor of social medicine at the University of Campinas and member of the CEBES nucleus in that city, took aim at the distinction commonly drawn between demographic control and family planning by advocates of the latter. Canesqui argued that this 'at best liberal' distinction, presented family planning as an extension of a humanitarian welfare state that assumed the obligation to present contraceptive methods and information to couples as a matter of redistribution. Ultimately, Canesqui contended, this framing abstracted the state from its entanglements with economic and political interests, including those of pharmaceutical corporations; and the doctor-patient consultation, from the structural contexts that led to this individualised exchange. This larger structural focus was particularly relevant because, as the feminist women's health activist Carmen Barroso (1984) observed at the time, a great number of tubal ligations performed in the country occurred 'not as the result of direct coercion or manipulation' but as a 'free' choice made by women as 'conscious moral agents,' though amid structural constraints that left very few alternatives (p. 172). Barroso explicitly framed her argument as an examination of problems that went beyond sterilisations without 'informed consent,' shedding light on the 'social determinative factors' that conditioned such consent, including women's position in the home and labour market, patriarchal culture, the commoditization of health and demographic policies (p. 179). Notably, this shared early feminist and *sanitarista* critique of social forces that overdetermined women's 'free' choice to get sterilised, which implied the need for intersectoral policies to foster greater social equity, would be reduced to measures designed to insure informed consent in the National Family Planning Law of 1996 by regulating the doctor-patient consultation.

The synergy between feminism and the *movimento sanitario* also had important policy and political repercussions. Dual militants active in both movements played a central role crafting and running the two most important early policy experiments in women's comprehensive healthcare, the Women's Health Program created in 1983 in São Paulo following the election of opposition Governor Franco Montoro, and PAISM at the national level. *Sanitaristas* also created institutional spaces that feminists would occupy. In addition to seats in various healthcare councils created under SUS as oversight bodies that incorporated civil society, the VIII National Healthcare Conference of 1986, where the architecture of SUS was hammered out, was followed by several thematic conferences, including the First National Conference on Women's Rights and Health, which followed municipal and state conferences to elect delegates. Thematic groups at the conference produced recommendations. The Group on the Rights of Human Reproduction called on the state to assume responsibility for making contraceptives and information available to women; to ban foreign involvement in national population policy; and to 'veto' the participation of individuals and organisations engaging in 'controlist practices' as Brazilian representatives in international forums. Black feminist organisations became a leading voice condemning such practices, and the Black Women's Identity Group called for the banning of sterilisation without expressed, informed consent, particularly in cases targeting racially and ethnically marginalised groups, and for punishment of such practices as genocide in other instances. Conference recommendations also reaffirmed the *sanitarista* project, calling for the institutionalisation of SUS and for comprehensive healthcare for women within it (Conferência Nacional de Saúde, 1987).

Politically, both movements also enunciated a forceful repudiation of the work of family planning organisations, particularly the most politically active, BEMFAM, which was seen as aligned with the global project of population control and the military government. For some years, BEMFAM had cultivated ties with political leaders. Between 1967 and 1988, it signed almost 2,000 contracts with state and municipal governments to provide family planning services (Fonseca Sobrinho, 1993). In the federal congress, BEMFAM promoted the creation of the Parliamentary Population and Development Studies Group, a cross-party caucus disproportionately composed of right-wing lawmakers, whose principal objective was to create a National Family Planning Program. The Group established a congressional inquiry commission in 1983 to look into 'problems related to population growth in Brazil.' The commission's final report included a bill to create such a programme and a national population council along the lines of Mexico's CONAPO. BEMFAM worked closely with the Armed Forces Chief of Staff and the congressional commission to produce the bill (BEMFAM, 1984). Reflecting striking contradictions within the state, it was in his testimony at these hearings that the Health Minister announced the launching of PAISM, which was intended to break not just with vertical family planning programmes but with the narrow focus on women's reproductive capacity of traditional programmes of maternal-child health. Both feminists and *sanitaristas* repudiated the commission's bill as 'controlist,' counterposing it to PAISM. These two opposing coalitions would clash around family planning until passage of the National Family Planning Law in 1996. Alongside these, a national Pro-Life movement took shape, articulated with a Church that was becoming more conservative as the country returned to formal democracy, in part due to Pope John Paul II's concerted efforts to weaken liberation theology in the region.

The contentious debates that produced the 1996 law reflected the persistent centrality of 'mass sterilization' on the feminist agenda and the government's failure to live up to its promise of comprehensive women's healthcare. While PAISM facilitated the development of noteworthy pilot projects, particularly where local women's organisations exercised oversight, it was never effectively implemented across the healthcare system, limited in part by the institutional shortfalls and underfunding that characterised the larger implementation of SUS (Almeida, 2005; Costa, 1992). Against this backdrop, the question of sterilisation persisted, with significant mobilisation around the issue by black feminist organisations in the late 1980s. This activism led to the creation of parliamentary inquiry commissions in three state assemblies, the City Council of Salvador, Bahia, and eventually one at the federal level, directed by Benedita da Silva, a federal deputy of the Workers Party and the first black woman elected to the post. That commission's report, written by the *sanitarista* feminist Ana Maria Costa, produced a proposal that would eventually become the Family Planning Law approved in 1996. That law and subsequent implementing regulations instituted several requirements designed to ensure informed consent for sterilisation procedures, including a minimum age of 25; at least two living children; a 60-day waiting period after the initial request, during which information on the implications of the procedure and reversible alternatives must be provided; a 42-day waiting period after childbirth except in medically prescribed circumstances; and consent of the partner or spouse. While it is beyond the scope of this article to fully examine the politics surrounding its passage, Caetano (2014) has found that its subsequent implementation has been, once again, spotty. According to a 2006 survey, for instance, despite the 42-day waiting period after childbirth, 58.7% of the procedures reported were performed during cesarean sections and another 9.0% after 'normal childbirth' (PNDS, 2006). Despite limitations in the law's material effects, its political effects were quite striking, effectively closing a decades-long debate and removing the issue from the feminist agenda.

The heated controversies around sterilisation that marked the history of family planning policy in Brazil are particularly noteworthy in comparison with Mexico. Undoubtedly Mexican feminists have periodically raised questions and presented complaints to human rights bodies involving abuses related to sterilisation in the country, recently framed around 'obstetric violence.' Perhaps most notably, the Tribunal to Defend Reproductive Rights organised by the Women's Health Network of the Federal District in 1996, a mock trial that heard 27 cases of violations of reproductive rights, included the case of a woman who had been sterilised without her consent in the public health system. Overall, however, the question never assumed the centrality it did in Brazil for feminists or on the political agenda more broadly (Menéndez, 2009). The difference is particularly striking when one considers that the Mexican government in fact implemented a much more neo-Malthusian project through the public health system, while the charges that feminists and *sanitaristas* levelled against the Brazilian government largely concerned sins of omission, particularly its lack of oversight over private-sector family planning organisations articulated with transnational networks.

## Conclusions

Full attention to all the reasons for these differences is beyond the scope of this piece. What this article has attempted to do, rather, is to use population policy as a window to explore how institutional contexts at the national level selectively condition the position and influence of TKNs mobilising around public policy, themselves understood in the plural.

Specifically, above I highlighted how the articulation of a counterhegemonic TKN mobilising around social medicine found different levels of influence and priorities in Mexico and Brazil –

particularly around women's health – in ways that responded to national-level institutional dynamics associated with gradual processes of formal democratisation. In Brazil, the institutional position of feminists and *sanitaristas* within a broad opposition movement to military rule reinforced both political synergies between the movements and the latter's influence on national healthcare policy and hence capacity to leverage knowledge. Such possibilities were largely precluded in Mexico, where the influence of social medicine has been constrained by the fate of the left and national healthcare policy has taken a radically different course (Pêgo & Almeida, 2004). Here, one might counterpose the project of social medicine with that of another TKN important to population policy. In Mexico, demographers more closely aligned with a global project of population control were able to leverage other forms of knowledge and ultimately shape the course of family planning policy, strengthened by institutional bases at CONAPO, the Federation for Population Studies and the Center for Economic and Demographic Studies at the Colegio de México. National actors, of course, are not mere mouthpieces for transnational networks (which themselves are internally diverse). This article, nonetheless, has highlighted how institutionalised fields of knowledge production at the national level constrain and channel opportunities for them to adapt, produce and ultimately mobilise applied knowledge.

## Notes

1. I would like to thank Francesca Degiuli, Hosu Kim, Jean Halley, Jaime Amparo Alves, as well as the reviewers of this article and the editors of *Global Public Health* for their very helpful feedback on earlier drafts of this piece.
2. United Nations Development Program, 'Other Funds and Programs: United Nations Funds for Population Activities - Proposed Projects and Programmes,' March 29, 1983, DP/FPA/PROJECTS/REC/8, http://web.undp.org/execbrd/archives/sessions/gc/30th-1983/DP-FPA-PROJECTS-REC-8.pdf, accessed January 25, 2018.
3. Dr. Susana Lerner, in discussion with author, January 23, 2017; Welti-Chanes, 2011.
4. IPPF/WHR, *Forty Years of Saving Lives with Family Planning: An Anniversary Publication*, New York: IPPF/WHR, Inc., pp. 11–12. Sophia Smith Collection, Smith College, Una Elizabeth Jacobs Papers, Box 3.
5. 'Editorial' *Salud Problema*, Oct. 1978, 3, p. 3.
6. Catalinas Eibenschutz, Professor of Social Medicine and one of the founders of the Masters Program at the UAM-Xochimilco in discussion with author, Mexico City, July 23, 2012.
7. CEBES, Programa de Trabalho do CEBES para 1978/79, *Saúde em Debate*, no. 6, Jan–Mar 1978, pp. 5–6; Editorial, *Saúde em Debate*, no. 7–8, Apr–Jun 1978, pp. 3–4.
8. 'Editorial,' *Saúde em Debate*, no. 9, Jan–Mar 1980, pp. 1–2.
9. Albertina Takiuti Duarte, in discussion with author, São Paulo, July 23, 2017.
10. Paulo de Almeida Machado, 'Despacho com o excelentíssimo senhor Presidente da República,' Nov. 3, 1977, Centro de Pesquisa e Documentação de História Contemporânea do Brasil, Fundação Getúlio Vargas, Ernesto Geisel Papers, EG pr 1974.04.25, Rio de Janeiro.
11. Sonia Fleury, in discussion with author, Rio de Janeiro, February 24, 2012.
12. Catalina Eibenschutz, in discussion with author, Mexico City, July 23, 2012.
13. Ana Maria Costa, in discussion with author, Brasilia, June 29, 2013.
14. 'Controle da natalidade em discussão' *Saúde em Debate*, no. 4 (Jul–Sept. 1977), pp. 84–85.
15. 'Editorial,' *Saúde em Debate*, no. 10, Apr–Jun 1980, pp. 3–4.

## Disclosure statement

No potential conflict of interest was reported by the authors.

## References

Almeida, C. (2005, July). *O movimento da reforma sanitária: Uma visão crítica*. Paper presented at the VI National Congress of Rede UNIDA, Belo Horizonte, Minas Gerais, Brazil.
Almeida, C. (2006). Reforma del sector salud en América Latina y el Caribe: El papel de los organismos internacionales al formular las agendas y al implementar las políticas. *Bienestar y Política Social*, 2(1), 135–175.
Bang, H., & Esmark, A. (2009). Good governance in network society: Reconfiguring the political from politics to policy. *Administrative Theory & Praxis*, 31(1), 7–37.

Barrett, D., Kurzman, C., & Shanahan, S. (2010). For export only: Diffusion professionals and population policy. *Social Forces, 88*(3), 1183–1207.

Barroso, C. (1984). Esterilização feminina: Liberdade e opressão? *Revista de Saúde Pública, 18*, 170–180.

BEMFAM. (1984 July). *A oficialização do planejamento familiar no Brasil* (Unpublished Mimeo). BEMFAM Documentation Center.

Berquó, E., & Baltar da Rocha, M. I. (2005). A Abep no contexto politico e no desenvolvimento da demografia nas décadas de 1960 e 1970. *Revista Brasileira de Estudos de População, 22*(2), 233–246.

Bertrand, J. T., Ward, V. M., & Santiso-Gálvez, R. (2015). *Family planning in Latin America and the Caribbean: The achievements of 50 years.* Chapel Hill, NC: MEASURE Evaluation. Retrieved from https://www.measureevaluation.org/resources/publications/tr-15-101

Caetano, A. J. (2010, September). *Ascensão e queda da laqueadura tubária no Brasil? Uma avaliação das Pesquisas de Demografia e Saúde de 1986, 1996 e 2006.* Paper presented at the XVII Encontro da Associação Brasileira de Estudos Populacionais, Caxambu, Minas Gerais, Brazil.

Caetano, A. J. (2014). Esterilização cirúrgica feminina no Brasil 2000–2006: aderência à lei de planejamento familiar e demanda frustrada. *Revista Brasileira de Estudos de População, 31*(2), 309–331.

Canesqui, A. M. (1981). Instituições de Saúde e o Planejamento Familiar. *Saúde em Debate, 12*, 35–40.

Conferência Nacional de Saúde. (1987). *Relatório final da Conferência Nacional de Saúde e Direitos da Mulher.* Brasilia: Centro de Documentação do Ministério da Saúde.

Connelly, M. (2003). Population control is history: New perspectives on the international campaign to limit population growth. *Comparative Studies in Society and History, 45*(1), 122–147.

Connelly, M. (2008). *Fatal misconceptions: The struggle to control world population.* Cambridge: Harvard University Press.

Costa, A. M. (1992). *O PAISM: Uma política de assistência integral à saúde da mulher a ser resgatada.* São Paulo: Comissão de Cidadania e Reprodução. National Archive, Brasilia, CNDM Collection, Code 210, Box 93, Document 1000002392.

Costa, A. M. (1999). Desenvolvimento e implementação do PAISM no Brasil. In K. Giffin & S. H. Costa (Eds.), *Questões da saúde reprodutiva* (pp. 319–335). Rio de Janeiro: Editora Fiocruz.

Crehan, K. (2017). *Gramsci's common sense: Inequality and its narratives.* Durham: Duke University press.

Duarte, E. (1991). Trayectoria de la medicina social en América Latina: Elementos para su configuración. In S. Franco, E. Nunes, E. Duarte, J. Breihl, E. Granda, J. Yépez, P. Costales, & C. Laurell (Eds.), *Debates en medicina social* (pp. 17–137). Quito: PAHO.

Felitti, K. (2012). Planificación familiar en Argentina de las décadas 1960 y 1970: ¿un caso original en América Latina? *Estudios Demográficos y Urbanos, 27*(1), 153–188.

Fonseca Sobrinho, D. (1993). *Estado e população: Uma história do planejamento familiar no Brasil.* Rio de Janeiro: Rosa dos Tempos & UNFPA.

Ilcan, S., & Phillips, L. (2008). Governing through global networks: Knowledge mobilities and participatory development. *Current Sociology, 56*(5), 711–734.

Kothari, A., McPherson, C., Gore, D., Cohen, B., MacDonald, M., & Sibbald, S. L. (2016). A multiple case study of intersectional public health networks: Experiences and benefits of using research. *Health Research Policy and Systems, 14*(11), doi:10.1186/s12961-016-0082-7

Laurell, A. C. (1982). Acerca de la reconceptualización de la epidemiología. *Salud Problema, 8*, 5–9.

Laurell, A. C. (2003). What does Latin American social medicine do when it governs? The case of the Mexico City government. *American Journal of Public Health, 93*(12), 2028–2031.

Márquez, V. B. (1984). La política de planificación familiar en México: Un proceso institucionalizado? *Revista Mexicana de Sociología, 46*(2), 285–310.

Menéndez, E. L. (2009). De racismos, esterilizaciones y algunos otros olvidos de la antropología y la epidemiología mexicanas. *Salud Colectiva, 5*(2), 155–179.

Mora Bravo, M. (1986). *El derecho a la planeación familiar: Marco jurídico.* México City: CONAPO.

Mora Bravo, M. (2017). *El derecho a la planeación familiar en México: Génesis del cambio.* Mexico City: CONAPO.

Natividad, M. D. F., Fiereck, K. J., & Parker, R. (2012). Knowledge networks for global public health. *Global Public Health, 7*(S1), S73–S81.

Navarro, F. A., & Manautou, J. M. (1986). *Inovaciones Administrativas del Programa de Planificación Familiar: Estudio de caso.* Mexico City: IMSS.

Nunes, E. D. (2015). Juan César García: Social medicine as project and endeavor. *Ciência & Saúde Coletiva, 20*(1), 139–144.

Nunes, E. D. (2016). La salud colectiva en Brasil: Analizando el proceso de institucionalización. *Salud Colectiva, 12*(3), 347–360.

Pesquisa Nacional de Demografia e Saúde da Criança e da Mulher (PNDS). (2006). *Relatório.* Brasilia: Ministry of Health.

Pêgo, R. A., & Almeida, C. (2004). Teoría y práctica de las reformas en los sistemas de salud: Los casos de Brasil y México. In C. Alba Vega & I. Bizberg (Eds.), *Democracia y Globalización* (pp. 335–380). Mexico City: CEI-COLMEX.

Potter, J. E. (1999). The persistence of outmoded contraceptive regimes: The cases of Mexico and Brazil. La persistance des methodes contraceptives depassees: Les cas du mexique et du bresil. La persistencia de las practicas anticonceptivas anticuadas: Los casos de Mexico y brasil. *Population & Development Review, 25*(4), 703–739.

Rodrigues, W. (1983, September). *Política populacional brasileira (alguns subsídios).* Paper presented at the I Congress of Maternal-Child Health and Family Planning, Rio de Janeiro, Brazil, Bemfam Documentation Center.

Secretariat de Salubridad y Asistencia (SSA). (no date). *Programas y proyectos.* Mexico City: SSA-Coordinación General de Planificación Familiar. Archivo General de la República, Mexico City.

Stone, D. (2013). *Knowledge actors and transnational governance: The private-public policy nexus in the global agora.* New York: Palgrave Macmillan.

Waitzkin, H., Iriart, C., Estrada, A., & Lamadrid, S. (2001). Social medicine in Latin America: Productivity and dangers facing the major national groups. *The Lancet, 358,* 315–323.

Welti-Chanes, C. (2011). La demografía en México, las etapas iniciales de su evolución y sus aportaciones al desarrollo nacional. *Papeles de población, 17*(69), 9–47.

Werneck Vianna, L. (1977). Leis Sociais e Demografia. *Estudos CEBRAP, 21,* 93–147.

Zarate Campos, M. S., & González Moya, M. (2013). Planificación familiar en la Guerra Fría. *História Crítica, 55,* 207–230.

# Latin American social medicine across borders: South–South cooperation and the making of health solidarity

Anne-Emanuelle Birn and Carles Muntaner

**ABSTRACT**
Latin American social medicine efforts are typically understood as national endeavours, involving health workers, policymakers, academics, social movements, unions, and left-wing political parties, among other domestic actors. But Latin America's social medicine trajectory has also encompassed considerable between-country solidarity, building on early twentieth century interchanges among a range of players who shared approaches for improving living and working conditions and instituting protective social policies. Since the 1960s, Cuba's country-to-country solidarity has stood out, comprising medic exchanges, training, and other forms of support for the health and social struggles of oppressed peoples throughout Latin America and around the world, recently via Misión Barrio Adentro in Venezuela. These efforts strive for social justice-oriented health cooperation based on horizontal power relations, shared political values, a commitment to social and economic redistribution, bona fide equity, and an understanding of the societal determination of health that includes, but goes well beyond, public health and medical care. With Latin America's left-wing surge now receding, this article traces the provenance, dynamics, impact, challenges, and legacy of health solidarity across Latin American borders and its prospects for continuity.

Over the past few decades, South–South health cooperation based on left-wing solidarity has thrived among various countries in Latin America (as well as other 'Global South' settings). These efforts both draw from and transcend longstanding Latin American social medicine (LASM) ideas and practices by incorporating social justice values into official foreign (health) policy. Here we lay out the origins of and connections between LASM and social justice-oriented health cooperation and examine the latter's contemporary practices, principles, perils, and prospects, focusing particular attention on the role of Cuba.

## Forerunners of social medicine (and its cross-border prospects) in Latin America

LASM – notwithstanding this regional label (Tajer, 2003) – is often examined as a collection of sim-ultaneous, albeit communicating, national endeavours (Franco, Nunes, Breilh, & Laurell, 1991; Hart-mann, 2016; Waitzkin, Iriart, Estrada, & Lamadrid, 2001a). To be sure, in Latin America, as elsewhere, social medicine has taken on different characteristics and trajectories in distinct contexts and time periods, as shaped by political movements, social conditions, and the role of medical experts, among other factors (Borowy & Hardy, 2008; Brown & Birn, 2013; Carter, 2018; Cueto &

Palmer, 2014). Here we loosely define social medicine as a realm of study, practice, and activism based on an understanding of health and disease as inherently rooted in social and political conditions and reflecting relations of power.

Especially in recent decades, there has been a vibrant parallel ambit to domestic experiences of LASM that is transnational, intergovernmental, and cooperative, in which government actors championing social medicine ideas have exchanged insights, expertise, experiences, and resources as a matter of official diplomacy based on mutually-held leftist values and aspirations for more egalitarian societies, and in some cases countering global capitalist power. Elsewhere, we have dubbed this endeavour social justice-oriented South–South health cooperation (SJSSC; not exclusive to Latin America). SJSSC is based on an understanding of the social and political underpinnings of health and disease (even as the content of cooperation may be biomedical) and a commitment to public, primary health care as a universal right.

The descriptor 'LASM across borders,' while also fitting, does not necessarily encompass official state actions in the way that SJSSC does. Brazil's 'structural cooperation in health' approach also overlaps with SJSSC given its attention to horizontal decision-making, institutional strengthening, and fostering sovereign capacity (Buss & Ferreira, 2010), but it 'does not perforce challenge the political and economic status quo' (Birn, Muntaner, & Afzal, 2017, p. 8). SJSSC pursues either shared socialist or social-democratic political principles: the first invoking an anti-hegemonic, anti-capitalist vision; the second an egalitarian approach that seeks to reform more than upend global capitalism.

Why have social medicine across borders – and SJSSC – unfolded so vibrantly in Latin America? While challenging to answer in an abbreviated fashion, here we track a few antecedents to contemporary developments in solidarity-oriented cooperation. These include: 1) an overlapping trajectory under – and struggles against – colonialism and subsequent forms of imperialism and repression; 2) longtime medical and health cooperation that was not necessarily social medicine-oriented but nonetheless helped forge mutual understanding among states and health and social welfare professionals; 3) labour militancy and social and political movements advocating working class, and sometimes rural agrarian, social welfare justice that spilled across the region (if often coopted or displaced by populist regimes); and 4) professional and political curiosity about, and/or commitment to, socialism and social medicine approaches implemented in the Soviet Union.

Typically traced to mid-nineteenth century Europe, when a wave of uprisings challenged state repression and the brutal working and living conditions of the Industrial Revolution, social medicine was crystallized in the thinking of Rudolf Virchow, who famously called for a devastating typhus outbreak in the impoverished Silesia region of Prussia to be addressed as a political and social problem, and who himself participated on the Berlin barricades of 1848 (Anderson, Smith, & Sidel, 2005; Waitzkin, 2006). Virchow's precepts were subsequently espoused, adapted, and reshaped across Europe and other regions (Brown & Birn, 2013; Porter, 2006), including Latin America (Iriart, Waitzkin, Breilh, Estrada, & Merhy, 2002).

Under Iberian rule, long before Virchow, the region even experienced a harbinger of sorts to social medicine in the figure of Eugenio Espejo, an erudite physician in colonial Quito of Indigenous background. Espejo's upbringing in a pauper institution, and the fact that his ancestors were enslaved, undoubtedly moulded his sensibilities. Commissioned in 1785 by the city's administrative council to identify a means of preventing frequent outbreaks of smallpox, Espejo pinpointed deficient sanitary and social conditions, as well as inept and self-interested colonial medical and religious authorities (Breilh Paz y Miño, 2001; Espejo, 1993). Like Virchow six decades later, Espejo was a political radical accused of subversion by imperial authorities, the former internally-exiled, the latter repeatedly imprisoned and persecuted by the Spanish Viceroy, along the way disseminating his anti-imperial convictions in Bogotá.

Beyond percolating ideas around social and political influences on health, a confluence of political, scientific, and professional factors in the 19th and 20th centuries shaped the region's receptiveness to social medicine more directly. Well before notions of Latin America as a region with shared features, problems, opportunities, and political leanings solidified under the Cold War (Bethell &

Roxborough, 1993), visions of Latin American distinctiveness emerged. First, a wave of liberation movements from 1810 to 1825, largely marshalled and inspired by revolutionary Simon Bolívar, resulted in the creation of independent republics across the region (except for Spain's Caribbean colonies), with Brazil remaining under imperial control until 1889. While European re-invasion of Mexico, internecine and inter-state wars, and border disputes persisted for over a century, the colonial legacy – and the Bolivarian movement for South American sovereignty/independence (Bolívar, 2003), together with ongoing shared experiences of European and North American economic domination and US political interference – helped engender a sense of regional identity and destiny. This was particularly the case among urban elites (with professionals and upper classes in Spain's former colonies speaking a common language), who were central to the state-building process (del Castillo, 2018).

By the late nineteenth century, tenets of Pan Americanism (regionwide cooperation, often, but not always, driven by US interests), as well as Latin American variants without US participation, burgeoned. A flurry of associations and meetings around political, commercial, cultural, technical, and scientific issues – facilitated by the rise of steamship and rail transport and communications advances – began to take shape, engaging multiple actors (García & Marichal, 2004; Sheinin, 2000). While most of these interchanges sought to further business and investment agendas across liberal republics, certain more radical ideas also flourished, drawing from the growing influence of Marxist ideas, anti-imperial struggles, and by the early twentieth century, the labour movement and new socialist political parties (Meade, 2016).

In the health, social welfare, and medical arenas, proliferating interactions stemmed from both the professionalisation of scientific disciplines – involving new journals, associations, scholarly networks, and conferences in areas such as hygiene and sanitation medicine, demography, eugenics,[1] and child well-being – and from the need to address conjoined health issues (Birn, 2005). These pressing and palpable problems included cross-border outbreaks (Chaves, 2009), domestic epidemics, infant mortality, and occupational diseases generated by miserable living and working conditions, urbanisation, migration, and heightened trade (Almeida, 2006).

Cooperative efforts to confront these issues were mostly hatched by those representing dominant political and commercial concerns. The Pan American Sanitary Bureau, founded in 1902 and for decades operated out of the US Public Health Service, held quadrennial regional congresses attended by high-ranking government officials in a position to negotiate legally binding international agreements, including the landmark 1924 Pan American Sanitary Code governing disease notification and epidemic control among all American republics (Cueto, 2007). For decades, it focused almost exclusively on safeguarding commercial interests, failing to respond to other priorities such as infant and maternal mortality (Birn, 2002). While Latin American sanitary treaties and most professional interchanges rarely constituted leftist solidarity, they did pave the way for intergovernmental and expert cooperation, and, occasionally, alternate players with more progressive views wielded influence.

Organised working class and other movements fighting for better living and working conditions were also salient to LASM across borders (and SJSSC later on). Struggles for health justice and social security involved a complex array of agrarian and industrial unions, Indigenous peoples, women militants, and other social movements. Mobilised against powerful and entrenched political and economic elites, these groups formed alliances with an assortment of leftwing political parties within their own countries, but also in communication with and inspired by militancy throughout Latin America (Carr, 2014; Chomsky, 2011; Herrera González, 2013). Activists pushed for social protections – including state-run health programmes – in several waves, starting in the Southern cone countries and extending to virtually the entire region by the late 1940s (Mesa-Lago, 1978; Ortúzar, 2013). With domestic reformers eyeing gains in neighbouring countries, legislative advances were peppered with solidarity at regional medical and welfare venues (Guy, 1998; Ramacciotti, 2015) and through (nationalist-minded) engagement with the social medicine-oriented League of Nations

Health Organisation and the more middle-ground International Labour Office (Borowy, 2009; Carter, 2018; Derecho Internacional Público, 2014; Weindling, 2006).

However, protective legislation was typically passed under populist or authoritarian, rather than socialist, regimes, as in Argentina, Brazil, and Chile, following Bismarck-style carrot-and-stick approaches of benefits for selected groups (while rejecting universal rights) even as repressive policies against labour and social activism were retained. In most settings, social security systems remained partial and heavily stratified, with urban industrial workers and civil servants enjoying the greatest benefits, while dependents and rural and informal workers lagged far behind (García, 1981; Marquez & Joly, 1986; Mesa-Lago, 1985). Coopting of social medicine ideas was evident in Uruguay, too, where advocates of 'childhood social medicine' marshalled adoption of a 'Código del Niño.' The code spelled out children's rights to health, welfare, education, housing, and other elements of well-being, but it came under a 1930s dictatorship, with the heavy hand of a repressive regime bent on disciplining juvenile 'delinquents' (Birn, 2012).

The early twentieth century founding of communist and socialist political parties in many Latin American countries served as a small yet relevant political harness for some social medicine activists (Angell, 1998; Concheiro, Modonesi, & Crespo, 2007; Löwy, 2007; Spenser, 1999), as did umbrella Popular Front coalitions motivated by the 'Second International' (international proletarian movement) and its Soviet successor Comintern, together with the USSR's social policies implemented following the Russian Revolution.[2] Starting in the 1930s, numerous Latin American experts – envisioning a Soviet welfare state utopia and seeking a blueprint for domestic reforms – were keen to witness the USSR's wide-reaching social policy accomplishments firsthand. Dozens of medical and public health professionals from Argentina, Brazil, Chile, Colombia, Cuba, El Salvador, Mexico, Uruguay, and Venezuela travelled to the Soviet Union (see, for instance, Zeno, 1933), a trend that accelerated after World War II (Viel, 1961). The books and popular articles these visitors penned about Soviet public health services, medical schools, and research institutes upon returning home entered into lively national and regional debates about how to shape policies and institutions, particularly as Latin American countries were positioning themselves in the Cold War (Rupprecht, 2015). Latin American nurses, physicians, and other medics were also active 'comrades in health' in the 1936–1939 Spanish Civil War, among the thousands of civilian volunteer health workers with the international medical brigades supporting the Republican cause against Franco's fascists (Baumann, 2009).

The larger political context and transnational interchanges engendered translation of ideas around both social medicine and socialised (or state) medicine into further political agendas. In mid 1930s Mexico, for example, the *nicolaítas*, a group of radical physician-advisors to socialist-leaning president Lázaro Cárdenas, elevated their proposals to government policy through the creation of mandatory physician service to rural areas and the resurrection of *Ejidos* (land collectives redistributed and returned to Mexico's large and increasingly organised peasant population) involving strong rural and community medicine components (Carrillo, 2005; Kapelusz-Poppi, 2001). Around the same time in Peru, social medicine practitioners sought to extend rural health campaigns to Indigenous populations in a community-based and more respectful manner than prior coercive interactions (Cueto, 1991).

It was in Chile that LASM came to political power most boldly (Waitzkin, 2005; Zárate Campos & Godoy Catalán, 2011). Salvador Allende, a social medicine devotee and committed socialist, rose to prominence in the 1930s: first as a medical student leader, and then as a young health minister for the Popular Front coalition elected in 1938 (Allende, 1939; Labra, 2000), setting the wheels in motion for Chile's milestone 1952 National Health Service (SNS) (Illanes, 1993). Allende, by then a Senator, helped shepherd the SNS proposal into law, convinced it would help 'prevent the tremendous injustices that arise due to the existence in this country of distinct social strata' (Allende, 1951, p. 1525). Both Allende and the SNS would become embroiled in Cold War ideological rivalries (Berlagoscky, 2013). In 1970, after multiple attempts – and embodying Virchow's idea of politics as (social) medicine at a grand scale – Allende was elected president on a platform of nationalisation and redistribution; the conservative physicians' association was among his fiercest opponents. Allende was deposed in a US-backed military coup in 1973, with dictator Augusto Pinochet systematically dismantling the SNS. Medical radicals (including social medicine advocates) were among the tens of thousands of Chileans tortured, executed, or 'disappeared' and the hundreds of thousands more forced into exile.

## LASM across borders and Cuba's SJSSC

The targeting of health leftists in Chile was not an isolated episode. The authoritarian regimes that swept across Latin America during the Cold War sidelined social medicine aspirations and subjected its advocates to persecution (Waitzkin, Iriart, Estrada, & Lamadrid, 2001b). These circumstances helped spur the founding of two key organisations: Associação Brasileira de Saúde Coletiva (ABRASCO), the Brazilian collective health movement, launched in 1979 amidst the 1964–1985 dictatorship and so-named to challenge the legitimacy of the repressive state to address the people's health; and the Latin American Social Medicine Association (ALAMES), begun in 1984 to foster solidarity and scholarly and policy interchange among leftist health professionals and academics and support those exiled. ABRASCO provided scaffolding to decades of political struggle to realise Brazil's unified national health system and social redistribution measures. Its members served in a range of policy (and prior to that, shadow policy) positions after the dictatorship ended (Lima & Santana, 2006), including in Brazil's South–South health cooperation. Today, both ABRASCO and ALAMES continue to hold periodic conferences, host publications, and participate in global health forums and domestic health and social policy activism (Granda, 2008). ALAMES consists of a network of social medicine academics and practitioners, albeit with palpable tensions, particularly around support for different varieties of leftist politics (e.g. socialist vs. social democratic). Various ALAMES members have been involved in building socially just health systems in locales such as Paraguay, Venezuela, and Mexico City (Laurell, 2003). ALAMES principles call for 'promot[ing] alliances for a radical defense of life among movements' (Torres Tovar, 2007); its members are most proud of the organisation's solidarity with revolutionary efforts, including ALBA[3] (Franco Agudelo, 2009). Despite being the region's most vibrant forum for LASM across borders, ALAMES has not incorporated SJSSC as an explicit part of its agenda.

Even before these developments, Cuba became the region's foremost champion of SJSSC, embarking on health solidarity efforts just a year after its 1959 revolution and heralding continuous engagement within and beyond Latin America (Cassells, 2016; Ojeda Medina, 2010). A few years earlier, the Soviet Union, German Democratic Republic, Romania, and other Eastern European countries had become involved in 'proletarian' health solidarity in North Korea and Vietnam (Hong, 2015; Iacob, 2017), making socialist health cooperation an instrument of the Soviet bloc's Cold War foreign policy, analogous to the disease campaigns and population control efforts operated by the US bloc (Packard, 2016). But Cuba's endeavours differed from the strategic alliance-making of the East–West geopolitical rivalry.

Before tracing Cuba's trajectory, a few conceptual points are merited. SJSSC differs from conventional development assistance for health (including mainstream South–South cooperation) in various ways. First, unlike most aid channels from high-income countries and multilateral agencies, it does not compromise sovereignty by imposing conditions as a quid pro quo for receiving aid. Indeed, SJSSC (not considered aid) is exercised on as equal terms as feasible, reducing, if not eliminating, power and resource differentials between parties. SJSSC responds to national and local demands for equity and draws from social rights approaches based on health-related human rights, for example in relation to universal, public comprehensive health care (Medicus Mundi, 2010). Thus, agenda-setting for cooperation is carried out mutually, decreasing overall dependency. Second, SJSSC cooperation aims to be transformative: for example, training local primary health care practitioners counteracts the brain drain; and investing in social infrastructure hand in hand with government agencies helps create lasting and equitable means of addressing human needs. Third, SJSSC seeks to be counter-hegemonic, that is, resist corporate, neoliberal capitalist forces as part of the project of building societies based on health and social justice, ideally following a bottom-up participatory approach of community-based democracy (Birn, Muntaner, et al., 2017).

Cuba's South–South medical cooperation began in 1960, when the government dispatched a team of emergency medicine experts to Chile in the aftermath of a major earthquake, even as half of Cuba's doctors were decamping to the United States and other countries. Disaster relief would continue to serve as a major component of Cuban health cooperation – enhanced by the establishment of its own civil defense system following a devastating 1963 hurricane.

Meanwhile, a more social medicine-oriented approach was underway, as articulated by Argentinean physician-turned-revolutionary Ernesto 'Che' Guevara, who famously fought side-by-side with Fidel Castro, later joining liberation movements in Congo and Bolivia. Echoing Virchow, he came to see political struggle as an extension of social medicine:

> integrating the doctor or any other health worker into the revolutionary movement [is essential], because … the work of educating and feeding the children … and … of redistributing the land from its former absentee landlords to those who sweat every day on that very land without reaping its fruits—is the grandest social medicine effort that has been done in Cuba (Guevara, 1960, p. 119).

In 1963 these ideas translated into Cuba's medical solidarity with Algeria, following its protracted war of independence from ruthless French colonial control (Gleijeses, 1996; Hatzky & Stites Mor, 2014; Johnson, 2015). A delegation of several dozen doctors, nurses, dentists, and technicians spent a year caring for the injured and working with Algeria's revolutionary government to rebuild health services for its shattered population. The next year, a replacement team of medics arrived, with similar missions participating in liberation movements in North Vietnam, the Congo, Guinea Bissau, Angola, and so on. Fidel's propensity to always say 'yes' to requests, regardless of the cost or consequences, at times angered the Soviets, who saw Cuban cooperation as trespassing on or distracting from their own efforts (Kirk, 2015).

One seeming paradox of Cuban domestic policies and SJSSC also marked Soviet approaches: because societal underpinnings of health were addressed through universal rights to housing, sanitation, employment, nutrition, education, elimination of poverty, and so on, the health sector focused more narrowly on medicine. The social and political dimensions of health were considered self-evident achievements of the socialist system; thus, the Soviets accorded priority to showcasing technological prowess and deploying universal access to biomedical care in their cooperative efforts (Venediktov, 1977). For Cuba, too, the social justice spirit of its approach to health has manifested in its advocacy of equitable, universal access to what is largely a biomedical approach, following a community-based, preventive care emphasis, both at home (Navarro, 1972) and abroad (Feinsilver, 2010).

Initially, Cuban cooperation was motivated by reciprocity with (and gratitude to) countries/peoples that had provided support during Cuba's revolution and/or that were engaged in similar struggles. Later, Cuba anchored both the domestic right to health care and a commitment to medical internationalism in its 1976 Constitution.

Other important solidarity activities involved supporting those targeted by authoritarian regimes across Latin America from the 1960s onwards. This involved rehabilitating leftist revolutionaries injured in Central America's violent civil wars in the 1980s, including medical comrades from Latin America and beyond who joined in El Salvador's prolonged struggle for a just society (Genaro & Gato, 2017). In the more hopeful situation across the border, a large Cuban medical brigade arrived just days after Nicaragua's 1979 Sandinista revolution, a steady presence in providing primary health care to long overlooked populations (Anderson, 2013; Garfield & Williams, 1992).

Another leading form of Cuban SJSSC has been its role in training medical personnel (Kirk & Erisman, 2009), which accelerated after the end of the Cold War. Since its founding in 1998, Cuba's Escuela Latinoamericana de Medicina (ELAM) has trained more than 26,000 students from throughout the Americas and globally – 123 countries in total (Loewenberg, 2016). Much of this training is free of charge for those coming from low-income countries (low-income and racialized backgrounds in the case of US students). ELAM thus constitutes Cuba's unique antidote to physician brain drain: trained in primary health care, tens of thousands of newly-minted physicians have now returned home to serve their communities.

Over time, Cuba's SJSSC – primary care provision and disaster relief to the tune of over 140,000 medical professionals serving across Latin America and in more than 100 countries, millions of cataract surgeries performed through 'Operación Milagro,' and establishment of almost a dozen medical schools abroad, in addition to its ELAM hub in Havana – has extended well beyond settings with active anti-hegemonic movements. Expanding since the demise of the Soviet Union, Cuba's cooperation with settings 'where no doctor has gone before' has made a significant impact around the world (Huish, 2013).

The principles, practices, and commitment to health equity domestically and to internationalism (or proletarian internationalism) (Brown & Birn, 2013; Featherstone, 2012) – with roots in socialist diplomacy constitutionally enshrined – are widely invoked as drivers of Cuba's health care cooperation (De Vos, De Ceukelaire, Bonet, & Van der Stuyft, 2007; Fitz, 2012; Kirk, 2015). Others cite humanitarian solidarity as the motor of the scope, reach, and durability of Cuba's health cooperation, which has arguably saved millions of lives and improved many more. In Guatemala alone, a stunning 35 million medical consults have been carried out spanning 15 years, serving millions of patients 'whose lives have been changed' by Cuba's programmes (Kirk, 2015, p. 273).

That said, Cuban SJSSC has also faced critiques. Domestically, the 50,000+ Cuban medical personnel (over half doctors) working in 66 countries in 2014,[4] resulted in physician shortages and resentment in parts of Cuba (Brotherton, 2013). There have also been defections, greatly exacerbated by the US State Department's 'parole' programme, which has incentivized over 1000 doctors to abandon Cuba (Kirk, 2015).

Mainstream responses to Cuba's SJSSC have been to ignore it (Novotny, Kickbusch, & Told, 2013), dismiss it (see Fitz, 2016), or cite it as a typical case study of soft power influence (Nye, 2009), in which health serves as an instrument of self-interested foreign policy (Kickbusch, 2011). To be sure, there are controversies surrounding Cuba's endeavours. Whereas in the past there was no quid pro quo, since 2006 under Raúl Castro over half of countries pay for medical services and training, bringing in over $8 billion annually in hard currency (Cuba's largest source of income – triple the earnings from tourism) (Benzi & Zapata, 2017). In Honduras doctors objected to the Cubans' presence but succumbed to pressure from populations left underserved. In 2014 Brazilian medical elites similarly protested the contracting of over 11,000 Cuban doctors to provide primary care where local doctors were 'unrecruitable' (Lidola & Borges, 2017; Walker & Kirk, 2017). Concerns about the low and deferred pay of internationalist doctors (cited as slave labour by some) have led to salary improvements (Oliveira et al., 2015).

A crucial question remains: how much of Cuba's SJSSC is truly social medicine-oriented? One facet has to do with its focus on disaster relief and medical training. Arguably, the problems faced by very low-income countries – such as the Central American countries struck by Hurricane Mitch in 1998, which killed or injured tens of thousands and displaced several million people – in dealing with sudden disasters makes long-term, infrastructure-oriented disaster relief a social medicine endeavour (as opposed to short-term charitable or humanitarian aid in this domain) (Buss & Ferreira, 2010). As far away as Pakistan, Cuban solidarity recovery and rebuilding efforts after the 2005 earthquake deeply inspired local populations, who reported having never witnessed such sustained, egalitarian attention from their own government or any other (Akhatar, 2006). Cuba's role in Haiti following the 2010 earthquake similarly stands apart: while other countries met with donor fatigue ex post facto, Cuban medics had already spent 11 years there engaged in cooperative and infrastructural activities, a situation downplayed by international media (Huish, 2013). In West Africa's 2014–2015 Ebola crisis, too, Cuba responded almost immediately with hundreds of health personnel, while the World Health Organization (WHO) and US government dithered.

By any account, Cuba's medical coverage at home and abroad are nothing short of extraordinary, even as accusations of propaganda or spying persist and many doctors may be as interested in adventure, earning cash, and advancing skills as they are in altruistic solidarity. Yet Cuba's *internacionalistas*, much as they might disparage the situation at home, have repeatedly recounted how shocked they were at the misery they saw abroad, including diseases they had only read about in textbooks (Garfield & Williams, 1992; Kirk, 2015).

Misleadingly, some consider Cuban medical solidarity to be the 'world's best kept secret' (Kirk, 2015). Yet it is hardly a secret to over 100 appreciative countries or to the US State Department actively monitoring these efforts. Still, Cuba's SJSSC is deliberately overlooked by most mainstream (Northern) observers, a classic 'threat of a good example' (Chomsky, 1992; Melrose, 1985).

Of late, the most well-known instances of Cuban medical cooperation have been in the Americas – especially Venezuela, Haiti, Central America, and Brazil, as well as a remarkable intersectoral door-to-door project to identify and address the health and social needs of hundreds of thousands of persons with disabilities in Ecuador (the Manuela Espejo mission; see Monje Vargas, 2013) and Bolivia.

## Contemporary SJSSC: expanding cooperation and integration against the grain

Cuba's early medical solidarity endeavours did not go unnoticed by its ideological opponents. The 1961 Charter of Punta del Este, which launched the US-led Alliance for Progress – a development approach aimed at preventing the proliferation of Cuba-like revolutions across the region – stimulated some inter-American efforts (excluding Cuba) around health planning and realisation of such goals as water and sanitation coverage, infectious disease control, and maternal and child health improvements. By 1978, and responding to the G-77's call for a New International Economic Order (stemming from a Third World movement against neocolonialism), the United Nations formally sought to stimulate technical cooperation between 'developing' countries. But this effort took place in the context of authoritarian regimes and debt crises, not as an expression of social solidarity (Birn, Pillay, & Holtz, 2017). Still, in the 1960s and 1970s, many Latin American governments set up foreign cooperation offices, creating an institutional framework that would serve subsequent, if politically divergent, objectives.

Since 2000, in conjunction with the Pink Tide (the wave of left-leaning governments elected in Central and South America), the region came to serve as a bona fide counter-hegemonic force in global (health) politics. For example, Latin America is the first and only subcontinent to have committed to remain free of nuclear arms (Musto, 2017). Three main developments made the expansion of SJSSC within Latin America possible: (1) from 2000 to 2015, over half of the region's 20 countries (plus Puerto Rico) elected social democratic or socialist governments with strong labour party and social movement backing that has reduced poverty and income inequality and expanded access to public health and social services (Cornia, 2014; Lustig, Lopez-Calva, Ortiz-Juarez, & Monga, 2016); (2) the rise in commodity prices enabling allocation of substantial sums to South–South cooperation generally and internally to social medicine-oriented reforms (e.g. Brazil, Venezuela) (Wilpert, 2007); and (3) Cuba's (re-) insertion into a new era of engagement in the region, driven by its economic and political relations with Venezuela (Morris, 2014; Muntaner et al., 2008).

Although such endeavours have been negatively affected by the 2008–2012 world financial crisis and, more recently, a shift in government regimes and policies (e.g. in Brazil, Argentina, Paraguay), other countries have sought to continue – some more effectively than others – to support SJSSC goals (Bolivia, Ecuador, Uruguay, Cuba, Nicaragua, El Salvador, and Venezuela), albeit amidst economic and political instability in many settings (Petras & Veltmeyer, 2016).

The emergence of Brazil as an economic powerhouse among middle-income countries (Prashad, 2013) helped spur the region's social medicine efforts domestically and across borders, partially building on Cuba's SJSSC model. Under president Lula's back-to-back Workers' Party administrations starting in 2003, Brazil's 'structural cooperation' involved training, health policy and health systems support, and 'horizontal' interchange with key counterparts in Latin America and former

Portuguese colonies (Ciência & Saúde Coletiva, 2017; Ferreira, Hoirisch, Fonseca, & Buss, 2016; Santos & Cerqueira, 2015). It has operated dozens of projects in sub-Saharan Africa – many coordinated by Fiocruz, Brazil's national health institute – ranging from capacity building for health care personnel (e.g. physicians, lab technicians), to disease control efforts, HIV drug donations, and an ARV factory in Mozambique (Carrillo Roa & Silva, 2015; Santana, 2011).

Like Cuba, Brazil has sought to prioritise the interests and needs of LMICs and refrained from imposing conditionalities – in some ways challenging the dominant political order – but its aggressive investments in African mining, construction, and other industries run parallel to its health diplomacy (Alden, Chichava, & Alves, 2017; Garcia & Kato, 2015; Ventura, 2013), with private corporate priorities trumping social solidarity. Within Latin America, Brazil's role has been more social medicine-oriented, focusing, for example, on equitable public health policy. Moreover, its leadership in challenging the pharmaceutical patent regime effectively resisted one of the most powerful corporate sectors in global health (Chan, 2015). Since 2014, however, Brazilian government commitment to South–South cooperation has cooled, and along with economic and political crises, civil society coordination and support has also lessened (Gómez & Perez, 2016).

Beyond bilateral efforts, the social justice orientation of many Latin American governments and their grassroots political movements (Harnecker, 2015; Karan & Sodhi, 2015) led to the creation of new organisations that favour SJSSC. Key among them are the Union of South American Countries (UNASUR), which has a permanent South American Health Council (involving member country health ministries) that strives for regional health care integration.[5] Heeding social medicine values, UNASUR has developed a mutual agenda emphasising universal access to health care and medicines, equity, and action on the social determinants of health. Its health research institute oversees research in these areas and helps craft common policies around disease surveillance, human resources for health, health systems development, health promotion, unified regional positions vis-à-vis WHO (Herrero & Tussie, 2015), and has rallied against the privatisation of medical care (Feo, 2012).

Even with much larger and well-financed players now participating, Cuba continues to be the most important SJSSC actor in Latin America (as well as around the globe) in terms of the volume and solidarity orientation of its health cooperation (Beldarraín Chaple, 2006; Feinsilver, 2010; Fitz, 2016; Huish, 2013).

## The threat of a good example: Barrio Adentro and Cuba-Venezuela SJSSC

Among the best-known examples of contemporary SJSSC is *Misión Barrio Adentro* (Inside the Neighbourhood), a primary health care programme developed under late Venezuelan president Hugo Chávez in 2003 to respond to the demands of poor urban and peri-urban slum residents chronically shunned by most physicians who prefer to serve wealthier patients (Castro, Gusmão, Martínez, & Vivas, 2006). Enabled by an agreement with the late Fidel Castro to furnish approximately 30,000 physicians – in return for much needed fuel supplies – plus thousands of other Cuban nursing and allied sciences professionals, including physical education specialist and dentists (Alvarado et al., 2006; Muntaner, Salazar, Rueda, & Armada, 2006), this exchange has had a combined ideological, political, and economic basis (Muntaner et al., 2008).

As is typical of Cuba's medical solidarity programmes, doctors are not treated as privileged consultants but are integrated into the neighbourhoods they serve, often living with local community members, who themselves help to plan and build health care clinics. Not wanting to generate reliance on Cuban health professionals, the agreement between Chávez and Castro also incorporated a training component for 10,000 Venezuelans from humble roots to receive medical and nursing education in Cuba before returning to practise in their communities. In order to further reduce dependence on Cuba, in 2010 the Venezuelan government launched an ambitious effort to train community physicians and nurses from low-income backgrounds in Venezuela: several new medical and nursing schools were established with Cuban support (Mahmood & Muntaner, 2013). As of March 2015, almost 19,000 Venezuelan physicians had graduated with degrees in Integral Community Medicine and begun working at Barrio Adentro facilities throughout the country (MPPS, 2015).

All told, according to Cuban officials, between 2003 and 2015 Barrio Adentro cared for more than 53 million patients, treating 1.7 million life-threatening emergencies amidst a quadrupling of health care facilities. Since its inception, Barrio Adentro has been integrated with other social programmes targeting nutrition, medications, poverty reduction, employment, and health education among other areas, enabling referrals and coordination across sectors (Castro et al., 2006; Muntaner, Chung, Mahmood, & Armada, 2011). Together, these efforts contributed to infant mortality declines from 21 deaths/1000 live births to 14; malnutrition reductions from 21% to 14% of the population (and accelerated child growth rates), and an increase in access to clean water from 80% to 94% of the population (Curcio, 2017).

It is important to note that the social medicine dimensions of Barrio Adentro reside in their integration into a larger commitment to public (non-market), universal, gratis, equitable social services in the context of overturning Venezuela's prior neoliberal capitalist state. In that sense, Cuban–Venezuelan SJSSC has centred on greatly expanded access to primary care for the majority of residents and training for prospective medical practitioners (especially from low-income communities) to ensure that the Barrio Adentro programme can last. Additionally, community support is managed at the local level by 'comités de salud' and 'consejos comunales.'

Notwithstanding the technical orientation of the programme itself, Barrio Adentro's initial leaders were aligned with the Latin American Marxist social medicine tradition represented by Salvador Allende, which seeks transformation of the capitalist social structure. Indeed, physician advocates of this tradition held high-level positions in Venezuela's Ministry of Health, early on producing scholarship on the role of imperialism and class power in shaping health inequities (Armada, Muntaner, & Navarro, 2001; Armada, Muntaner, Chung, Williams-Brennan, & Benach, 2009).

This helps explain why the content of Venezuelan physician training (like its Cuban counterpart) has not focused significant attention on the social determinants of health or policies aimed at reducing health inequities (MPPS, 2013): these dimensions are understood to be addressed by the overall political commitment to policies advancing well-being and diminishing economic and social inequities. In this context, a focus on biomedical and behavioural dimensions does not replace political and social understandings of health but is corollary to the larger societal commitment to human welfare and equality. Advocates of Cuba's SJSSC hold that providing support for the attainment of universal access to public, comprehensive, and equitable medical care shared among sister nations is the epitome of solidarity (Fitz, 2012). Yet some believe that a vision of social medicine that appears apolitical and centred on individual care risks ignoring social injustice and may end up conflated with mainstream humanitarian cooperation approaches (Saney, 2009).

The fate of the Barrio Adentro programme (and of the Venezuelan state) cannot be understood without an account of ongoing internal and external opposition and the effects of Venezuela's 'resource curse' – being an export-oriented country with the world's second largest oil reserves (Amin, 2014; Spronk & Webber, 2015). One useful distinction is between the 'early years' (Armada et al., 2009) – before the 2008 global financial crisis dramatically lowered the price of oil – and the aftermath of the crisis, which is still generating political and economic turmoil. The first years witnessed an impressive surge in access to health care, reaching about 17 million more Venezuelans than before (some 60% of the population at the time) and improvements in several avoidable causes of child hospitalisation and mortality (Aguirre, 2010; Armada et al., 2009; Castro et al., 2006; Ubieta Gómez, 2007). In 2005, Chávez expanded the programme to cover diagnostic and medical technology and rehabilitation centres, also ensuring emergency primary care access around the clock (Aguirre, 2010; Castro et al., 2006).

Well before the recent unrest, news of abandoned primary care centres and defecting Cuban doctors was used by opponents of Venezuela's Bolivarian government to discredit Barrio Adentro and announce its imminent demise (e.g. Ceaser, 2007). While instances of defection, neglect, and corruption undoubtedly occurred to some extent, as in most health care systems (Birn, Pillay, et al., 2017), that they have been gleefully cited as an SJSSC failure by the mainstream anti-Cuban press (e.g. the Miami Herald) and newspapers with economic interests in Venezuela (e.g. El País, El Universal) casts doubt on such claims. Still, some of these journalistic concerns (Carroll, 2013) have also been voiced from within the Bolivarian camp (Feo Istúriz, 2017), albeit in a more nuanced manner.

In spite of the popularity of Barrio Adentro among Venezuelans (Walker, 2015), certain problems are evident. The relationship between the Cuban mission and Chávez was hermetic, often alienating not only mainstream Venezuelan doctors but even those supportive of the programme, who had little input into its policies. A further challenge has been the inability to integrate Barrio Adentro into the existing state public health system (the two operate in parallel) and to fund community health workers who currently work as volunteers (Cooper, 2015).

Without discounting the damage caused by shortages of medications and corruption and poor maternal and child health outcomes, since 2015 other problems affecting medical supplies, equipment, health care infrastructure, and personnel can be traced to a protracted 'civil war' conducted via hoarding, boycotts, and deliberate outside interference (Bolton, 2016; Curcio, 2017; Hetland, 2017). Due to these external factors, Barrio Adentro has not become the stable institution that it was meant to be, with members of the opposition even reportedly destroying some Barrio Adentro facilities (Watsup Americas, 2017).

Political scientists critical of the Bolivarian Revolution have found parallels between Chávez and charismatic populists who governed Latin American countries in the mid-twentieth century (e.g. Getúlio Vargas in Brazil and Juan Perón in Argentina), as well as contemporaries including Bolivia's Evo Morales and Ecuador's Rafael Correa (Huber & Stephens, 2012; López-Maya & Lander, 2011). All of these leaders have engaged in populist and anti-capitalist rhetoric, direct contact with poor and working classes, and strong control of state institutions. At the same time, their de facto policy records have been less egalitarian than promised, representing class compromise, continuation of capital accumulation among elites, and inadequate changes to the tax structure. Chávez's populism may also reflect the difficulties of establishing strong welfare state institutions in many extractive economies (Acemoglu & Robinson, 2013). Yet unlike some leftwing populists of Latin America's past, Chávez strove to implement long-term policy changes (e.g. Barrio Adentro), with institutionalisation undergirded by a strong political party pursuing these political objectives beyond its tenure (Huber & Stephens, 2012). It is too early to tell whether the beleaguered Bolivarian Revolution will achieve these historical ambitions (Ellner, 2017). Still, importantly, Chávez's support for a socialist programme mounted rather than retreated after the 2003 coup attempt against him (Gott, 2011; Wilpert, 2007), expressed in a range of comprehensive universalist health policies (Barrio Adentro, plus dental and eye care, services excluded from some national health systems in the Global North). This redoubled commitment distinguishes Chávez from the typical ideological contradictions of populist leaders, whose pledge to public programmes often diminishes after they have consolidated their power.

In sum, Barrio Adentro embodies the virtues of SJSSC: an exchange of low-cost Venezuelan oil for Cuban expertise in primary care and intersectoral action for health. That the programme survived the Great Recession years, the violent boycott of the Venezuelan opposition, and declining oil revenues is in itself proof of the resistance of Cuban–Venezuelan solidarity, further sustained by the ongoing training of thousands of doctors and continued presence of clinics in poor neighbourhoods. Moreover, the grassroots support for the programme remains strong. Barrio Adentro's popularity as the centrepiece of Venezuelan social protection (Muntaner et al., 2011) provides ample justification as to why the Bolivarian government has continued to enjoy electoral support from the country's poor, working class, and sections of the middle class (Ulmer & Chinea, 2017).

Still, a key question is whether the cooperation can endure amidst the unrelenting hostile national, regional, and global context against the Bolivarian Revolution and whether Barrio Adentro's adaptation of Cuba's health care system remains relevant as an SJSSC exemplar for other settings seeking equity and health justice.

## Conclusion – SJSSC at a crossroads: a reversion to LASM across borders?

In the wake of conservative forces gaining control of major countries in the region (Brazil, Argentina, Chile), with others embattled (Venezuela, Ecuador, El Salvador, Nicaragua, Uruguay), the foreseeable future for SJSSC in the region is uncertain. Might Cuba, given its own changes towards a market economy, continue to hold the torch, or will SJSSC in Latin America revert to the domain of civil society cooperation (LASM across borders) as part of an ongoing large-scale struggle against global capitalism and imperialism?

Returning to Barrio Adentro, despite current turbulence, Venezuela's prior trajectory under Chávez – and the country's ongoing commitment to universal, community-based public health care for millions of previously disenfranchised people perennially ignored by physicians and politicians alike (Walker, 2015) – helps demystify why so many Venezuelans are seeking to preserve the Chavista legacy even in the face of still unfolding political and economic problems. This remarkable, though certainly not flawless, programme is one of the most dynamic instances of SJSSC in recent years – all the more so because Venezuela has long been capable, resource-wise, of meeting population health needs (Buxton, 2016).

In seeking to explain why the region's experience of SJSSC has been both longstanding and fruitful, it is useful to briefly compare it to BRICS countries' (Brazil, Russia, India China, South Africa) engagement in cooperation. Brazil's dual model of social justice actions combined with mainstream foreign aid/foreign policy objectives, illuminates this question. BRICS cooperation, like SJSSC approaches, seeks long-term sustainability, sovereignty, and horizontality in decisionmaking. But Brazil, like China (which also stresses the lack of conditionalities in its aid), India, and Russia, also treats South–South cooperation as an avenue for advancing capitalist development and corporate interests (Garcia & Kato, 2015; Ventura, 2013).

Notwithstanding deleterious political conditions, perhaps there remains hope: the new players and expanded activities of recent decades, at least partly generated by 'barrio democracy' (Canel, 2010), suggests that SJSSC aspirations may help drive a long-term effort for current and future generations to mobilise their energies, skills, imagination, and commitment in favour of social (medicine) justice and in solidarity with the struggles of the *pueblos* of Latin America and well beyond.

## Notes

1. As in other countries, many Latin American public health specialists and social medicine adherents in the early 20th century also advocated different forms of eugenics, mostly favouring 'positive' measures to foster healthy reproduction and child-rearing (Leyton, Palacios, & Sánchez, 2015; Miranda & Vallejo, 2005; Stepan, 1992; Turda & Gillette, 2014).
2. In 1926 anarcho-feminist Menshevik turned Bolshevik Alexandra Kollontai, the First People's Commissar for Social Welfare, became the Soviet Ambassador to Mexico. Her short-lived and controversial stay animated Mexico's post-revolutionary discussions around social welfare; however, Mexico's increasingly influential Communist Party was banned in 1929.
3. The Alianza Bolivariana para los Pueblos de Nuestra América (ALBA – originally Bolivarian 'Alternative') for the Americas) was created in 2004 and now includes Venezuela, Bolivia, Cuba, Ecuador, Nicaragua and several Caribbean island states.
4. This would be equivalent to 25% of US doctors involved in overseas cooperation.
5. Other new regional bodies whose relation to health is more indirect include ALBA and the 33 country-strong Comunidad de Estados Latinoamericanos y Caribeños (CELAC), which maintain explicit goals of Latin American and Caribbean integration and reducing US influence in the region.

## Acknowledgements

We are grateful to the anonymous reviewers for their stimulating, thoughtful, and thorough suggestions and to Mariajosé Aguilera for her editing expertise.

## Disclosure statement

No potential conflict of interest was reported by the authors.


## Funding

Funding for this research was provided by the Canadian Institutes of Health Research [CIHR grant # EOG-126976] Ethics Office. This funder had no other role in the writing of the article or in the decision to submit for publication. The ideas expressed herein are the authors' alone.


## References

Acemoglu, D., & Robinson, J. A. (2013). *Why nations fail: The origins of power, prosperity, and poverty*. New York, NY: Random House.

Aguirre, V. (2010). *Tecnologías en salud: Desafíos de las políticas, Venezuela (1989–2006)*. Caracas: Ministerio de Ciencia y Tecnología.

Akhatar, A. S. (2006). Cuban doctors in Pakistan: Why Cuba still inspires. *Monthly Review, 58*(6), 49–55. Retrieved from https://monthlyreview.org/2006/11/01/cuban-doctors-in-pakistan-why-cuba-still-inspires/

Alden, C., Chichava, S., & Alves, A. C. (2017). *Mozambique and Brazil: Forging new partnerships or developing dependency?* Johannesburg: Jacana Media.

Allende, S. (1939). *La realidad médico-social chilena*. Santiago: Ministerio de Salubridad Pública.

Allende, S. (1951). *Sesión 33.a, en jueves 6 de septiembre de 1951. Diario de sesiones del senado*. Santiago: Biblioteca del Congreso Nacional de Chile.

Almeida, M. (2006). Circuito aberto: Idéias e intercâmbios médico-científicos na América Latina nos primórdios do século XX. *História, Ciências, Saúde-Manguinhos, 13*(3), 733–757. doi:10.1590/S0104-59702006000300010

Alvarado, C., Arismendi, C., Armada, F., Bergonzoli, G., Borroto, R., Castellanos, P. L., ... Vivas, S. (2006). *Derecho a la salud e inclusión social en Venezuela*. Caracas: OPS-OMS para Venezuela.

Amin, S. (2014). Latin America confronts the challenge of globalization: A burdensome inheritance. *Monthly Review, 66*(7), 29–34. Retrieved from https://monthlyreview.org/2014/12/01/latin-america-confronts-the-challenge-of-globalization/

Anderson, K. C. (2013). Doctors within borders: Cuban medical diplomacy to Sandinista Nicaragua, 1979–1990. In V. Garrard-Burnett, M. A. Lawrence, & J. E. Moreno (Eds.), *Beyond the eagle's shadow: New histories of Latin America's Cold War* (pp. 200–225). Albuquerque, NM: University of New Mexico Press.

Anderson, M. R., Smith, L., & Sidel, V. W. (2005). What is social medicine? *Monthly Review, 56*(8), 27–34. Retrieved from https://monthlyreview.org/2005/01/01/what-is-social-medicine/

Angell, A. (1998). The left in Latin America since c. 1920. In L. Bethell (Ed.), *Latin America: Politics and society since 1930* (pp. 75–14). Cambridge, MA: Cambridge University Press.

Armada, F., Muntaner, C., Chung, H., Williams-Brennan, L., & Benach, J. (2009). Barrio Adentro and the reduction of health inequalities in Venezuela: An appraisal of the first years. *International Journal of Health Services, 39*(1), 161–187. doi:10.2190/HS.39.1.h

Armada, F., Muntaner, C., & Navarro, V. (2001). Health and social security reforms in Latin America: The convergence of the World Health Organization, the World Bank, and transnational corporations. *International Journal of Health Services, 31*(4), 729–768. doi:10.2190/70BE-TJ0Q-P7WJ-2ELU

Baumann, G. G. (2009). *Los voluntarios latinoamericanos en la guerra civil Española*. Cuenca: Ediciones de la Universidad de Castilla-La Mancha. Retrieved from: http://www.brigadasinternacionales.uclm.es/wp-content/uploads/2014/06/Los-voluntarios-latinoamericanos-en-la ... .pdf

Beldarraín Chaple, E. (2006). La salud pública en Cuba y su experiencia internacional (1959–2005). *História, Ciências, Saúde-Manguinhos, 13*, 709–716. doi:10.1590/S0104-59702006000300008

Benzi, D., & Zapata, X. (2017). Good-bye Che?: Scope, identity, and change in Cuba's South–South cooperation. In I. Bergamaschi, P. Moore, & A. B. Tickner (Eds.), *South-South cooperation beyond the myths: Rising donors, new aid practices?* (pp. 79–106). London: Palgrave Macmillan UK.

Berlagoscky, F. (2013). Entrevista a la historiadora Dra. Jadwiga Pieper Mooney. Encuentros con biografia e historia: El Dr. Benjamin Viel y las políticas de la salud pública. *Revista Chilena de Salud Pública, 17*(1), 63–67. Retrieved from http://www.revistasaludpublica.uchile.cl/index.php/RCSP/article/viewFile/26647/28222

Bethell, L., & Roxborough, I. (Eds.). (1993). *Latin America between the Second World War and the cold war: Crisis and containment, 1944–1948*. Cambridge, MA: Cambridge University Press.

Birn, A.-E. (2002). "No more surprising than a broken pitcher"? Maternal and child health in the early years of the Pan American Sanitary Bureau. *Canadian Bulletin of Medical History, 19*(1), 17–46. doi:10.3138/cbmh.19.1.17

Birn, A.-E. (2005). Uruguay on the world stage: How child health became an international priority. *American Journal of Public Health, 95*(9), 1506–1517. doi:10.2105/AJPH.2004.038778

Birn, A.-E. (2012). Uruguay's child rights approach to health: What role for civil registration? In K. Breckenridge & S. Szreter (Eds.), *Registration and recognition: Documenting the person in world history* (pp. 415–447). Oxford: Oxford University Press for the British Academy.

Birn, A.-E., Muntaner, C., & Afzal, Z. (2017). South-South cooperation in health: Bringing in theory, politics, history, and social justice. *Cadernos de Saúde Pública, 33*(Suppl. 2), S37–S52. doi:10.1590/0102-311x00194616

Birn, A. E., Pillay, Y., & Holtz, T. H. (2017). *Textbook of global health.* New York, NY: Oxford University Press.

Bolívar, S. (2003). D. Bushnell (Ed.), *El Libertador: Writings of Simón Bolívar.* (F. Fornoff, Trans.). New York, NY: Oxford University Press.

Bolton, P. (2016). *The other explanation for Venezuela's economic crisis.* Washington, DC: Council on Hemispheric Affairs.

Borowy, I. (2009). *Coming to terms with world health: The League of Nations Health Organisation 1921–1946.* Frankfurt: Peter Lang.

Borowy, I., & Hardy, A. (2008). *Of medicine and men: Biographies and ideas in European social medicine between the world wars.* Frankfurt: Peter Lang GmbH, Internationaler Verlag der Wissenschaften.

Breilh Paz y Miño, J. (2001). *Eugenio Espejo: La otra memoria (Nueva lectura de la historia de las ideas científicas).* Cuenca: Universidad de Cuenca.

Brotherton, S. (2013). Fueling la revolución: Itinerant physicians, transactional humanitarianism, and shifting moral economies. In N. J. Burke, (Ed.), *Health travels: Cuban health(care) on the island and around the world* (pp. 127–151). San Francisco, CA: University of California Press.

Brown, T. M., & Birn, A.-E. (2013). The making of health internationalists. In A.-E. Birn & T. M. Brown (Eds.), *Comrades in health: U.S. health internationalists, abroad and at home* (pp. 15–42). New Brunswick, NJ: Rutgers University Press.

Buss, P. M., & Ferreira, J. R. (2010). Critical essay on international cooperation in health. *RECIIS–Eletr Rev of Com Inf Innov Health, 4*(1), 86–97. doi:10.3395/reciis.v4i1.350en

Buxton, J. (2016). Venezuela after Chávez: Interview. *New Left Review, 99,* 5–25. Retrieved from https://newleftreview.org/II/99/julia-buxton-venezuela-after-chavez

Canel, E. (2010). *Barrio democracy in Latin America: Participatory decentralization and community activism in Montevideo.* University Park, PA: Pennsylvania State University Press.

Carr, B. (2014). Pioneering transnational solidarity in the Americas: The movement in support of Augusto C. Sandino 1927–1934. *Journal of Iberian and Latin American Research, 20*(2), 141–152. doi:10.1080/13260219.2014.939122

Carrillo, A. M. (2005). Salud pública y poder en México durante el Cardenismo, 1934–1940. *Dynamis: Acta Hispanica ad Medicinae Scientiarumque Historiam Illustrandam, 25,* 145–178. Retrieved from http://www.raco.cat/index.php/Dynamis/article/view/114016

Carrillo Roa, A., & Silva, F. R. B. (2015). Fiocruz as an actor in Brazilian foreign relations in the context of the community of Portuguese-speaking countries: An untold story. *História, Ciências, Saúde-Manguinhos, 22*(1), 153–169. doi:10.1590/S0104-59702015000100009

Carroll, R. (2013). *Comandante: Hugo Chávez's Venezuela.* London: Penguin.

Carter, E. D. (2018). Social medicine and international expert networks in Latin America, 1930–1945. *Global Public Health.* Advance online publication. doi:10.1080/17441692.2017.1418902

Cassells, E. D. (2016). Cuba: Still punching above its weight. In J. A. Braveboy-Wagner (Ed.), *Diplomatic strategies of nations in the global south* (pp. 319–344). New York, NY: Palgrave Macmillan US.

Castro, A., Gusmão, R., Martínez, M. E., & Vivas, S. (Eds.). (2006). *Barrio Adentro: Derecho a la salud e inclusión social en Venezuela.* Caracas: Pan American Health Organization.

Ceaser, M. (2007). Cuban doctors working abroad defect to the USA. *The Lancet, 369*(9569), 1247–1248. doi:10.1016/S0140-6736(07)60577-7

Chan, J. (2015). *Politics in the corridor of dying: AIDS activism and global health governance.* Baltimore, MD: Johns Hopkins University Press.

Chaves, C. L. (2009). Políticas internacionais de saúde: O primeiro acordo sanitário internacional da América (Montevidéu, 1873). *Locus-Revista de História, 15*(2), 9–27. Retrieved from https://locus.ufjf.emnuvens.com.br/locus/article/viewFile/917/787

Chomsky, A. (2011). Labor history as world history: Linking regions over time. In L. Fink (Ed.), *Workers across the Americas: The transnational turn in labor history* (pp. 23–32). New York, NY: Oxford University Press.

Chomsky, N. (1992). *What uncle Sam really wants.* Berkeley, CA: Odonian Press.

Ciência & Saúde Coletiva. (2017). Desarrollo, desigualdad y cooperación internacional en salud, [special issue]. *Ciência & Saúde Coletiva, 22*(7), 2094–2319. doi:10.1590/1413-81232017227.08972017

Concheiro, E., Modonesi, M., & Crespo, H. (Eds.). (2007). *El Comunismo: Otras miradas desde América Latina.* México: UNAM–CEIICH.

Cooper, A. (2015). What does health activism mean in Venezuela's Barrio Adentro program? Understanding community health work in political and cultural context. *Annals of Anthropological Practice, 39*(1), 58–72. doi:10.1111/napa.12063

Cornia, G. A. (Ed.). (2014). *Falling inequality in Latin America: Policy changes and lessons.* Oxford: Oxford University Press.

Cueto, M. (1991). 'Indigenismo' and rural medicine in Peru: The Indian Sanitary Brigade and Manuel Nuñez Butrón. *Bulletin of the History of Medicine, 65*(1), 22–42. Retrieved from https://www.ncbi.nlm.nih.gov/pubmed/2021691

Cueto, M. (2007). *El valor de la salud. Historia de la Organización Panamericana de la Salud.* Washington, DC: Pan American Health Organization.

Cueto, M., & Palmer, S. (2014). *Medicine and public health in Latin America: A history.* Cambridge, MA: Cambridge University Press.

Curcio, P. (2017). *Indicadores de calidad y bienestar social en Venezuela.* Caracas: Universidad Bolivariana de Venezuela.

del Castillo, L. (2018). *Crafting a republic for the world: Scientific, geographic, and historiographic inventions of Colombia.* Lincoln, NE: University of Nebraska Press.

Derecho Internacional Público. (2014, January 18). Primera Conferencia Interamericana de Seguridad Social. Santiago de Chile, 10–16 de septiembre de 1942. *Derecho Internacional Público.* Retrieved from https://www.dipublico.org/101526/primera-conferencia-interamericana-de-seguridad-social-santiago-de-chile-10-16-de-septiembre-1942/

De Vos, P., De Ceukelaire, W., Bonet, M., & Van der Stuyft, P. (2007). Cuba's international cooperation in health: An overview. *International Journal of Health Services, 37*(4), 761–776. doi:10.2190/HS.37.4.k

Ellner, S. (2017). Venezuela's fragile revolution: From Chávez to Maduro. *Monthly Review, 69*(5), 1. Retrieved from https://monthlyreview.org/2017/10/01/venezuelas-fragile-revolution/

Espejo, E. (1993). Estrella, E. (Ed.), *Reflexiones acerca de un método para preservar a los pueblos de viruelas.* Quito: Nueva Editorial.

Featherstone, D. (2012). *Solidarity: Hidden histories and geographies of internationalism.* London: Zed Books.

Feinsilver, J. (2010). Fifty years of Cuba's medical diplomacy: From idealism to pragmatism. *Cuban Studies, 41*, 85–104. Retrieved from https://muse.jhu.edu/article/413140

Feo, O. (2012). *La crisis mundial y su impacto sobre la salud y la vida.* Paper presented at the first national meeting against health privatization, Alianza Interinstitucional por la Salud, Cali.

Feo Istúriz, O. (2017, October 28). El deterioro de la salud en Venezuela. *Aporrea.org.* Retrieved from https://www.aporrea.org/contraloria/a254438.html

Ferreira, J. R., Hoirisch, C., Fonseca, L. E., & Buss, P. M. (2016). International cooperation in health: The case of Fiocruz. *História, Ciências, Saúde-Manguinhos, 23*(2), 267–276. doi:10.1590/S0104-59702016000200002

Fitz, D. (2012). Cuba: The new global medicine. *Monthly Review, 64*(4), 37–46. Retrieved from https://monthlyreview.org/2012/09/01/cuba-the-new-global-medicine/

Fitz, D. (2016). Cuba's medical mission. *Monthly Review, 67*(9), 54–61. Retrieved from https://monthlyreview.org/2016/02/01/cubas-medical-mission/

Franco, S., Nunes, E., Breilh, J., & Laurell, A. C. (1991). *Debates en medicina social.* Quito: Non Plus Ultra, OPS/ALAMES.

Franco Agudelo, S. (2009). On the 25th anniversary of ALAMES. *Social Medicine, 4*(4), 199–203.

Garcia, A., & Kato, K. (2015). The story of the hunter or hunted? Brazil's role in Angola and Mozambique. In P. Bond & A. Garcia (Eds.), *BRICS: An anti-capitalist critique* (pp. 117–134). London: Pluto Press.

García, A. G., & Marichal, C. (2004). *Construcción de las identidades latinoamericanas: Ensayos de historia intelectual, siglos XIX y XX.* México: El Colegio de México.

García, J. C. (1981). La medicina estatal en América Latina, 1880–1930. *Revista Latinoamericana de Salud, 1*, 73–104. Retrieved from http://scielo.sld.cu/scielo.php?script=sci_arttext&pid=S0864-34662016000100015

Garfield, R., & Williams, G. (1992). *Health care in Nicaragua: Primary care under changing regimes.* New York, NY: Oxford University Press.

Genaro, J., & Gato (Eds.). (2017). *Dos pueblos a los que amar, un mundo por el que luchar.* Retrieved from http://marcialteniarazon.org/documentos-historicos/libros/dos-pueblos-que-amar-un-mundo-por-que-luchar

Gleijeses, P. (1996). Cuba's first venture in Africa: Algeria, 1961–1965. *Journal of Latin American Studies, 28*(1), 159–195. Retrieved from http://www.jstor.org/stable/157991

Gott, R. (2011). *Hugo Chávez and the Bolivarian revolution.* London: Verso Books.

Gómez, E., & Perez, F. A. (2016). Brazilian foreign policy in health during Dilma Rousseff's administration (2011–2014). *Lua Nova: Revista de Cultura e Política, 2*, 171–197. doi:10.1590/0102-6445171-197/98

Granda, E. (2008). Algunas reflexiones a los veinticuatro años de la ALAMES. *Medicina Social, 3*(2), 217–225. Retrieved from http://www.medicinasocial.info/index.php/medicinasocial/article/view/177

Guevara, E. (1960). Discurso a los estudiantes de medicina y trabajadores de la salud. In M. D. C. Ariet Garcia & D. Deutschmann (Eds.), *Che Guevara presente: Una antología mínima* (pp. 118–127). Melbourne: Ocean Press.

Guy, D. J. (1998). The Pan American child congresses, 1916 to 1942: Pan Americanism, child reform, and the welfare state in Latin America. *Journal of Family History, 23*(3), 272–291. doi:10.1177/036319909802300304

Harnecker, M. (2015). *A world to build: New paths toward twenty-first century socialism.* New York, NY: Monthly Review Press.

Hartmann, C. (2016). Postneoliberal public health care reforms: Neoliberalism, social medicine, and persistent health inequalities in Latin America. *American Journal of Public Health*, *106*(12), 2145–2151. doi:10.2105/AJPH.2016.303470

Hatzky, C., & Stites Mor, J. (2014). Latin American transnational solidarities: Contexts and critical research paradigms. *Journal of Iberian and Latin American Research*, *20*(2), 127–140. doi:10.1080/13260219.2014.939121

Herrera González, P. (2013). La Confederación de Trabajadores de América Latina y la implementación de su proyecto sindical continental (1938–1941). *Trashumante. Revista Americana de Historia Social*, *2*, 136–164.

Herrero, M. B., & Tussie, D. (2015). UNASUR health: A quiet revolution in health diplomacy in South America. *Global Social Policy: An Interdisciplinary Journal of Public Policy and Social Development*, *15*(3), 261–277. doi:10.1177/1468018115599818

Hetland, G. (2017, May 14). Why is Venezuela spiraling out of control? *Jacobin*. Retrieved from https://www.jacobinmag.com/2017/05/venezuela-crisis-maduro-opposition-violence-elections-economy

Hong, Y. S. (2015). *Cold War Germany, the third world, and the global humanitarian regime*. Cambridge, MA: Cambridge University Press.

Huber, E., & Stephens, J. D. (2012). *Democracy and the left: Social policy and inequality in Latin America*. Chicago, IL: University of Chicago Press.

Huish, R. (2013). *Where no doctor has gone before: Cuba's place in the global health landscape*. Waterloo: Wilfrid Laurier University Press.

Iacob, B. C. (2017, June). *Trial-runs for internationalizing socialist health: North Korea and Vietnam*. Paper presented at the workshop boundaries of socialist medicine, University of Exeter, Exeter, UK.

Illanes, M. A. (1993). *'En el nombre del pueblo, del estado y de la ciencia … ': Historia social de la salud pública, Chile 1880–1973 (hacia una historia social del Siglo XX)*. Santiago: Colectivo de Atención Primaria.

Iriart, C., Waitzkin, H., Breilh, J., Estrada, A., & Merhy, E. E. (2002). Medicina social latinoamericana: Aportes y desafíos. *Revista Panamericana de Salud Pública/Pan American Journal of Public Health*, *12*(2), 128–136. Retrieved from https://www.scielosp.org/scielo.php?pid=S1020-49892002000800013&script=sci_abstract

Johnson, J. (2015). *The battle for Algeria: Sovereignty, health care, and humanitarianism*. Philadelphia, PA: University of Pennsylvania Press.

Kapelusz-Poppi, A. M. (2001). Physician activists and the development of rural health in postrevolutionary Mexico. *Radical History Review*, *80*(1), 35–50. Retrieved from https://muse.jhu.edu/article/30175

Karan, A., & Sodhi, G. (2015). *Protecting the health of the poor: Social movements in the South*. London: Zed Books.

Kickbusch, I. (2011). Global health diplomacy: How foreign policy can influence health. *BMJ: British Medical Journal*, *342*, d3154–d3154. doi:10.1136/bmj.d3154

Kirk, J. M. (2015). *Healthcare without borders: Understanding Cuban medical internationalism*. Gainsville, FL: University Press of Florida.

Kirk, J. M., & Erisman, H. M. (2009). *Cuban medical internationalism: Origins, evolution, and goals*. New York, NY: Palgrave Macmillan.

Labra, M. E. (2000). Política e medicina social no Chile: Narrativas sobre uma relação difícil. *História, Ciência, Saúde-Manguinhos*, *7*(1), 23–46. doi:10.1590/S0104-59702000000200002

Laurell, A. C. (2003). What does Latin American social medicine do when it governs? The case of the Mexico city government. *American Journal of Public Health*, *93*(12), 2028–2031. doi:10.2105/AJPH.93.12.2028

Leyton, C., Palacios, C., & Sánchez, M. (Eds.). (2015). *Bulevar de los pobres: Racismo científico, higiene y eugenesia en Chile e Iberoamérica, siglos XIX y XX*. Santiago: Ocho Libros Editores.

Lidola, M., & Borges, F. T. (2017). Negotiating horizontality in medical South–South cooperation: The Cuban mission in Rio de Janeiro's urban peripheries. *Global Public Health*, *13*(3), 355–368. doi:10.1080/17441692.2017.1395470

Lima, N. T., & Santana, J. P. (Eds.). (2006). *Saúde coletiva como compromisso: A trajetória da Abrasco*. Rio de Janeiro: Editora Fiocruz.

Loewenberg, S. (2016, March 14). Can Cuban medicine help solve American inequality? *The Development Set*. Retrieved from https://thedevelopmentset.com/

López-Maya, M., & Lander, L. (2011). Venezuela's presidential elections of 2006: Towards 21st century socialism? In T. Ponniah & J. Eastwood (Eds.), *The revolution in Venezuela: Social and political change under Chávez* (pp. 131–154). Cambridge, MA: Harvard University Press.

Löwy, M. (2007). *El marxismo en América Latina: Antología, desde 1909 hasta nuestros días*. Santiago: Lom Ediciones.

Lustig, N., Lopez-Calva, L. F., Ortiz-Juarez, E., & Monga, C. (2016). Deconstructing the decline in inequality in Latin America. In K. Basu & J. E. Stiglitz (Eds.), *Inequality and growth: Patterns and policy* (pp. 212–247). Basingstoke: Palgrave Macmillan UK.

Mahmood, Q., & Muntaner, C. (2013). Politics, class actors, and health sector reform in Brazil and Venezuela. *Global Health Promotion*, *20*, 59–67. doi:10.1177/1757975913476902

Marquez, P. V., & Joly, D. J. (1986). A historical overview of the ministries of public health and the medical programs of the social security systems in Latin America. *Journal of Public Health Policy*, *7*, 378–394. doi:10.2307/3342464

Meade, T. A. (2016). *History of modern Latin America: 1800 to the present*. Chichester: Wiley.

Medicus Mundi. (2010). *La participación social en salud: El reto de pasar del discurso a la práctica marco legal, estratégico y de políticas públicas que dan énfasis en los procesos de participación e incidencia social existente en los sistemas públicos de salud de la región centroamericana.* Madrid: Ministerio de Asuntos Exteriores y de Cooperación/Medicus Mundi/AECID.

Melrose, D. (1985). *Nicaragua: The threat of a good example?* Oxford: Oxfam.

Mesa-Lago, C. (1978). *Social security in Latin America: Pressure groups, stratification, and inequality.* Pittsburgh, PA: University of Pittsburgh Press.

Mesa-Lago, C. (1985). *El desarrollo de la seguridad social en América Latina.* Santiago: United Nations.

Ministerio del Poder Popular para la Salud (MPPS). (2013). *Medicina integral comunitaria.* Caracas: MPPS.

Ministerio del Poder Popular para la Salud (MPPS). (2015). Se incrementa en Venezuela la matrícula de médicos comunitarios. Retrieved from https://www.mppeuct.gob.ve/actualidad/noticias/se-incrementa-en-venezuela-la-matricula-de-medicos-comunitarios

Miranda, M., & Vallejo, G. (Eds.). (2005). *Darwinismo social y eugenesia en el mundo latino.* Buenos Aires: Siglo XXI.

Monje Vargas, J. (2013). Misión 'Manuela Espejo', paradigma de la solidaridad convertida en política de Estado en Ecuador. *Revista Cubana de Salud Pública, 39*(3), 598–608. Retrieved from http://www.bvs.sld.cu/revistas/spu/vol39_3_13/spu14313.htm

Morris, E. (2014). Unexpected Cuba. *New Left Review, 88,* 5–45. Retrieved from https://newleftreview.org/II/88/emily-morris-unexpected-cuba

Muntaner, C., Armada, F., Chung, H., Rosicar, M., Williams-Brennan, L., & Benach, J. (2008). Venezuela's Barrio Adentro: Participatory democracy, South-South cooperation and health care for all. *Social Medicine, 3*(4), 232–246. Retrieved from http://www.socialmedicine.info/index.php/socialmedicine/article/view/250

Muntaner, C., Chung, H., Mahmood, Q., & Armada, F. (2011). History is not over: The Bolivarian revolution, 'Barrio Adentro,' and health care in Venezuela. In T. Ponniah & J. Eastwood (Eds.), *The revolution in Venezuela: Social and political change under Chávez* (pp. 225–256). Cambridge, MA: Harvard University Press.

Muntaner, C., Salazar, R. M. G., Rueda, S., & Armada, F. (2006). Challenging the neoliberal trend: The Venezuelan health care reform alternative. *Canadian Journal of Public Health, 97*(6), I19–I24. doi:10.17269/cjph.97.792

Musto, R. A. (2017). 'A desire so close to the hearts of all Latin Americans': Utopian ideals and imperfections behind Latin America's nuclear weapon free zone. *Bulletin of Latin American Research.* Advance online publication. doi:10.1111/blar.12557

Navarro, V. (1972). Health services in Cuba: An initial appraisal. *New England Journal of Medicine, 287*(19), 954–959. doi:10.1056/NEJM197211092871904.

Novotny, T. E., Kickbusch, I., & Told, M. (Eds.). (2013). *21st century global health diplomacy (Vol. 3).* Singapore: World Scientific Publishing.

Nye, J. S. (2009). *Soft power: The means to success in world politics.* New York, NY: PublicAffairs.

Ojeda Medina, T. (2010). Cuba, 50 años de solidaridad con el sur. In B. Ayllón & J. Surasky (Eds.), *La cooperación sur-sur en Latinoamérica* (pp. 132–155). Madrid: La Catarata.

Oliveira, F. P. D., Vanni, T., Pinto, H. A., Santos, J. T. R. D., Figueiredo, A. M. D., Araújo, S. Q. D., … Cyrino, E. G. (2015). 'Mais Médicos': A Brazilian program in an international perspective. *Interface-Comunicação, Saúde, Educação, 19*(54), 623–634. doi:10.1590/1807-57622014.1142.

Ortúzar, D. (2013). Legislación y medicina en torno a los accidentes del trabajo en Chile 1900–1940. *Nuevo Mundo Mundos Nuevos. Nouveaux mondes mondes nouveaux-Novo Mundo Mundos Novos-New world New worlds.* doi:10.4000/nuevomundo.66007

Packard, R. (2016). *A history of global health: Interventions into the lives of other peoples.* Baltimore, MD: Johns Hopkins University Press.

Petras, J., & Veltmeyer, H. (2016). *What's left in Latin America?: Regime change in new times.* New York, NY: Routledge.

Porter, D. (2006). How did social medicine evolve, and where is it heading? *PLoS Medicine, 3*(10), e399. doi:10.1371/journal.pmed.0030399

Prashad, V. (2013). *The poorer nations: A possible history of the global south.* Brooklyn, NY: Verso Books.

Ramacciotti, K. I. (2015). Diálogos transnacionales entre los saberes técnicos e institucionales en la legislación sobre accidentes de trabajo, primera mitad del siglo XX. *História, Ciências, Saúde-Manguinhos, 22*(1), 201–219. doi:10.1590/S0104-59702015000100012

Rupprecht, T. (2015). *Soviet internationalism after Stalin: Interaction and exchange between the USSR and Latin America during the Cold War.* Cambridge, MA: Cambridge University Press.

Saney, I. (2009). Homeland of humanity: Internationalism within the Cuban revolution. *Latin American Perspectives, 36*(1), 111–123. Retrieved from http://www.jstor.org/stable/27648164

Santana, J. P. D. (2011). An overview of South-South cooperation on health. *Ciência & Saúde Coletiva, 16*(6), 2993–3002. doi:10.1590/S1413-81232011000600037

Santos, R. de F., & Cerqueira, M. R. (2015). South-South cooperation: Brazilian experiences in South America and Africa. *História, Ciências, Saúde-Manguinhos, 22*(1), 23–47. doi:10.1590/S0104-59702015000100003

Sheinin, D. (Ed.). (2000). *Beyond the ideal: Pan Americanism in inter-American affairs*. Westport, CT: Praeger Publishers.

Spenser, D. (1999). *The impossible triangle: Mexico, Soviet Russia, and the United States in the 1920s*. Durham, NC: Duke University Press.

Spronk, S. J., & Webber, J. R. (Eds.). (2015). *Crisis and contradiction: Marxist perspectives on Latin America in global political economy*. Leiden: Brill.

Stepan, N. (1992). *'The hour of eugenics': Race, gender, and nation in Latin America*. Ithaca, NY: Cornell University Press.

Tajer, D. (2003). Latin American social medicine: Roots, development during the 1990s, and current challenges. *American Journal of Public Health, 93*(12), 2023–2027. doi:10.2105/AJPH.93.12.2023

Torres Tovar, M. (2007). ALAMES: Organizational expression of social medicine in Latin America. *Social Medicine, 2* (3), 125–130.

Turda, M., & Gillette, A. (2014). *Latin eugenics in comparative perspective*. London: Bloomsbury.

Ubieta Gómez, E. (2007). *Venezuela rebelde: Solidaridad vs dinero*. Caracas: Casa Editora Abril.

Ulmer, A., & Chinea, E. (2017, 16 October). Venezuela's opposition refuses to recognise surprise win for Maduro in regional elections. *The Independent*. Retrieved from http://www.independent.co.uk/news/world/americas/venezuela-election-nicolas-maduro-socialists-chavez-result-a8003221.html

Venediktov, D. D. (1977). *Mezhdunarodnye problemy zdravookhraneniia*. Moscow: Meditsina.

Ventura, D. (2013). Public health and Brazilian foreign policy. *SUR International Journal on Human Rights, 10*(19), 95–113. Retrieved from https://ssrn.com/abstract=2446162

Viel, B. (1961). *La medicina socializada y su aplicación en Gran Bretaña, Unión Soviética y Chile*. Santiago: Editorial Universidad de Chile.

Waitzkin, H. (2005). Commentary: Salvador Allende and the birth of Latin American social medicine. *International Journal of Epidemiology, 34*(4), 739–741. doi:10.1093/ije/dyh176

Waitzkin, H. (2006). One and a half centuries of forgetting and rediscovering: Virchow's lasting contributions to social medicine. *Social Medicine, 1*(1), 5–10. Retrieved from http://www.socialmedicine.info/index.php/socialmedicine/article/view/6

Waitzkin, H., Iriart, C., Estrada, A., & Lamadrid, S. (2001a). Social medicine then and now: Lessons from Latin America. *American Journal of Public Health, 91*(10), 1592–1601. doi:10.2105/AJPH.91.10.1592

Waitzkin, H., Iriart, C., Estrada, A., & Lamadrid, S. (2001b). Social medicine in Latin America: Productivity and dangers facing the major national groups. *The Lancet, 358*(9278), 315–323. doi:10.1016/S0140-6736(01)05488-5

Walker, C. (2015). *Venezuela's health care revolution*. Halifax: Fernwood.

Walker, C., & Kirk, E. J. (2017). Alternatives–Pitfalls of polarized internationalism: protest against Cuban medical solidarity. *Studies in Political Economy, 98*(1), 82–92. doi:10.1080/07078552.2017.1297045

Watsup Americas. (2017, April 17). Denuncian en Vzla. que opositores destruyen consultorios comunitarios. *Watsup Americas*. Retrieved from http://bolivia.watsupamericas.com/news/denuncian-en-vzla-que-opositores-destruyen-consultorios-comunitarios/

Weindling, P. (2006). The League of Nations Health Organisation and the rise of Latin American participation, 1920–40. *História, Ciências, Saúde-Manguinhos, 13*(3), 555–570. doi:10.1590/S0104-59702006000300002

Wilpert, G. (2007). *Changing Venezuela by taking power: The history and policies of the Chávez government*. London: Verso Books.

Zárate Campos, M. S., & Godoy Catalán, L. (2011). Madres y niños en las políticas del Servicio Nacional de Salud de Chile (1952-1964). *História, Ciências, Saúde-Manguinhos, 18*, 131–151. doi:10.1590/S0104-59702011000500008

Zeno, L. (1933). *La medicina en Rusia, con un prefacio del profesor Sergio Judine*. Buenos Aires: Librerías Anaconda.

# Collective health and regional integration in Latin America: An opportunity for building a new international health agenda

María Belén Herrero ⓘ , Jorgelina Loza ⓘ and Marcela Beatriz Belardo ⓘ

**ABSTRACT**

From its origins, the Latin American Social Medicine and the Collective Health (LASM/CH) movements have focused on thinking about health from and for the region. After the implementation of neoliberal policies, social improvements and the geopolitical strengthening of the region became the roots of new regional integration projects in South America. The objective of this article is twofold. First, we explore the legacy of long-standing efforts in the region that address the social and political dimensions of health, associated with the LASM/CH movements and their influence on the contemporary regional health agenda. Second, we analyze the UNASUR Health policy, its role in the construction of a regional health agenda, and the principles of South-South cooperation it supports. In order to accomplish this, a qualitative analysis was conducted, involving primary and secondary data. Through UNASUR, a new framework of regional health integration and regional health diplomacy emerged in South America and a 'window of opportunity' opened for the ideas of Social Medicine and Collective Health to occupy a dominant place on the regional health agenda. It is possible to observe a confluence between the principles and values of these movements and those of the main constituent bases of UNASUR Health.

## Introduction

The implementation of neoliberal policies increased social inequalities, inequities in health, and social exclusion in Latin America. Inadequate access to medical care and drugs remains a problem, particularly among the most vulnerable population groups in this region. Both access to medical care and access to medicines are recognised as social determinants of poor health outcomes and living conditions. To face this, a decade later, with the coming to power of leftist and progressive governments in most South American countries social policy has gained ground as a central principle for Latin American governments (Riggirozzi & Tussie, 2012). Furthermore, a more horizontal and solidary international cooperation between these countries has emerged as a strategy to increase power so that these countries may stop being mere receivers of the most traditional international cooperation and become cooperators in order to meet local social needs (Vance, Mafla, & Bermudez, 2016).

Social improvements and the geopolitical strengthening of the region became the roots of this new project in the region (Sanahuja, 2011). Good health improves living conditions, while better living conditions contribute to good health. Thus, social policies, and particularly health policies, have become essential strategies for the fight against poverty and for reducing inequalities on a regional scale in Latin America (Herrero, 2017). Likewise, health has acquired an important place in international relations and has come to play a key role in a regional policy agenda over the last decade. A key expression of this process was the founding of the South American United Nations (UNASUR 2008) in 2008 and particularly the creation of its Health Council. A special feature of the UNASUR Health Council is the fact that regional identity is based on health sovereignty and does not require that the member countries delegate any degree of national sovereignty. However, through the Health Council, UNASUR has incorporated the issue of social determinants, the right to health, and universal access to health systems into the debate on regional health policies.

In this paper we show that the approach of the Latin American Social Medicine and the Collective Health (LASM/CH) movements had considerable influence on many of UNASUR Health's principles and values. Both intellectual traditions address the problems of disease, health and medical care of populations. These traditions are considered not only a field of scientific knowledge but also of political action. From this perspective, health is examined through different disciplines such as medicine, epidemiology, anthropology, sociology, history and political science (Paim & de Almeida Filho, 1998). From its origins, LASM/CH has focused on thinking about health from the region and for the region (Galeano, Trotta, & Spinelli, 2011). It is a field of knowledge and practice that claims the collective realisation of the right to health and universal and public health systems (Iriart, Waitzkin, Breilh, Estrada, & Merhy, 2002). It also focuses on the social determination of health, inequities and inequalities in health, and the social production of the health and disease process (Breilh, 2013).

Indeed, it is possible to observe a confluence between the principles and values of these trajectories and the main constituent bases of UNASUR Health (evident in its structure and explicit in its constitutive treaty). We argue that a window of opportunity was opened in the region that allowed LASM/CH to influence the principles and values of the new projects of regional integration. And, at the same time, this way of looking at the region and understanding regional integration contributed to strengthening new ways of South-South Cooperation (SSC) in Latin America. Importantly, the creation of this new project of regional integration in 2008 – UNASUR with its ministerial sectoral councils – is one of the most significant recent experiences of SSC in the region (Vance et al., 2016).

The objectives of this article are twofold. First, we explore the legacy of long-standing efforts in the region that address the social and political dimensions of health, those associated with the LASM/CH movements and their influence on the health agenda of some states, as well as at the regional level. Second, we analyze regional-level politics and the UNASUR Health policy, its role in the construction of a regional health agenda and the principles of SSC it supports. In order to accomplish this analysis, a qualitative study was conducted, including primary and secondary data. Secondary data was based on a review of bibliography and was systematized in relation to the history and main principles of these health traditions in the region. Primary data was collected through semi-structured interviews among key actors related directly to UNASUR and others working in public health in Argentina, Bolivia, Brazil, Ecuador, Uruguay and Paraguay. Fieldwork was carried out during 2014 and 2015, including more than 35 interviews with Health Ministers, former officials in charge of health public policies and representatives of regional and national organisations. In this article, the identity of the interviewees remains anonymous.

The paper explores how the participation of the South American Health Council in the international arena has thus far tangibly contributed to building a shared agenda, and the contribution that these trajectories of thought can make in a new regional context that seems to be taking a new direction. Our goal here is to contribute to the understanding of the principles on which international health cooperation has been built in Latin America, the role that regional organisations such as UNASUR have played in laying the foundations for health and the contribution of this organism to the promotion of a renewed form of south-south cooperation.

## Latin American social medicine and collective health movements and their contributions in the field of health

A variety of theoretical and methodological perspectives have converged in a specific intellectual tradition called Latin American Social Medicine, or Collective Health, as Brazilians have called it. This intellectual tradition emerged in the 1970s from academics, researchers and social movements concerned about the economic, social and political consequences of military dictatorships. That decade was also characterised in several regions by a strong tension in the medical field because the medical profession was going through a deep crisis of confidence. For example, the governments of the United States and Great Britain began to question the enormous expenditures on medical technologies that did not seem to produce a substantial improvement in the quality of life of the population – or at least that was the argument for the adjustment of the public health expenditure. The strong reaction was against not only the increasingly obvious inequity in health and differential access to health services but, fundamentally, to hegemonic thinking that was more concerned with cure than prevention. At the time, interventions were focused exclusively on medical care, underestimating the powerful role of social factors (apart from medical care) in shaping health.

The LASM/CH tradition has had varying degrees of influence on health policy agendas according to the particular historical moment in question. Latin America has long been a place in which trade unions and social and political movements have played a central role in national politics. In the last decades of the twentieth century, social movements in the region struggled especially for the fulfilment of basic social rights, including the right to health, equity in access to health services and improvement of living conditions. This long history of struggle in the region coupled with political reform processes in the 1990s in health (as in other spheres) facilitated the transnationalization of social movement action across the region. This led to a growing visibility of experiences of transnational collective action.

Latin American Social Medicine has two basic principles. First, it recognises the social nature of disease, the historical and political character of the disease/health process, and the impact of inequities and social differences. This political-intellectual trajectory gives particular importance to the social determinants[1] of health and health as a human right. Second, it recovers the primary responsibility of the state in the solution of health-disease problems. From the LASM/CH perspective, it is assumed that health issues are linked to political issues, that is, to collective and individual decisions. In this way, the social determinants of health perspective, as understood by LASM/CH becomes a useful tool to make visible the structural aspects of health. It brings greater political content to discourse on the right to health (as part of the whole of economic, social, cultural and environmental rights), making clear that its guarantee requires structural changes to the way societies are organised for an equitable distribution of economic resources, power, and knowledge. The LASM/CH approach encourages the values of solidarity and cooperation in the agendas of the struggles of social and cultural movements and in the public action of progressive local and national governments. In this sense, it focuses on strengthening a continental and global movement for equity in health, inscribed within the broad framework of regional and global struggles for the right to health (Granda, 2003; López Arellano, Escudero, & Carmona, 2008).

Over time, there has been significant growth in this arena of thought, which insists on overcoming the matrix exported from developed countries. This exported matrix observes public health problems from the perspective of developed countries, their own interests, and their own recipes – what Anibal Quijano (2005) called the 'coloniality of power and knowledge' that extends through economic and geopolitical interests.

## Globalisation and health in the international agenda

Global health governance solidified and diversified after World War II and new concepts appeared with the 1948 establishment of the World Health Organization (WHO) (Fidler, 2010). During the period of the Cold War the field of international health suffered tensions of political and ideological rivalries of the two most important blocks of that time: the one that represented capitalism and the other that represented communism; and health was not immune to this dispute. When the Soviet Union and the communist countries decided to withdraw in 1949 from the UN and, therefore, from the WHO, this body was clearly controlled by the interests of the Western block, particularly the United States, stimulating professionalism and bureaucratic growth, and carrying out global campaigns and technically oriented to the control or elimination of specific diseases in vertical programmes, operating with an approach similar to that of the Rockefeller Foundation imposed as a model since the beginning of the century (Brown, Cueto, & Fee, 2006). Two health approaches in permanent tension characterised this stage: one based on social and economic approaches that determine the health of the population and the other more focused on technologies and diseases. Both approaches remained over time with different emphases, increasing or decreasing (Brown et al, 2006) depending on the strong relationships of the countries and the interests of international actors. The 1960s and 1970s were marked by the emergence of decolonised African nations, the expansion of socialist and nationalist movements and new theories of development with an emphasis on economic and social growth. A milestone was the Alma Ata Declaration in 1978 which posits health as a fundamental human right that must be achieved by integrated social and health policies. Behind the movement for primary health care was a series of successful experiences of non-governmental organisations in Latin America, Africa and Asia that acted together with local populations. The response to Alma-Ata was the Bellagio Conference (Italy) influenced by the United States, funded by the Rockefeller Foundation, and supported by the World Bank. The meeting launched the concept of 'selective primary health care'. That is, the implementation of technical interventions, low cost and small scale, with UNICEF leading the initiative in the 1980s. However, retrenchment and neoliberal policies were strongly felt in the WHO, which began to rely increasingly on contributions. In the 1990s, World Bank loans for the health sector surpassed the total budget of the WHO (Brown et al., 2006). The WHO subsequently lost credibility and in order to strengthen its global image began to employ the concept of 'global funds' and 'global partnerships'. Its agenda was reduced to specific goals such as fighting Malaria or Tuberculosis (Stop TB) or improving access to new and underused vaccines for children living in the world's poorest countries (GAVI). These programmes are public-private partnerships, the Bill and Melinda Gates Foundation being one of the largest funders. Partnerships with the commercial sector clearly limit the objectives of the universal right to health, through a limited approach focusing on 'priority diseases' (Buse & Waxman, 2001).

The so-called process of globalisation has generated an unprecedented hike in funding while also growing the influence of policymakers, activists, and philanthropists who claim health as a foreign policy issue of first-order importance. Likewise, this increasing role of health in the foreign policy agenda gave rise to the emergence of new actors with renewed flags and perspectives.

Amidst market globalisation, health emerged during the twenty-first century on the global political agenda as an issue that could only be effectively addressed through cooperative efforts. In this context, health has acquired an important place in international relations and has come to play a key role in foreign policy agendas in the last decade. The fields of international health and health diplomacy owe much of their growth and development, during the twentieth century, to the processes of economic expansion (Gómez-Dantés & Khoshnood, 1991). The Declaration of the Millennium Development Goals in the year 2000 also revealed the central role of health in the international debate on social policy. The WHO Commission on Social Determinants of Health, formed in 2005, injected further momentum. Fidler (2010) has called this moment the global health 'revolution' to denote the increasing role of health in foreign policy (Fidler, 2010; Labonté y Gagnon, 2010). That 'revolution' generated an unprecedented increase in funding and a rise in the influence of policymakers, activists, and philanthropists who claim health as a foreign policy issue of first-order importance. As a result, global health became an essential part of the equation of international relations (Fidler, 2001; 2010).

While in the past globalisation has often been seen as a more or less an economic process, it is increasingly understood as a more comprehensive phenomenon, fashioned by a multitude of factors and events that are reshaping our society as well (Huymen, Martens, & Hilderink, 2005). Through migration, war, and epidemics, health has transcended national boundaries, causing political and economic impacts on a global scale. Better life and good health are both essential elements towards the quality of civic life, peace, security, and governance. In this way, health has become a multi-dimensional topic that could be linked to global action. Accordingly, in the field of international relations there is now greater awareness of the scope of health issues and about the consequences of the rapid pace of scientific and technological development. Despite this and while there have been major advances in life expectancy over the past century, health inequalities, lack of access to health systems and social exclusion persist within and between countries. In this scenario, we argue that future prospects for health improvements depend increasingly on the relative new directions of the globalisation processes, international cooperation, and regional integration.

Latin America was a leading region in the promotion and practice of social medicine since 1970. It was swiftly reasserted when the process of re-democratization picked up in the early 1980s (Mariani, 2007), but along with the green shoots of democratisation, international financial institutions, and in particular the World Bank gained the upper hand in policy writ large. In the social sectors, reforms effectively removed the idea of equity and universalism as an organising principle for national social policy. Although these ideas were pushed aside during health reforms that were carried out in this period, they remained the organising principle of the overtly politically strategy of the Movimiento Sanitarista (Sanitation Movement). The Social Medicine and the Collective Health movements (especially in Brazil) continued to work to develop an approach linked to social epidemiology and to assert the ambitious goal of collective health and social determination of health to address the causes of ill health: social inequalities (Breilh, 2013).

## Recovering the region: The influence of Latin-American social medicine on UNASUR

After the Washington Consensus, by the early 1990s neoliberalism had taken hold as a political and economic paradigm in Latin America. As a result of neoliberal policies the regional picture was becoming increasingly weak, challenging the notion of Latin America as an independent region given the influence of US-led liberal governance. The market orientation of neoliberal policies led to a selective focus in public policies, resulting in a series of simple and often low-quality benefits for the poor, which had a serious impact on the health sector and particularly on primary care (Giovanella, 2015). Access to more complex health care increasingly became associated with the ability to pay. Vertical programmes targeting populations or specific problems through the creation of targeted health insurance were strengthened, deepening the segmentation of health systems while poverty rates and income inequality increased region-wide (Soares, 2001).

In the 2000s, leftist and progressive governments gained power in most countries in the region and attempted to counteract the effects of neoliberal policies. The region itself also began to emerge as a territorial unit capable of intervening in struggles for power and symbolic resources. Subsequent attempts at the constitution of regional organisations under progressive and left-leaning governments (including UNASUR, The Community of Latin American and Caribbean States – CELAC-, The Bolivarian Alliance for the Peoples of Our America –ALBA-) have represented a conglomerate of commercial, political, and social projects that revolve around new principles of solidarity and regional autonomy and have provided the opportunity to synchronise policy at multiple scales.

The effort to recover South America's potential for development was a clear manifestation of a historical change, a 'change of era' (rather than simply an era of change), in accordance with the statements by the President of Ecuador, Rafael Correa, in his inaugural speech in January 2007. This change of era was characterised by the formulation of political practices rooted in social development, community, and new practices of regional action.

Social and health policies were key axes of the Welfare State in many South American countries. After the results of neoliberal policies, in a context of increased social inequalities, lack of access to health systems and expansion of social exclusion, social policy rose to a high priority of countries. Thus, social policies, and particularly health policies, become essential strategies to combat poverty and reduce inequalities. Health is a prime example of an ongoing quiet revolution in the regional political economy of cooperation and diplomacy. New catalysts, at the national and international level, forged new opportunities to redefine objectives of regional political economy and forms of collective action.

Health is a paradigmatic example of regional cooperation, as a possibility of expanding chains of public policy (Riggirozzi, 2014). As argued by Riggirozzi (2014, p. 434), the attention to health policies shows a 'social turn' in the life of Southern regional organisations and their mission to cooperate in order to meet high-profile social demands. An expression of that is the emergence of the South American Health Council of UNASUR. The appearance of UNASUR is a paradigmatic case that shows not only important changes in the form and content of regional governance and the structure of opportunities for social inclusion through health, but also on the principles and particular values that have permeated this agenda..

The member countries of UNASUR assumed the political commitment to give prominence to the health sector as never before. This commitment acquired different characteristics compared to the principles and actions carried out by traditional international organisations such as WHO and PAHO. Traditional international cooperation usually develops specific programmes for diseases, for example, against malaria, HIV / AIDS and tuberculosis through specific funds. These are 'vertical' programmes that do not take into account neither the specificities nor the participation of the population. In contrast, UNASUR has attempted to modify this traditional approach and has tried to understand health from a more political perspective and from an approach based on human rights. This paradigm shift has resulted in different actions such as the promotion of a joint work of public health schools, the strengthening of national health systems and the encouragement of regional studies of the social determinants of health (Herrero & Loza, 2018). All the interviewees argued that the UNASUR Health Council put on agenda the social determinants of health in regional health policies.

Our results show that, since its creation, UNASUR Health has changed the traditional paradigm in health due to the influence of regional actors such as the Latin American Association of Social Medicine (LASM). Moreover, the creation of UNASUR Health was driven by this movement that designed its structure and drafted its fundamental principles and values. This critical political movement, which was always excluded from the state proposals, had an opportunity with the progressive and left-wing governments of the 2000s. Further, an interviewee who played a central role in the founding of the Health Council stated that it was relatively easy to strategically impact on UNASUR because of the long previous experience of working together in ALAMES[2] (AL04, personal interview. October 9th, 2014). This is a key point, considering that other of the interviewees (who participated at the time of the constitution of the Health Council of UNASUR and has been coordinator of ALAMES) said that the experience of ALAMES (and so of LASM/CH) and many of its members facilitated the conformation of the Health Council and its main values and principles (AL04, personal interview. October 9th, 2014). When UNASUR was formed, the resolution to set up the Health Council was already drafted (AL04, personal interview. October 9th, 2014). Another interviewee mentioned that the creation of the Health Council of UNASUR was strategically connected to the political shift in the region toward giving back centrality to the public sphere, the recovery of certain perspectives focused on social rights and a new regional integration and south-south cooperation (AL08, personal interview. June 24th, 2014).

The interviewees clearly pointed out that the creation of the Health Council was also due to the influence of some health ministers who took advantage of the opportunity when the Defense Council was built (AL08, personal interview, June 24, 2014). The Health Council was the second to be created and had much more dynamism than the Defense Council.

In my personal opinion, I believe that countries increasingly understand the role of regional integration processes. It is better understood that there are shared needs and challenges and also that there are asymmetries that must be reduced to achieve common goals. (PY02, personal interview. October 23rd, 2014)

Other interviewee mentioned that UNASUR decided to support Universal Health Systems instead of Universal Health Coverage, after a heated debate[3] (AL04, personal interview, October 9, 2014). In that decision the representatives of ALAMES had a fundamental influence. UNASUR agreed on this position and discussed it at a meeting of PAHO health ministers. In 2014, Brazil, Chile, Ecuador and Paraguay occupied the Executive Board of PAHO. Finally, it was approved at the 53rd session of the PAHO Directors Board (CD 53/5) with the following denomination: coverage and universal access to health, trying to contain different positions. That common positioning was then taken to the WHO World Health Assembly in 2015. 'This is a very important success for UNASUR because it ended up taking a joint position (…) since there are more opportunities at some moments than others and that must be taken advantage of' (AL04, personal interview, October 9, 2014).

The previous one was not the only joint position in the international scene. UNASUR strives for obtaining a voice in global health, gaining political prominence through two parallel movements highly relevant in terms of health diplomacy. To do so, UNASUR has taken its position to the global arena in which there has been an increase in health issues on the agenda (Rio + 20, ICPD + 20, World Conference on SDH, etc.). These scenarios are permeated by two different global movements, one linked to the opening and globalisation of the health market and the other linked to rights (related to Alma-Ata, forums such as Health in All Policies, the Framework Convention Snuff Control). Beyond these two movements that pervade the stage, there is also a change with the emergence of debates on the agenda of health and development in the World Trade Organization (WTO) and World Intellectual Property Organization (WIPO), among others (Coitiño, 2014). Gaining a voice in global diplomacy, UNASUR is a central driving force that also allows regional identity building. For example, it was able to negotiate as a block in the 67th World Health Assembly (WHA) over the report submitted by the Health Development Advisory Panel on Research (ISAGS, 2014). In this case, UNASUR member States took a common position on ten issues: vaccines, disabilities, monitoring of the Millennium Development Goals, Post-2015 Agenda, repercussion of the exposure to mercury, health contribution to social and economic development, access to essential medicines, strengthening of the regulation systems and follow-up of the Recife Political Declaration on human resources and of the report presented by the Consultative Expert Working Group on Research and Development (ISAGS, 2014). Thus, the participation of the Health Council in this kind of international forum was central to the mission of building a shared agenda. An example of this has been the mapping of experiences of primary care in the Americas carried out by the ISAGS that accounts for the various models of comprehensive health care adopted over time and that was submitted to the WHA. The initiative aims to provide governments with information to identify strategic policies for local or regional action, facilitating decision-making.

In its 'Five Year Plan' (2010–2015), UNASUR adopted the social determinants approach and a transversal perspective in its policies, promoting the development of partnerships and networks with civil society. It also proposes to increase the number of countries in the region that reorient their health systems towards a focus on social determinants. In this way, the central role that health took in the region-building process helped to position social inclusion within the regional agenda. References to health as a human right and emphasis on addressing social determinants of health are not simply rhetorical in the Five Year Plan. The conformation – and the actions – of the Five Technical Groups (Health Surveillance and Response, Development of Universal Systems, Universal Access to Medicines, Health Promotion and Action on Social Determinants of Health, Development and Management of Human Resources) speak to a real intention to uphold those principles. Likewise, the need to reinforce cooperation mechanisms among countries of the region promoted joint actions and the strengthening of integration, under the recognition of national sovereignties.

Teixeira (2017) argues that the process of regional integration and cooperation carried out by UNASUR contributes to the promotion of regional health sovereignty, while strengthening the national health sovereignties of each member country. In this line, Mario Rovere (ALAMES member and sanitary specialist in Social Medicine) argues that health sovereignty is achieved by strengthening the capacity of the state to guarantee the right to health and to provide public goods, which is an axis for redefining health policies and through which to build new negotiating capacities within the framework of alternative international health, where the state is the central actor (Rovere, 2011). Thus, the regional project strengthens and broadens the capacity to negotiate and defend its interest in multilateral spaces, in front of the market and other international and transnational organisations, which in turn generates greater autonomy for the countries involved in the process of regional integration.

Health is itself a privileged field for the construction of foreign sovereignty through cooperation, since it can engage continental and global multilateral spaces of negotiation and exercise of sovereignty, spaces which other social areas do not possess (Teixeira, 2017). UNASUR also emerged as a feasible space for the promotion of south-south cooperation (from here, SSC), as countries sought to reduce regional inequities through the creation of spaces for exchange and collaborative action (Vance et al., 2016).

SSC in this arena was early fostered at the Bandung Conference, held in 1955 to promote greater articulation among developing countries to stimulate their own growth (Buss & Ferreira, 2010). SSC is initiated, organised and managed by developing countries themselves, with governments often playing a lead role. SSC can include different sectors and its nature might be bilateral, multilateral, subregional, regional or interregional (Vance et al., 2016). The SSC agenda and initiatives must be determined by the countries of the South, guided by the principles of respect for national sovereignty, national ownership and independence, equality, non-conditionality, non-interference in domestic affairs and mutual benefit. Accordingly, SSC became a fundamental strategy for South American countries based on a horizontal relationship and on cooperation between equals. The creation of UNASUR in 2008 and its ministerial sectorial councils in the following years is one of the most recent experiences of SSC in the region.

UNASUR encouraged the values of SSC through its declarations and, according to our fieldwork, it also fortified a continental as well as a global position for new health diplomacy. This cooperation is also evident in the South American Health Council, its Technical Groups and Structuring Networks, and the South American Institute of Government in Health[4] (ISAGS). UNASUR's Five-Year Plan (2010–2015) provided for the creation of the ISAGS, as a centre for high-level study, critical reflection and training of strategic personnel. The intention was to promote the construction of a South American vision and to reinforce critical reflection on global health, aligning positions and fostering a cooperative circle (Vance et al., 2016).

Both UNASUR and ISAGS propose a horizontal model, in which all members contribute to the identification of problems and the development of solutions. For example, ISAGS acts by facilitating the processes of cooperation in health through its spaces of debate (thematic workshops, conferences and courses). Moreover, in accordance with the principles of SSC, the regional block has strict regulations regarding its financing, which does not allow any type of economic support outside of the member countries without the prior approval of its Council of Ministers of Foreign Affairs (Vance et al., 2016).

This regulation seeks to protect the decisions, actions and strategies of the entity against external interests that may oppose the public interest. In this way, the resources that are handled come from the member states. The decision for UNASUR to be financed exclusively through the contributions of its member countries, placing strong restrictions on third-party funds (except those on which all foreign ministers decide otherwise) has also been a wise decision. The fact that decisions are adopted by consensus has generated decisions that acquire greater political weight and legitimacy (Belardo, 2018). We could see a quiet revolution in health diplomacy in the region that promotes a movement towards horizontal cooperation and technical support, away from what its leaders view as an out-dated vertical model of donors and recipients (Herrero, 2017).

## Conclusion

In Latin America, health, education, employment, and the struggle for land and housing have been long-standing social demands, strongly linked to the concept of citizenship in the XXth century (Roberts & Portes, 2005). LASM/CH are intellectual traditions and political movements committed to the living conditions of the popular majorities. Insofar as they recognise the social and political dimension of diseases, they have given great importance to studying – and reporting – the social determinants of health and disease processes and to considering health as a human right.

With the consequences of neoliberal policies and the deepening of social inequality, representatives of the Social Medicine and Collective Health movements fought for the need to recover the role of the State. With the emergence of leftist and progressive governments in the region, a 'window of opportunity' was opened for the ideas of Social Medicine and Collective Health to occupy a dominant place on the agenda of some States, as well as at the regional level. In this scenario, and from its origins, UNASUR has understood health as a right for all and a duty of States. That is why UNASUR has embraced the principles of solidarity, social justice and equity and focuses on the social determinants of health and the struggle for universal health systems. The construction of new blocks in the Latin American region (as UNASUR, CELAC or ALBA) revived the idea of Simon Bolivar of the construction of a Great Fatherland (the 'Patria Grande' project) to recover our sovereignty.

UNASUR represents an attempt to establish an alternative paradigm for the integration of the twelve countries of the region. The creation of this international organisation responded to a geopolitical vision based on principles such as independence, sovereignty, solidarity and complementarity among the member countries. This eminently political and intergovernmental initiative emerged with the aim of generating regional autonomy in a great diversity of aspects (health, defense, infrastructure, energy, education, social and cultural development), enhancing the scale of individual efforts, and with the purpose of setting common positions on the world stage.

Ten years after the emergence of UNASUR, we can affirm that health had a prominent place in its agenda. The values, principles and alternative approaches in health were incorporated into the organisation's policies thanks to the intellectual and militant efforts of a group of committed professionals, belonging to the long tradition of Latin American Social Medicine / Collective Health, who visualised an opportunity to influence both nationally and regionally. This conceptual framework allows UNASUR to discuss health policy guidelines instead of 'programs' for specific diseases, as traditionally done by PAHO, which resulted in the imposition of programmes designed in Washington to our countries.

However, some of its strengths can become weaknesses or limits. The fact that policy decisions are adopted unanimously gives greater power and legitimacy to the measures. But when the political representation of the member countries changes significantly, necessarily UNASUR, in a context of different interests and conflicting ideological visions, can enter a situation of stagnation. That is the situation that UNASUR is going through now.[5] Another weakness of UNASUR is that as a regional organisation, it aims to harmonise public policies but not to implement them or their recommendations. Then, there may be a general consensus, but each country implements that consensus in a different, even opposite, way. For example, there is a general consensus about the need for universal health. However, countries interpret this universalisation in a very different way. This translates into different national health systems. Finally, despite the fact that several articles of the Constitutive Treaty of UNASUR proclaim citizen participation in health, this popular participation has not been made effective or institutionalised (Belardo, 2018).

Despite the mentioned weaknesses, UNASUR has been considered an example of political-technical cooperation between countries without requiring members to relinquish individual sovereignty and to establish consensual cooperation agreements. UNASUR is also demonstrating that regional integration is possible without supranational governance. And finally, the Health Council, its Technical Groups and Structuring Networks, and ISAGS are spaces for strengthening integration and SSC recognising that health is a bridge to peace and the development of peoples.

After a decade of work in favour of integration, the experience of UNASUR is threatened by the emergence of conservative leaders in the region and the recent decision of Argentina, Brazil, Chile, Colombia, Paraguay and Peru to leave the bloc. This decision jeopardises the continuity of joint plans and projects in the area of health, weakening the initiative of integration.

## Notes

1. LASM/CH promoted the analysis of the category of social determination of health (Breilh, 2013). This differs from the concept of social determinants, used above all by PAHO and WHO. The concept of Social Determination of Health had a great importance in the development of LASM/CH. For the purposes of this article we will not delve into this debate since, to our knowledge, UNASUR has used both concepts interchangeably, and more frequently that of 'social determinants of health'. Also, for more information authors recommend this lecture: ALAMES (2015).
2. The Latin American Association of Social Medicine (ALAMES) is a political organisation made up of people linked to different fields of theory and practice of Social Medicine/Collective Health in Latin America. It was formally constituted in 1984 during the 3rd Latin American Seminar on Social Medicine, held in Ouro Preto, Brazil.
3. Universal health coverage and universal health systems are two different and opposed ways of understanding the right to health. The first is supported by the WHO, the World Bank and the IMF and is also supported by the Rockefeller and Bill and Melinda Gates foundations. The second is supported by the movements of collective health and social medicine in Latin America. Both currents of thought are framed in the need for health reforms but the proposals are different. Universal health coverage proposes the entry of the market into the health sector and for this purpose opts for 'insurance' or 'coverage' with multiple administrators, buyers and providers of health services and the channelling of fiscal subsidies to support it. The most important Latin American examples are the reforms of Chile, Colombia and Mexico. The other current raises a public health system. It is inspired by the Social State where health services are public precisely to guarantee equal and free access to the services required of the entire population, thus guaranteeing the right to health. This approach claims the redistributive role of the State in the form of providing social services. The most prominent Latin American examples are Cuba and Brazil.
4. ISAGS is a centre of high studies and debate of public policies, its actions contribute for the development of governance and leadership in health in South America. The headquarters of the Institute are in Rio de Janeiro, Brazil.
5. In the current context of conservative's governments other visions of regional integration begin to gain strength, even with agreements that overlap as the alliances linked to the interests of the United States as well as the rapprochement between the Pacific Alliance and MERCOSUR or the attempts of alliance between the European Union and MERCOSUR.

## Acknowledgements

The authors gratefully acknowledge to all the participants, who kindly shared their experiences, knowledge, and opinions and made this study possible. Also, warmly thanks to Adriana Greco for her comments to the early versions of this paper. Finally, we want to especially thank the editorial board of this journal for an invaluable contribution with their careful review and the assistance in the edition of the final draft.

## Disclosure statement

No potential conflict of interest was reported by the authors.

## Funding

The field work mentioned in this article was carried out with support from the UK Economic and Social Research Council (ESRC), Grant Ref. ES/L005336/1. The article and does not necessarily reflect the opinions of the ESRC.

## ORCID

*María Belén Herrero* ⬤ http://orcid.org/0000-0002-6941-0580
*Jorgelina Loza* ⬤ http://orcid.org/0000-0003-1442-5782
*Marcela Beatriz Belardo* ⬤ http://orcid.org/0000-0001-9032-3919

## References

ALAMES. (2015). Taller Latinoamericano sobre determinantes sociales de la salud. Retrieved from http://www.uasb. edu.ec/UserFiles/376/File/ponencias_Taller%20Determinantes%20Sociales.pdf

Belardo, M. (2018). Una década en la integración de Sudamérica: límites y perspectivas en salud. 15 de febrero. Retrieved from https://sincopa- sv.blogspot.com/2018/02/una-decada-en-la-integracion-de.html

Breilh, J. (2013). La determinación social de la salud como herramienta de transformación hacia una nueva salud pública (salud colectiva). *The Revista Facultad Nacional de Salud Pública, 31*(1), S13–S27.

Brown, T. M., Cueto, M., & Fee, E. (2006). The World Health Organization and the transition from International to Global public health. *American Journal of Public Health, 96*(1), 62–72.

Buse, K., & Waxman, A. (2001). Public-private health partnerships: A strategy for WHO. *Bulletin of the World Health Organization, 79*, 748–754.

Buss, P., & Ferreira, J. R. (2010). Ensaio crítico sobre a cooperação internacional em saúde. *RECIIS, 4*(1), 93–105.

Coitiño, A. (2014). Análisis del fenómeno de los procesos regionales de integración en salud como actores emergentes de la diplomacia de la salud global: el caso UNASUR (pp. 1–32, Unpublishedmimeo). Programas de Líderes de Salud Internacional OPS/OMS (PLSI). Washington, DC: PanAmerican Health Organisation.

Fidler, D. (2001). The globalization of public health: The first 100 years of international health diplomacy. *Bulletin of the World Health Organization, 79*(9), 842–849.

Fidler, D. (2010). *The challenges of global health governance.* New York: Council on Foreign Relations, 2010. Retrieved from http://www.cfr.org/global-governance/challenges-global-health-governance/

Galeano, D., Trotta, L., & Spinelli, H. (2011). Juan César García y el movimiento latinoamericano de medicina social: notas sobre una trayectoria de vida. *Salud Colectiva, 7*(3), 285–315. Retrieved from http://www.scielo.org.ar/scielo. php?script=sci_arttext&pid=S1851-82652011000400002&lng=es&tlng=es

Giovanella, L., compiler. (2015). *Atención primaria de salud en Suramérica.* Rio de Janeiro: ISAGS UNASUR.

Gómez-Dantés, O., & Khoshnood, B. (1991). La Evolución de la Salud Internacional en el Siglo XX. *Salud Pública Mexicana, 33*(4), 314–339.

Granda, U. E. (2003). *A qué llamamos salud colectiva hoy?* Ponencia presentada en el VII Congreso Brasileño de Salud Colectiva, Brasilia.

Herrero, M. B. (2017). Moving towards South-South international health: Debts and challenges in the regional health agenda. *Ciência & Saúde Coletiva, 22*(7), 2169–2174. doi:10.1590/1413-81232017227.03072017

Herrero, M. B., & Loza, J. (2018). Building a regional health agenda: A rights-based approach to health in South America. *Global Public Health, 13*(9), 1179–1191.

Huymen, M., Martens, P., & Hilderink, H. (2005). The health impacts of globalization: A conceptual framework. *Globalization and Health, 1*, 14.

Iriart, C., Waitzkin, H., Breilh, J., Estrada, A., & Merhy, E. E. (2002). Latin American social medicine: Contributions and challenges. *Revista Panamericana de Salud Pública, 12*, 128–136.

ISAGS. (2014, June). *Posiciones comunes de UNASUR hacen avanzar la agenda de Salud Global. Newsletter.* Rio de Janeiro: Author. Retrieved from http://www.isagsunasur.org/uploads/eventos/v%5B282%5Dling%5B2%5Danx% 5B257%5D.pdf

Labonté, R., & Gagnon, M. L. (2010). Framing health and foreign policy: Lessons for global health diplomacy. *Globalization and Health, 6*(14), 1–19.

López Arellano, O., Escudero, J. C., & Carmona, L. D. (2008). Los determinantes sociales de la salud. Una perspectiva desde el Taller Latinoamericano de Determinantes Sociales de la Salud. *ALAMES Medicina Social, 3*(4), 323–335.

Mariani, R. (2007). *Democracia/Estado/Ciudadanía: Hacia un Estado de y para la Democracia en América Latina (Coord).* Lima: Sede PNUD.

Paim, J. S., & de Almeida Filho, N. (1998). Saúde coletiva: uma "nova saúde pública" ou campo aberto a novos paradigmas? *Revista de Saúde Pública, 32*(4), 299–316.

Quijano, A. (2005). *Colonialidad del poder, eurocentrismo y América Latina in Lander, E. (comp) La colonialidad del saber: eurocentrismo y ciencias sociales.* Buenos Aires: CLACSO and UNESCO. 201–246.

Riggirozzi, P. (2014). Regionalism through social policy: Collective action and health diplomacy in South America. *Economy and Society, 43*(3), 432–454.

Riggirozzi, P., & Tussie, D. (compilers) (2012). *The rise of Post-hegemonic Regionalism: The case of Latin America.* Dordrecht: Springer.

Roberts, B., & Portes, A. (2005). *Enfrentando la ciudad del libre mercado. La acción colectiva urbana en América Latina, 1980–2000.* en A. Portes, B. R. Roberts, & A. Grimson (Eds.), *Ciudades latinoamericanas. Un análisis comparativo en el umbral del nuevo siglo* (pp. 509–556). Buenos Aires: Prometeo.

Rovere, M. (2011). Organismos Internacionales de Salud y la Argentina. *Voces en el Fénix, 2*(7), 21–24.

Sanahuja, J. A. (2011). Multilateralismo y regionalismo en clave suramericana: el caso de UNASUR. Los desafíos del multilateralismo en américa latina. Edición especial: CRIES – Universidad de Guadalajara – Universidad Iberoamericana, p 115.

Soares, L. T. R. (2001). *Ajuste neoliberal e desajuste social na América Latina.* Petrópolis: Vozes.

Teixeira, M. F. (2017). *O Conselho de Saúde da Unasul e os desafios para a construção de soberania sanitária* (doctoral thesis). FundaçãoOswaldo Cruz, Brasil.

UNASUR. (2008). South American union of nations constitutive treaty. Retrieved from http://www.comunidadandina.org/unasur/tratado_constitutivo.htm

Vance, C., Mafla, L., y Bermudez, B. (2016). La cooperación Sur-Sur en Salud: la experiencia de UNASUR. *Línea Sur, Revista de Política Exterior, 3*(12), 89–102.

# Revisiting the social determinants of health agenda from the global South

Elis Borde ⓘ and Mario Hernández

**ABSTRACT**

In an effort to provide an overview of the conceptual debates shaping the mobilisation around social determinants of health and health inequities and challenge the apparent consensus for equity in health, this essay compares two of the most influential approaches in the field: the WHO Commission on Social Determinants of Health approach (CSDH), strongly influenced by European Social Medicine, and the Latin American Social Medicine and Collective Health (LASM-CH) 'Social determination of the health-disease process' approach, hitherto largely invisibilized. It is argued that the debates shaping the equity in health agenda do not merely reflect conceptual differences, but essentially different ethical-political proposals that define the way health inequities are understood and proposed to be transformed. While the health equity agenda probably also gained momentum due to the broad political alliance it managed to consolidate, it is necessary to make differences explicit as this allows for an increase in the breadth and specificity of the debate, facilitating the recognition of contextually relevant proposals towards the reduction of health inequities.

## Introduction

One of the most marked characteristics of the global social structure is the existence of substantial inequalities in wealth and income, which also find expression in differences in health between countries and between social groups within countries (Berkman, Kawachi, & Glymour, 2014; Dorling & Barford, 2007). While many countries have experienced sharp reductions in absolute poverty and excess mortality (Victora et al., 2011), inequities in health persist across countries and reflect historically defined and territorially specific expressions of structural conflictuality in the capitalist accumulation and production regime (Piketty, 2014; Sanahuja, 2013; Wallerstein, 2011) along the lines of class, race/ethnicity and gender as well as the global North/South divide. This patterning is evident in infant mortality rates varying between 2 per 1000 live births in Iceland and over 120 per 1000 live births in Mozambique, the 28 year difference in life expectancy at birth for men of two Glasgow neighbourhoods or the fact that in the United States, 886,202 deaths could have been averted between 1991 and 2000 if mortality rates between white and African Americans were equalised, contrasted to 176,633 lives saved in the US by medical advances in the same period, just to name a few examples (CSDH, 2007).

In recent decades, international health agendas have tended to oscillate between two main approaches: (1) narrowly defined, technology-based medical and public health interventions; and (2) an understanding of health as a social phenomenon, proposing more complex forms of intersectoral policy action, and sometimes linked to a broader social justice agenda (Solar & Irwin, 2010). The latter found expression in the celebrated Alma Ata Conference from 1978 and the Primary Health Care Agenda, the Ottawa Charter for Health Promotion (1986), and more recently, in the work of the WHO Commission on Social Determinants of Health (CSDH), the adoption of the Rio Political Declaration in 2011, following the World Conference on Social Determinants of Health in Rio de Janeiro as well as in the Health in All Policies Framework and the Lancet-University of Oslo Commission on Global Governance for Health. Although health and social security system reforms over the last two decades have been dictated by a neoliberal agenda shaped by the convergence of the World Health Organization, international financial institutions, and transnational corporations (Armada, Muntaner, & Navarro, 2001; Hernández, 2003), particularly in Latin America, and strict fiscal austerity following the 2008 economic crisis currently strain and erode Southern European health and social security systems (Karanikolos et al., 2013), the health equity question is notably present in the international health agenda and public discourse.

The publication of the final report of the WHO CSDH in 2008 evinced the renewed interest and political will to address health inequities, constituting a crucial advance in the mobilisation for health equity by making a case for the urgent need for comprehensive action and by drawing attention to government responsibility. The conceptual framework of the Commission and policy directions for action implied by the proposed SDH approach became a key reference and driver of the global health equity agenda (Birn, 2009; Cabrera et al., 2011); also because it offered an overdue and yet not overly radical critique of the prevailing social, economic and political order at a time when it was no longer possible to hide away or deny the negative consequences the growth oriented development model – at the core of the prevalent social, economic and political order - has for human well-being, environment and health.

Nonetheless and despite the fact that the SDH approach was presented and celebrated as a globally consented proposal and new opportunity to improve health and tackle inequities (Friel & Marmot, 2011; Solar & Irwin, 2006), three alternative declarations were published following the adoption of the Rio Political Declaration in 2011, which several commentators (Birn, 2009; Borde, Porto, & Hernández, 2015; Breilh, 2011b; Cabrera et al., 2011) understand as an expression of the dissatisfaction, and primarily, of differences in the way social determinants of health and health inequities are understood. That is to say, different ethical-political proposals on social justice, equity, policy action and emancipation, that define how social determinants of health and health inequities are conceived, conceptualised, researched and proposed to be transformed, and consequently mobilise different political, social and economic agendas.

The declarations respectively emitted by the International Federation of Medical Student Associations (IFMSA), the People's Health Movement (PHM) and the *Asociación Latinoamericana de Medicina Social* (ALAMES)/*Centro de Estudos Brasileiros sobre a Saúde* (CEBES), in this regard made the existence of alternative proposals visible and showed how the call for health equity is less unequivocal than it may seem. Furthermore, it was shown that it is necessary to better differentiate to further qualify the debate and to provide a critical historical perspective on the proposed scope and concrete opportunities for action on social determinants of health and health inequities.

In an effort to provide an overview of the conceptual debates shaping the mobilisation around social determinants of health and health inequities and challenge the apparent consensus for equity in health, this essay exemplary compares and contrasts two of the most influential approaches in the field: the WHO Commission on Social Determinants of Health approach (CSDH), strongly influenced by European Social Medicine, and the Latin American Social Medicine and Collective Health (LASM-CH) 'social determination of the health-disease processes' approach, hitherto largely invisible in the dominant global agenda for health equity and in the mobilisation around SDH and health inequities.

## Methods

The essay draws on a review of published and unpublished literature on social determinants of health and health inequities in English, Spanish and Portuguese, retrieved between February 2015 and December 2017 from the following automated search engines: PubMed, LILACS, VHL, Google Scholar and Scielo. Furthermore, bibliography was manually selected based on the criteria of the authors.

We begin by providing an overview of the conceptual debates shaping the dominant equity in health agenda and introduce the WHO Social Determinants of Health (SDH) approach to illustrate how social determinants of health and health inequities are conceived, conceptualised, researched and proposed to be transformed according to this agenda. In the second part, the WHO SDH approach is compared and contrasted with the Latin American Social Medicine and Collective Health (LA SM-CH) 'Social determination of the health-disease-care process' or short, 'social determination of health' approach, which has been developing over the last 50 years in Latin American Social Medicine and Collective Health and has been discussed and recognised as an alternative and yet mostly undervalued and invisibilized approach to address health inequities (Birn, 2009; Borde et al., 2015; Spiegel, Breilh, & Yassi, 2015; Tajer, 2003).

## Debates shaping the dominant equity in health agenda

Several developments, debates and theories have shaped the mobilisation around social determinants of health and health inequities over the years and constituted a global health equity agenda. Apart from external economic, social and political pressures that defined the scope and relative dominance of the agenda for health equity at different points in time, the agenda expresses internal mediations and, essentially, choices on ontological, epistemological and praxiological proposals. These choices, and more so the relative dominance of specific ontological, epistemological and praxiological stances in the global agenda for health equity are rarely discussed and often limited to rather linear accounts on the historical development of a specific agenda or a specific field of research. In this regard, it seems necessary to recognise the dialectics of dominance/subalternity and visibility/invisibility in the global agenda for health equity and in science in general, recognising differences and conflicts between different approaches to better understand the apparently subtle discursive and theoretical shifts that orchestrate often profound political, social and economic changes.

In the following, we will review theories and approaches that are recognised in and have defined the global health equity agenda and will then exemplify the discussion in relation to two approaches. In this regard, we will critically analyze the way social determinants of health and health inequities are conceived, conceptualised, researched and proposed to be transformed according to the dominant SDH approach promoted by the WHO CSDH and will then contrast it with the LA SM-CH 'social determination of the health-disease process' approach, addressing key concepts and discussions that have shaped this approach and LA SM-CH in general.

It is important to note that despite the fact that we are proposing to compare and contrast the SDH approach and the LA SM-CH 'social determination of the health-disease process' approach, both approaches share the recognition of health as a human and social right and goal, the need for intersectoral action for health and the condemnation of health inequities, amongst others, and although to different degrees, both constitute a rupture in relation to more traditional, conservative public health approaches based on narrowly defined, technology-based interventions and the naturalisation of health inequities based, for example, on biological essentialism consisting of a belief that certain phenomena are natural, inevitable and biologically determined.

## Defining the dominant global health equity agenda

The CSDH conceptual framework recognises three not necessarily mutually exclusive theoretical directions in current social epidemiology which seek to elucidate principles capable of explaining social inequalities in health: (a) psychosocial approaches, (b) ecosocial theory and related multi-level frameworks; and (c) social production of disease/political economy of health (Solar & Irwin, 2010, p. 15). Psychosocial approaches proposed by Cassels (1976) and Wilkinson & Pickett (2006), amongst others, ascribe the existence of health inequalities to the direct or indirect effects of stress, arguing that the exposure to adverse psychosocial environments, for example at the workplace (high demands, low control and or effort-reward imbalances), elicits sustained stress reactions with negative (long-term) consequences for health (Kawachi, Subramanian, & Almeida-Filho, 2002; Solar & Irwin, 2010). Direct and indirect effects of stress are recognised and it is suggested that the exposure to daily adverse life circumstances creates wear and tear on the organism through allostatic loads. Furthermore, stress may affect health by promoting a more adverse profile of behaviours such as smoking and excessive alcohol consumption (Kawachi et al., 2002). It is argued that these exposures are likely to be experienced more frequently among lower socioeconomic groups and that the extent of the effects on health produced by such exposures may be greater in lower socioeconomic groups, which are considered more vulnerable and less resistant to stressors due to arguably weaker social cohesion and disintegration of social bonds. Krieger (2001b) accordingly concludes that a psychosocial framework

'directs attention to endogenous biological responses to human interactions. Its focus is on responses to "stress" and on stressed people in need of psychosocial resources. Comparatively less attention is accorded both theoretically and empirically to: (1) who and what generates psychosocial insults and buffers, and (2) how their distribution – along with that of ubiquitous or non-ubiquitous pathogenic physical, chemical, or biological agents – is shaped by social, political and economic policies'. (Krieger, 2001b, p. 670)

The ecosocial approach and related multi-level frameworks integrate social and biological factors and propose a dynamic, historical and ecological perspective to develop new insights into determinants of population distribution of disease and inequities in health (Solar & Irwin, 2010). Analyses of population patterns of health, disease and well-being are analyzed in relation to different levels of biological, ecological and social organisation and embrace a social production of disease perspective while aiming to complement macro-level analyses with biological and ecological analysis.

"Thus, more than simply adding "biology" to "social" analyses, or "social factors" to "biological" analyses, the ecosocial framework begins to envision a more systematic integrated approach capable of generating new hypotheses, rather than simply reinterpreting factors identified by one approach (e.g. biological) in terms of another (e.g. social)'. (Krieger, 2001b, p. 673)

Krieger's notion of 'embodiment' is central to this approach and describes how the material and social world finds expression in and shapes our biology. According to this approach pathways of embodiment are structured by (a) societal arrangements of power and property and patterns of production, consumption and reproduction as well as by (b) constraints and possibilities of biology, shaped by evolution, the ecological context and individual and family trajectories of biological and social development (Krieger, 2001a).

In social production of disease/political economy of health approaches, economic and political determinants of health and disease are emphasised, understanding inequalities in health between social groups as expressions of the social organisation characteristic of the capitalist accumulation and production regime and related processes of exploitation, oppression and marginalisation (Kaplan, Pamuk, Lynch, Cohen, & Balfour, 1996; Lynch et al., 1998). In this regard, it is recognised that diseases are socially produced and distributed and that the very way in which disease is treated is itself an aspect of capitalist society in the sense that disease is individualised and depoliticised and essentially geared towards the generation of profit. The social organisation and the processes that produce and reproduce this organisation accordingly become central to the analyses proposed by these approaches, addressing questions such as: 'how does prioritizing capital accumulation over human need affect health, as evinced through injurious workplace organization and exposure to occupational hazards, inadequate pay scales, profligate pollution, and rampant commodification of virtually every human activity, need, and desire?' (Krieger, 2001b, p. 670). The underlying hypothesis is that economic and political institutions and decisions that create, enforce, and perpetuate economic and social privilege and inequality along the lines of class, gender and ethnicity/race are root causes of social inequalities in health (Krieger, 2001b, p. 670), which implies that reducing inequalities in health requires changes in the social and economic order.

While the Latin American Social Medicine and Collective Health 'social determination of the health disease-process' approach is often subsumed under social production of disease/ political economy of health approaches (Krieger, 2001a, 2001b; Solar & Irwin, 2010), though rarely properly recognised or referenced in English language publications, we argue that the LA SM-CH approach constitutes a different theoretical direction, which synthesises social production of disease/ political economy of health approaches and ecosocial approaches but introduces yet other constructs and ways of addressing inequities in health – ontologically, epistemologically and praxiologically – which do not neatly fit into the previously outlined theoretical directions. This is particularly so as the Latin American Social Medicine and Collective health approaches developed in Latin America – with other geo-cultural and epistemological references that developed within a distinct and largely subordinated genealogy of critical thought, undoubtedly strongly influenced by Marxist approaches but also by the works of Bourdieu and Foucault, particularly in Brazil.

The WHO CSDH or SDH approach, in contrast, does not constitute a radical rupture but rather synthesises the above outlined theoretical directions and essentially, the Anglo-Saxon European Social Medicine, primarily based on the CSDH´s chair Sir Michael Marmot and his colleague's work. While this is not explicitly recognised and the SDH approach has substantially defined the global equity in health agenda, it has been noted by several commentators (Breilh, 2011b; Guzmán, 2009; Lynch et al., 1998; Morales-Borrero, Borde, Eslava-Castañeda, & Concha-Sánchez, 2013) and is evident in the ontological, epistemological and praxiological proposals that constitute the SDH approach. In the following, the CSDH SDH approach will be critically analyzed and contrasted with the LA SM-CH SD approach.

## The dominant equity in health agenda and the SDH approach

In recent years, the dominant health equity agenda particularly found expression in the WHO SDH approach. The SDH approach and the final report of the CSDH make several important contributions and have undoubtedly strengthened the global health equity agenda, documenting the existence and consequences of health inequities within and between countries. Nonetheless, there are several shortcomings that will be discussed in the following and in the next section contrasted to alternatives invoked by the LA SM-CH social determination of the health-disease-care process approach.

The CSDH proposes a model which differentiates between two types of social determinants of health: structural determinants and intermediary determinants. Structural determinants are those that generate or reinforce social stratification in the society and that define individual socioeconomic position, configuring health opportunities of social groups based on their placement within hierarchies of power, prestige and access to resources (economic status) (Solar & Irwin, 2010, p. 30). The socioeconomic position is primarily shaped by occupational status, educational achievement and income level and also the role of gender and ethnic/racial discrimination is recognised, which are all proposed to be measured at individual, household and neighbourhood level and at different points of the lifespan. The authors of the CSDH conceptual framework further recognise contextual factors including: culture and social values, public policies on education, medical care, water and sanitation, social policies affecting factors such as labour, social welfare, land and housing, macroeconomic policies, governance mechanisms related to the definition of needs, patterns of discrimination, civil society participation, accountability and transparency in public administration, and epidemiological conditions including epidemics that alter the social structure, such as HIV/Aids (Solar & Irwin, 2010, p. 25).

The intermediary determinants of health flow from the configuration of underlying social stratification and determine differences in exposure and vulnerability to health-compromising conditions and include the following factors: material circumstances; psychosocial circumstances; behavioural and/or biological factors; and the health system itself (Solar & Irwin, 2010, p. 36). Material circumstances are linked to the physical environment such as housing, consumption potential and the physical working and neighbourhood environment. Psychosocial circumstances refer to different degrees of exposure to experiences and life situations that are perceived as threatening and difficult according to socioeconomic status, including job strain, high debt and lack of social support. The authors of the CSDH conceptual framework further recognise social differences in behavioural/lifestyle factors related to nutrition, physical activity, tobacco and alcohol consumption (Solar & Irwin, 2010, p. 39). The health care system is recognised as a social determinant of health in the sense that it can directly address differences in exposure and vulnerability by improving equitable access to health care and promote intersectoral action to improve health status, as the authors of the CSDH conceptual framework note (Solar & Irwin, 2010, p. 40).

While the SDH approach identifies social conditions in which people are born, live and work and claims that 'social injustice is killing people on a grand scale' (CSDH, 2007), the CSDH analysis and conceptual framework concentrate on what society produces in terms of inequalities and reduce the scope of the critique to what is more than evident, particularly in the global South and increasingly in the global North, failing to clarify the causes of the 'causes of the causes', that is, the processes that historically created and systematically reproduce inequities (Birn, 2009; Navarro, 2009). In this regard, the final report extensively documents inequalities in health between and within countries and provides scientific foundation for appreciating the role of social factors in health, but does not make explicit why and in which way educational achievement, income level, racial/ethnic discrimination, occupational status and gender discrimination structurally determine health across the world. Considered as an 'interplay between the socioeconomic-political context, structural mechanisms generating social stratification and the resulting socioeconomic position of individuals' (CSDH, 2007), the 'social determinants of health inequities', that is, 'structural determinants of health' remain vague, decontextualised and essentially individual, conveying an idea of social 'risk' factors that affect individuals according to their position in the social hierarchy and engender in what the CSDH euphemistically calls 'market-driven globalization'. Accordingly, health outcomes are associated with social stratification and specifically with structural determinants such as income level, ethnicity/race and educational achievement but in the absence of a comprehensive analysis of society, of power relations in society and the processes in which these determinants develop and are reproduced, barely serve as markers of inequities between individuals rather than social groups and become descriptive factors rather than analytical categories of societal characteristics (Breilh, 2011a; Starfield, 2006).

In this regard and although market forces and globalisation are recognised as social determinants of health inequities, the CSDH consistently 'refrains from referring to global capitalism' (Birn, 2009, p. 179) and in this same line, transforms 'social class' into 'socioeconomic status' or 'income level' and 'racism' into ethnic and racial 'discrimination', just to name a few examples. While the CSDH conceptual framework (Solar & Irwin, 2010) does offer theoretical foundations for each of the social determinants proposed in the SDH model, there is no discussion on political struggle, oppression and exploitation, that is, social processes that generate and substantiate unequal power relations in capitalist development models, let alone alternatives to capitalist development. The market and globalisation accordingly appear as obscure and abstract forces that present failures and produce inequalities (Cabrera et al., 2011), which can, however, be corrected with redistributive policies, good governance and by making the market responsible (CSDH, 2007). The CSDH in this regard proposes to 'heighten public health representation in economic policy negotiations, anchored by the institutionalization of health equity impact assessment (HEIA) in all national and international policies and economic treaties' (Birn, 2009, p. 173). Both proposals certainly make interesting and yet blatantly insufficient proposals that imply a rather random, accidental and unforeseen impact of 'the market' on health and health equity, omitting the systematic pattern of social determination engendered in the context of the extreme exploitation of labour and of nature in capitalist accumulation and production regimes. In this regard, there is no recognition of the incompatibility of this regime with healthy lives and the CSDH is content with improvements in an inherently unjust system (Breilh, 2011a). The horizon of transformation is accordingly limited to the correction of distortions that the system presents, without contesting and confronting it (Breilh, 2011a, p. 48), reserving a privileged role for redistributive government policies.

The CSDH imagines a social mobilisation for equity in health and departs from the supposition that the recognition of the scope of inequalities in health is reason enough to mobilise local and national authorities and civil society. This conveys a rather naïve understanding of policy making and of drivers of societal change, which is particularly evident in the discussion of the Northern European welfare states in the CSDH final report, presented and glorified with no mention of the political struggles that were needed to consolidate such systems, let alone the historically shaped structures of exploitation, contributing to the viability and acceptance of such systems in these parts of the world, while similar efforts are being systematically eroded in the global South. Similarly, following Birn (2009), the low and middle income countries that have achieved a level of good health and managed to reduce inequities despite their level of national income and are proposed as examples by the CSDH, all passed through

> long-term political struggle whether arising from armed revolution (in the case of Cuba), [...] a long and ongoing struggle for left-wing political parties to be elected and re-elected to office (in Kerala); or strong populist and labor movements favoring social protections, an end to military spending following a brutal civil war, and the fending off of imperialist interests (in Costa Rica). (Birn, 2009, p. 175)

These omissions seriously hamper a comprehensive understanding of the structural drivers of health equity and weaken the call for 'social participation' and 'empowerment', central to the SDH approach. In this regard, both concepts remain superficial and fixed to an idea of civil identity, liberty and autonomy, subject to a similarly vain understanding of 'political will'. The history of public health and even the review of historical trajectories forging the equity in health agenda proposed in the CSDH conceptual framework (Solar & Irwin, 2010) and in the final report (CSDH, 2007) show social mobilisation to be the key factor that has rendered governments accountable and responsive and has brought about societal transformations, the SDH approach continues to privilege technical solutions focusing on policy makers, questions of governance and a strong belief in the possibility of and need for 'win-win' solutions, driven by false pragmatism and a skewed understanding of politics that render politics apolitical and naturalise relationships shaped by asymmetrical power relations. Similarly, the role of social movements is downplayed and reduced to a functional and hollow understanding of civil society participation (Breilh, 2011a).

The CSDH is unequivocal in the defense of universal health systems and calls for resurrecting the state's role in providing health services, invoking the government responsibility to respect, protect and fulfil the human right to health (Birn, 2009) – a claim that has also mobilised Latin American SM-CH. And yet, contradictory or not, several of the CSDH commissioners have been at the forefront of the universal health *coverage* (UHC) agenda (Andrade et al., 2015; Marmot, 2013), transforming the call for universal health systems into a call for universal health coverage, which represents a significant retreat and implies essentially different ethical-political proposals, as Heredia et al. (2015) point out. In this regard Heredia et al. (2015) argue that it is critical to distinguish forms of health insurance – be they voluntary or compulsory and public or private – from a unified tax-funded public health system and contrast the experiences in Chile, Mexico and Colombia with that of Brazil and Cuba and, more recently, Venezuela, Bolivia and Ecuador, which adopted constitutionally guaranteed reform models amidst broad social mobilisation, and in the case of Bolivia and Ecuador in the phase of rethinking and restructuring the State according to an alternative development paradigm anchored in the indigenous principle of 'living well' (Sumak Kawsay) (Breilh, 2010; Breilh & Muñoz, 2009), with all the contradictions that this transition involves (Radcliffe, 2012).

These discursive shifts are not a minor issue and in the context of the historical retreat, for example, from Primary Health Care to Selective Primary Health Care, they underline the need to carefully differentiate and dissect the ethical-political foundations of the respective proposals. This requires an analysis of the concrete possibilities that actors, commissions and reports have, which would, for example, explain but not necessarily justify why the CSDH final report is notably more politically timid than the CSDH conceptual framework. Further, and as recognised by Birn (2009, p. 174) in relation to the way the CSDH addresses the role of the private sector and the lack of accountability of large philanthropies, this may imply understanding that it 'may be too impolite and impolitic' for the WHO CSDH to explicitly call for the disempowerment of the private sector and political allies to wield 'benign' influence. And yet, Birn (2009) rightly asserts that the report could and 'should certainly refrain from its assertion that health equity will be achieved with the collaboration of private actors' (Birn, 2009, p. 174).

Nonetheless, the CSDH conception seems to reflect a conviction and wish of health equity advocates shaping the dominant equity in health agenda, that it is possible and necessary to get the private sector on board and furthermore, to generate win-win scenarios, coherent with the consistent failure to match groups needing empowerment against those who wield excessive power and to seriously engage with the dialectics of oppressor-oppressed and privilege-benefit, amongst others, and to transcend polarizations, deemed outdated and unrealistic (Birn, 2009).

## Social determination of the health-disease-care process

The Social Determination of the Health-Disease-Care Process is developing as part of Latin American Social Medicine and Collective Health (LA SM-CH), a stream of thought and a movement that evolved in three phases, with the *early formative period* dating back to the 1960s and 1970s (Almeida-Filho & Paim, 1999; Breilh, 2008; García, 1994; Laurell, 1994) and being primarily influenced by labour health demands as well as critical analyses of the epistemological foundations of modern epidemiology and traditional public health. Cecilia Donnangelo (Donnangelo & Pereira, 1976), Jaime Breilh (1986), Sergio Arouca (2003), Edmundo Granda (1989), Asa Cristina Laurell (1979) and Ricardo Bruno Mendes-Gonçalves (Santos & Ayres, 2017) arguably made the most notable contributions during that phase, addressing issues as diverse as medical practice and formation, workers' health and the epistemology of modern epidemiology. Breilh (2008) self-critically recognises these early works, particularly those of himself and his direct colleagues, as being overtly state-centered and based on a unicultural theoretical matrix, possibly necessary to position social class inequity in epidemiological and public health research agendas, but clearly insufficient to capture processes of social determination of the health/disease/care process. In the advent of neoliberalism and structural adjustment programmes during the 1980s and 1990s, the need for organisational structures became evident and LA SM-CH organised around national organisations such as ABRASCO, CEBES, CEAS and particularly around the *Asociación Latinoamericana de Medicina Social* (ALAMES), which was founded in 1984, premised on the defense of health as a public good and civil right and as a social, political, and academic movement. In this period it was recognised that it was necessary to diversify the study of inequity and understanding the linkages between social class, ethnic and gendered power relations shaped by macro-economic processes and the social determination of health (|Breilh, 1986, 2008), evolving into a *second period*. Regarding this period Breilh (2008) notes that 'an immediate challenge was to deconstruct the official discourse of conservative multiculturalism and of culturally relativistic interpretations of health problems, which worked parallel to the neoliberal political economy to justify the dissolution and decentralization of public health epidemiological programmes' (Breilh, 2008, p. 747). The Brazilian health reform undertaken during the 1980s and culminating in the consolidation of the constitutionally guaranteed Unified Health System (*Sistema Único de Saúde* – SUS) in 1988, became an important inspiration for the Latin American SM-CH and essentially represented a synthesis of the proposals of the movement (Escorel, 2009). During the last decade and *third period*, the idea of an alternative subjectivity and of critical interculturality matured, integrating indigenous people's movement demands for emancipatory intercultural knowledge and the Marxist concept of subjectivity that recognises the subject as historically conditioned and at the same time a maker of history (Tajer, 2003). During that time graduate and postgraduate programmes in Social Medicine and Collective Health were consolidated across the region, particularly in Brazil, Argentina, Ecuador, Colombia, Venezuela and Mexico.

Although it is clear that LA SM-CH does not constitute a single, monolithic block and has rather been characterised by constant renovation and diversity, there are some unifying and distinctive elements, that will be outlined in the following.

LA SM-CH movement has historically recognised the need to intertwine processes of transformation on ontological, epistemological and praxiological level – rethinking health and health inequities as theoretical objects; innovating the way these are conceptually and methodologically addressed and projected in praxis. In this regard, there have been comprehensive efforts to rethink health, seeking to overcome the dichotomy of biomedically defined health and disease towards an understanding of health as a complex, multidimensional and essentially social process (Almeida-Filho, 2001; Coelho & Almeida-Filho, 2002), translating into the 'consideration of the dialectic relation between being healthy, being sick, and health care practices, not as unrelated situations but as a historical process described as the health-disease-care process' (Tajer, 2003, p. 2024). Consequently, LA SM-CH has proposed to understand health as a complex social process in as far as it cannot be disconnected from the societal arrangements within which these processes evolve. Rather than an association between society and individual-level biology, the health-disease-care process is understood and conceptualised as part and expression of society. It is in this regard that Breilh (2010) speaks of the 'social determination of health and life', arguing that measures to improve health will not be complete unless they are articulated with the defense of life, primarily the environmental integrity necessary for human survival. Breilh (2010, 2013) accordingly speaks of the ethics of life and health based on the four 'Ss' of a healthy life (sustainability, sovereignty, solidarity and health/holistic biosecurity), which leads the author to affirm that the prevailing capitalist accumulation and production regime is incompatible with health and life. This applies as

> 'the contemporary capitalist logic not only exerts itself through the extraction of surplus value from workers and the traditional market mechanisms, but now depends heavily on truly predatory forms of practice, fraud and violent extraction, which are imposed by taking advantage of inequalities and power asymmetries to dispossess weaker countries or vulnerable groups directly. (Breilh, 2005)

Capitalist societies are accordingly recognised as being shaped by a concentration of power and particularly by a 'triple inequity', which defines the intersection of class, gender and ethnicity/race oppressions that shape social structure and define the quality and scope of oppression, exploitation and marginalisation individuals and social groups suffer under this regime. It is argued that only by considering these processes can categories like gender, ethnicity and social class have analytical value and can individual specificities such as sex, age, income level or educational achievements have explanatory relevance. This is intimately linked to the ontology of health inequities and inversely the way equity in health is understood, remitting to ethical considerations around justice.

The liberal notion of justice has been dominant during the last 30 years (Hernández, 2003, 2011) and has shaped and reproduced the capitalist accumulation and production regime, particularly driving 'market fundamentalism' as social, economic and cultural rights are not strictly considered as rights, but rather as commodities. This also applies to health, defined as a private responsibility and to health care, understood as a private good. Justice accordingly primarily translates into the respect for the rights of individuals, namely property and possession rights as well as the right to freedom, particularly to be at liberty to make rational choices. In this same line of reasoning, society is understood as a set of individuals or rational agents, essentially ahistorical subjects without socio-cultural roots (Benhabib, 1992), which interact and seek to maximise personal utility.

The WHO CSDH distances itself from the liberal notion of justice and following Amartya Sen, recognises health as a 'special good'. Inequalities in health are thus recognised as 'inequalities in people's capability to function' which substantiates the conceptualisation of health equity as the absence of unfair and avoidable/remediable differences in health among social groups (Solar & Irwin, 2010). Health is accordingly seen as a prerequisite for individual agency and freedom and reversely, greater agency and freedom are considered to yield better health (Solar & Irwin, 2010, p. 12). By explicitly assuming 'the human rights framework as the appropriate conceptual structure within which to advance towards health equity through action on SDH' (Solar & Irwin, 2010, p. 12), the CSDH removes actions to promote health equity from the voluntary realm of charity to the domain of law and calls on national governments to assume the responsibility for protecting and enhancing health equity. In this light, reversing inequities in health translates into equipping individuals with greater 'possibilities of control over their health' (Solar & Irwin, 2010). Equity in health accordingly requires minimising avoidable disparities in health and its determinants between groups of people who have different levels of underlying social advantage due to their position in society and in practices translates into actions seeking to affect educational attainment, occupational status and income inequality. The notion of 'avoidability' is central to this approach and conditions the notion of justice/injustice.

The social egalitarian notion of justice, that is dominant in the social determination of health approach of the LA SM-CH recognises health inequalities as unfair as these are produced by an improper and essentially unjust appropriation of means that reproduce and reinforce an unfair social and economic order shaped by power asymmetries along the lines of social class, gender and race/ethnicity. Rather than a 'rational agent', a 'historical subject' shaped by social relations and within concrete societal arrangement is recognised (Hernández, 2011, p. 182). This same subject is further recognised as a political subject capable of adopting emancipatory praxis instead of passively waiting for state or philanthropic interventions.

Another important distinctive and unifying element of LA SM-CH and ultimately also of the social determination of health approach is that it recognises that 'the science of epidemiology, like "any other symbolic operation [...] is a transformed, subordinate, transfigured and sometimes unrecognizable expression of the power relations of a society"' (Breilh, 2008, p. 745). LA SM-CH proposals for transformations on epistemological level have therefore explicitly challenged the epistemological foundations of dominant epidemiological and public health research. In this regard, Naomar Almeida-Filho has produced some of the most refined epistemological and historical analysis about health and epidemiological reasoning, unveiling the limitations implicit in the notions of causality and validity adopted in dominant epidemiological and public health research (Almeida-Filho, 1989, 2000) and proposing an alternative general theory of health (Almeida-Filho, 2001). Ricardo Ayres, Luis David Castiel and Jaime Breilh amongst others proposed an extensive critique of the notion of 'risk' (Ayres, 1997; Breilh, 2003; Castiel, 1999, 2010) and the risk-factor logic that fragments the understanding of social processes and has been emphasised also in the critique of the CSDH SDH approach. This critique has driven extensive work on the concept of 'vulnerability', particularly in the field of HIV/Aids and generally linked to human rights frameworks, radically questioning the traditional epidemiological risk-factor logic that mechanically transformed abstract epidemiological research categories with elevated risk for certain diseases into social identities and ultimately, into target groups (Ayres, 1997; Paiva, Ayres, & Buchalla, 2012). Thereby heterogeneous groups of individuals were reduced to 'risk groups', that undoubtedly influenced highly stigmatising and mostly ineffective prevention campaigns and, as in the case of the HIV/Aids epidemic, isolation measures, for example, directed at men who have sex with men. This critique has not exclusively been formulated by researchers and activists linked to LA SM-CH, but has undoubtedly taken new stances in Latin America, for example, by situating the critique in more structural revisions of the epistemological foundations of modern epidemiology and by incorporating a critique of the notion of 'risky behavior', that is recognised as a mean to depolitize and individualise disease occurrence and distribution, emphasising the need to rather study vulnerability and, this is particularly evident in the 'social determination of the health-disease-care process' approach, on processes of vulnerabilization, looking into the complex configuration of processes that turn certain social groups and individuals more vulnerable to certain conditions.

The writings of Juan Samaja (1998) have concerned issues of epistemology, semantics and method, providing important insights on social dialectics and the movement between the collective social order and the individual, which has been relevant for overcoming the notorious difficulty to address 'the social', evident in the dominant health equity agenda and particularly the SDH approach, which has resulted in models that establish links between social factors and average health outcomes, but limit the analysis to individual-level expressions, unidirectional links and essentially external associations between factors. The notion of 'subsumption' proposed by Jaime Breilh is central in this regard, takes up Samaja's work and dialogues with the eco-social approach and particularly the notion of 'embodiment' proposed by Nancy Krieger (2001b). Originally applied by Karl Marx to explain the internal and external subjugations operating in the labour process under capitalism, Breilh, following Bolívar Echeverría, incorporates the notion of 'subsumption' to substantiate the idea of social determination. He differentiates

> formal subsumption of the capitalist mode that changes the conditions of property and production/consumption and affects, externally, the relationships between the system of consumption needs and the system of production capacities; and secondly, the real subsumption, or "substantial" subsumption, in which the social internalization of this mode disrupts, from within, the dialectics between needs and capacities. (Breilh, 2011b, p. 394)

Essentially, it describes how the capitalist materiality marks the general, particular and singular level processes and consequently shapes the social-environmental metabolism, 'modes of life' and finally, on singular level, individual-level biological processes and lifestyles.

Jaime Breilh has proposed an early critique of positivism and causation, which unchained a methodological and conceptual search culminating in the pioneering proposal of the category of 'social determination', the previously discussed notion of 'subsumption' as well as the notion of 'modes of life' as a structured and dynamic dimension of the 'epidemiological profile' (Breilh, 2003), which articulates on a 'particular' level, social class, ethnic/racial and gendered power relations ('triple inequity') in correspondence with the ontological understanding of capitalist societies being structured by processes of exploitation, marginalisation and domination, systematically privileging upper class, white, European and male subjects and collectivities (Breilh, 1996). The 'Social determination of the health-care-disease process' approach as proposed by Jaime Breilh accordingly synthesises and expresses the cumulative and yet dynamic interplay between historically, spatially and socially shaped processes of exposure/imposition, susceptibility and resistance.

These ontological and epistemological considerations translate into praxiological imperatives that have shaped the SM-CH praxis as expressed in government experiences (Hernández, Forero, & Torres, 2005; Laurell, 2003), curricular reforms, action-research proposals (Breilh et al., 2005; Soliz, 2014) and constitutional reforms amongst others. The notion of 'praxis' as the articulation between theory and political practice has been central in this regard. In this sense, Latin American SM-CH, influenced by Italian Marxist philosopher Antonio Gramsci, understands theory as contributing to efforts tending towards social change, but at the same time nourished by these efforts. Consequently, research activities of SM-CH practitioners are often developed together with social and political movements, trade unions, community organisations and explicitly support their struggles in correspondence to the ontological understanding of health and health inequities – implying a break with conventional postures of scientific 'neutrality' (Tajer, 2003) and rather considering that 'the generation and transmission of knowledge is a tool for change', as Deborah Tajer puts it (2003, p. 2024).

LA SM-CH certainly finds inspiration in several sources, particularly Marxist critical thought and authors like Bourdieu and Foucault. Its main driving force, however, is a continued reflection on Latin American social, cultural and political reality, including the subaltern knowledge of exploited and oppressed social groups. If dependency theory (Cardoso & Faletto, 1979; Santos, 1979), liberation theology (Boff, 1987; Gutiérrez, 1975), decolonial theory (Castro-Gómez & Grosfoguel, 2007; Escobar, 2007; Grosfoguel, 2010; Lander, 2005) and participatory action research (Fals-Borda, 1987) can be said to have been the most original contributions of Latin American critical thought in the twentieth century (Bialakowsky, 2012), the LA SM-CH emerges as heir to this tradition (Waitzkin, Iriart, Estrada, & Lamadrid, 2001) and makes major contributions to the field, which can and should no longer be ignored or undervalued. This said, it is important to note that LA SM-CH and its 'social determination of health' approach are, without a doubt, result of transcultural dialogue, within the global South but also with the global North. Apart from its clear dialogue with early European Social Medicine, including works of Virchow and Engels, many representatives of the LA SM-CH pursued postgraduate studies in the global North and in other Latin American countries, which definitely shaped the approaches and the references of LA SM-CH.

## Conclusions

In an effort to challenge the apparent consensus for equity in health, this essay offered an overview of the debates shaping the global health equity agenda and compared and contrasted two of the most influential approaches: the WHO SDH approach, strongly influenced by European Social Medicine, and the LA SM-CH 'social determination of the health-disease-care process' approach, hitherto largely invisibilized. Apart from external economic, social and political pressures that have defined the scope and relative dominance of the agenda in relation to agendas placing emphasis on narrowly defined, technology-based interventions, the global health equity agenda is shaped by internal mediations that have defined the way inequities in health are understood, conceptualised and proposed to be transformed. In this regard, and although the approaches ascribing to the health equity agenda are rather heterogenic, we argued that there is a dominant agenda with specific ontological, epistemological and praxiological features, which in recent years has been driven by the WHO SDH approach. The apparent consensus for health equity, which has accompanied the consolidation of the dominant health equity agenda and was reinforced by a systematic invisibilization of alternative approaches and dissent voices, for example in the final report of the CSDH (2007), which contains none but one reference to LA SM-CH, has accordingly consolidated a false universality that annihilates historical trajectories and dilutes the debate.

In the context of the historical and recurrent retreats we discussed for example in relation to the shift from primary health care to selective primary health care but also from universal health systems to universal health coverage, this differentiation seems more necessary than ever as it allows to reveal the often implicit ethical and political proposals and in that way qualifies the debate. While Irwin and Scali (2005, p. 25) seem to welcome the 'relatively more consensual climate' in the international health and development field, moving beyond some of the 'ideologically charged' polarizations of the 1990s, we insist on the need to evince differences and conflicts and are opposed to false consensus backed by discursive adaptations as this seems to weaken the health equity agenda – both the dominant and subalternalized agendas. In order to avoid a 'light' SDH approach substituting the already rather timid WHO SDH approach in the dominant global health equity agenda, its principles and ethical-political foundations need to be clarified in order to avoid an apparently subtle and firstly merely discursive betrayal of its principles. In this regard it seems necessary to question the strong believe in win-win solutions invoked by the dominant health equity agenda and ask whether the gap can truly be closed in one generation, as the CSDH proclaims, if there is no willingness to accept that those who have historically won will have to lose, even if this translates into regression and currency devaluation, which are presently framed as negative and unacceptable scenarios – not to mention a true transformation of social class, ethnic/racial and gendered power relations, the choice for degrowth, non-capitalist economies and what has been referred to as the 'alternatives to (capitalist) development' (Escobar, 2011).

As outlined above, it is necessary and high time to seriously engage with hitherto invisibilized approaches and research traditions as this will broaden and at the same time specify the debate, facilitating the recognition of contextually relevant proposals towards a systematic reduction of health inequities, the appraisal of processes that shape concrete social realities, history and territory and – rather than the result of a linear association between social factors and individual-level biology – understand the processes that shape differences in health, define the quality of death and suffering and recognise the health-disease-care process as an integral part and expression of social processes and the configuration of power in specific territories.

## Disclosure statement

No potential conflict of interest was reported by the authors.

## Funding

This work was supported by Departamento Administrativo de Ciencia, Tecnología e Innovación: [grant number Colciencias 727].

## ORCID

Elis Borde    http://orcid.org/0000-0001-5560-6956

## References

Almeida-Filho, N. (1989). *Epidemiologia sem números*. Rio de Janeiro: Editora Campus.
Almeida-Filho, N. (2000). *La ciencia tímida. Ensayos de deconstrucción de la epidemiologia*. Buenos Aires: Lugar Editorial.
Almeida-Filho, N. (2001). For a general theory of health: Preliminary epistemological and anthropological notes. *Cadernos de Saúde Pública, 17*(4), 753–770.
Almeida-Filho, N., & Paim, J. S. (1999). La crisis de la salud pública y el movimiento de la salud colectiva en Latinoamérica. *Cuadernos Médico Sociales, 75*, 5–30.
Andrade, L. O. M., Pellegrini Filho, A., Solar, O., Rígoli, F., de Salazar, L. M., Serrate, P. C. F., … Atun, R. (2015). Social determinants of health, universal health coverage, and sustainable development: Case studies from Latin American countries. *The Lancet, 385*(9975), 1343–1351.
Armada, F., Muntaner, C., & Navarro, V. (2001). Health and social security reforms in Latin America: The convergence of the world health organization, the World Bank, and transnational corporations. *International Journal of Health Services, 31*(4), 729–768.
Arouca, S. (2003). *O dilema preventivista. Contribuição para uma compreensão e crítica da medicina preventiva*. São Paulo: Editora UNESP.
Ayres, J. R. (1997). *Sobre o risco*. São Paulo: Hucitec.
Benhabib, S. (1992). *El ser y el otro en la ética contemporánea. Feminismo, comunitarismo y posmodernismo*. Barcelona: Gedisa.
Berkman, L. F., Kawachi, I., & Glymour, M. (2014). *Social epidemiology*. Oxford: Oxford University Press.
Bialakowsky, A. (2012). *Latin American critical thought: Theory and practice*. Buenos Aires: CLACSO.
Birn, A. E. (2009). Making it politic(al): closing the gap in a generation: Health equity through action on the social determinants of health. *Social Medicine, 4*(3), 166–182.
Boff, L. (1987). *Introducing liberation theology*. New York: Orbis Books.
Borde, E., Porto, M. F. S., & Hernández, M. (2015). Uma análise crítica da abordagem dos Determinantes Sociais da Saúde a partir da medicina social e saúde coletiva latino-americana. *Saúde em Debate, 39*(106), 841–854.
Breilh, J. (1986). *Epidemiología: medicina, economía y política*. México: Editora Fontamara.
Breilh, J. (1996). *El Género Entrefuegos: Inequidad y Esperanza*. Quito: Ediciones CEAS.
Breilh, J. (2003). *Epidemiología Crítica. Ciencia emancipadora e intercultural*. Buenos Aires: Universidad Nacional de Lanus, Lugar Editorial.
Breilh, J. (2005). Floriculture and the health Dilemma: Towards fair and ecological flower production. In J. Breilh (Ed.), *Alternative Latin American health report*. Quito: Global Health Watch; CEAS. Retrieved from http://repositorio.uasb.edu.ec/handle/10644/3390
Breilh, J. (2008). Latin American critical ('social') epidemiology: New settings for an old dream. *International Journal of Epidemiology, 37*(4), 745–750.

Breilh, J. (2010). Las tres 'S'de la determinación de la vida: 10 tesis hacia una visión crítica de la determinación social de la vida y la salud. In R. P. Nogueira (org.)., *Determinação social da saúde e reforma sanitária* (pp. 87–125). Rio de Janeiro: Cebes. Retrieved from http://www.cebes.org.br/media/File/Determinacao.pdf.

Breilh, J. (2011a). La subversión del buen vivir (rebeldía esclarecida para el siglo XXI: una perspectiva crítica de la obra de Bolívar Echeverría). *Salud colectiva, 7*(3), 389–397.

Breilh, J. (2011b). Una perspectiva emancipadora de la investigación e incidencia basada en la determinación social de la salud. In C. Eibenschutz, R. Tamez, & R. González (Eds.), *¿Determinación social o determinantes sociales de la salud? Memoria del Taller Latinoamericanos sobre Determinantes Sociales de la Salud.* Ciudad de México: Editora Universidad Autónoma Metropolitana, Abate Faria.

Breilh, J. (2013). La determinación social de la salud como herramienta de transformación hacia una nueva salud pública (salud colectiva). *Rev Fac Nac Salud Pública, 31*(Suppl 1), 13–27.

Breilh, J., & Muñoz, Y. T. (2009). *Aceleración global y despojo en Ecuador: el retroceso del derecho a la salud en la era neoliberal.* Quito: Univ. Andina Simón Bolívar.

Cabrera, A., Camacho, I., Cortés, N., Eibenschutz, C., González, R., Ortiz, L., … Tamez, S. (2011). Por una discussion acerca de la CDSS desde la perspectiva de la medicina social latinoamericana. In C. Eibenschutz, S. Tamez, & R. González (Eds.), *¿Determinación social o determinantes sociales de la salud? Memoria del Taller Latinoamericanos sobre Determinantes Sociales de la Salud.* Ciudad de México: Editora Universidad Autónoma Metropolitana Abate Faria.

Cardoso, F. H., & Faletto, E. (1979). *Dependency and development in Latin America.* San Francisco: Univ of California Press.

Cassel, J. (1976). The contribution of the Social environment to host resistance. *American Journal of Epidemiology, 104*(2), 107–23.

Castiel, L. D. (1999). *A medida do possível … saúde, risco e tecnobiociências.* Rio de Janeiro: Editora Fiocruz.

Castiel, L. D. (2010). *Correndo o risco: Uma introdução aos riscos em saúde.* Rio de Janeiro: Editora Fiocruz.

Castro-Gómez, S., & Grosfoguel, R. (2007). *El giro decolonial: reflexiones para una diversidad epistemológica más allá del capitalismo global.* Bogotá: Siglo del Hombre Editores.

Coelho, M. T., & Almeida-Filho, N. (2002). Conceitos de saúde em discursos contemporâneos de referência científica. *História, Ciências, Saúde-Manguinhos, 9*(2), 315–333.

Commission on Social Determinants of Health (CSDH). (2007). *Final report: Closing the gap in a generation. Health equity through action on the social determinants of health. Commission on social determinants of health.* Geneva: World Health Organization.

Donnangelo, C., & Pereira, L. (1976). *Saúde e sociedade.* São Paulo: Duas Cidades.

Dorling, D., & Barford, A. (2007). Shaping the world to illustrate inequalities in health. *Bulletin of the World Health Organization, 85*(11), 890–893.

Escobar, A. (2007). Worlds and knowledges otherwise 1: The Latin American modernity/coloniality research program. *Cultural Studies, 21*(2-3), 179–210.

Escobar, A. (2011). *Encountering development: The making and unmaking of the third world.* Princeton University Press.

Escorel, S. (2009). História das Politicas de Saúde no Brasil de 1964 a 1990: do golpe militar á reforma sanitária. In L. Giovanella, S. Escorel, L. V. C. Lobato, & J. C. Noronha (Eds.), *Carvalho, A.I. Políticas e Sistema de Saúde no Brasil* (pp. 385–434). Rio de Janeiro: Fiocruz, CEBES.

Fals-Borda, O. (1987). The application of participatory action-research in Latin America. *International Sociology, 2*(4), 329–347.

Friel, S., & Marmot, M. G. (2011). Action on the social determinants of health and health inequities goes global. *Annual Review of Public Health, 32*, 225–236.

García, J. C. (1994). Ciencias sociales en salud en América Latina. In J. C. García (Ed.), *Pensamiento social en salud en América Latina* (pp. 184–191). México DF: Organización Panamericana de la Salud, Interamericana-McGraw Hill.

Granda, E. (1989). *Saúde na sociedade.* São Paulo: Abrasco.

Grosfoguel, R. (2010). Para descolonizar os estudos de economia política e os estudos pós-coloniais: Transmodernidade, pensamento de fronteira e colonialidade global. In B. S. Santos, & M. P. Meneses (Eds.), *Epistemologias do Sul* (pp. 455–491). São Paulo: Editora Cortez.

Gutiérrez, G. (1975). *Teologia de la liberación.* Ediciones Sigueme: Salamanca.

Guzmán, R. G. (2009). La medicina social ante el reporte de la Comisión sobre los Determinantes Sociales de la Salud, Organización Mundial de la Salud. *Medicina Social, 4*(2), 135–143.

Heredia, N., Laurell, A. C., Feo, O., Noronha, J., González-Guzmán, R., & Torres-Tovar, M. (2015). The right to health: What model for Latin America? *The Lancet, 385*(9975), e34–e37.

Hernández, M. (2003). Neoliberalismo en salud: desarrollos, supuestos y alternativas. In D. I. Restrepo (Ed.), *La falacia neoliberal: Crítica y alternativas. Bogotá: Vicerrectoría Académica y Sede Bogotá* (pp. 347–361). Universidad Nacional de Colombia.

Hernández, M. (2011). Desigualdad, inequidad e injusticia en el debate actual en salud: posiciones e implicaciones. In C. Eibenschutz, S. Tamez, & R. González (Eds.), *¿Determinación social o determinantes sociales?* Ciudad de México: Editora Universidad Autónoma Metropolitana. Abate Faria.

Hernández, M., Forero, L., & Torres, M. (2005). The experience of Bogota D.C.: A public policy to Guarantee the right to health. In J. Breilh (Ed.), *Alternative Latin American health report*. Quito: Global Health Watch; CEAS. Retrieved from http://repositorio.uasb.edu.ec/handle/10644/3390.

Irwin, A., & Scali, E. (2005). *Action on the social determinants of health: Learning from experience*. Geneva: CSDH, WHO.

Kaplan, G. A., Pamuk, E. R., Lynch, J. W., Cohen, R. D., & Balfour, J. L. (1996). Inequality in income and mortality in the United States: Analysis of mortality and potential pathways. *BMJ, 312*(7037), 999–1003.

Karanikolos, M., Mladovsky, P., Cylus, J., Thomson, S., Basu, S., Stuckler, D., ... McKee, M. (2013). Financial crisis, austerity, and health in Europe. *The Lancet, 381*(9874), 1323–1331.

Kawachi, I., Subramanian, S. V., & Almeida-Filho, N. (2002). A glossary for health inequalities. *Journal of Epidemiology and Community Health, 56*(9), 647–652.

Krieger, N. (2001a). A glossary for social epidemiology. *Journal of Epidemiology & Community Health, 55*(10), 693–700.

Krieger, N. (2001b). Theories for social epidemiology in the 21st century: An ecosocial perspective. *International Journal of Epidemiology, 30*(4), 668–677.

Lander, E. (Ed.). (2005). *A colonialidade do saber: eurocentrismo e ciências sociais. Perspectivas latino-americanas. Colección Sur-Sur*. Buenos Aires: CLACSO.

Laurell, A. C. (1979). Work and health in Mexico. *International Journal of Health Services, 9*(4), 543–568.

Laurell, A. C. (1994). Sobre la concepción biológica y social del proceso salud-enfermedad. In M. I. Rodríguez (coord.)., *Lo biológico y lo social. Su articulación en la formación de personal de salud. Serie Desarrollo de Recursos Humanos N° 101* (pp. 1–12). Washington, DC: OPS/OMS.

Laurell, A. C. (2003). What does Latin American social medicine do when it governs? The case of the Mexico City government. *American Journal of Public Health, 93*(12), 2028–2031.

Lynch, J. W., Kaplan, G. A., Pamuk, E. R., Cohen, R. D., Heck, K. E., Balfour, J. L., & Yen, I. H. (1998). Income inequality and mortality in metropolitan areas of the United States. *American Journal of Public Health, 88*(7), 1074–1080.

Marmot, M. (2013). Universal health coverage and social determinants of health. *The Lancet, 382*(9900), 1227–1228.

Morales-Borrero, C., Borde, E., Eslava-Castañeda, J. C., & Concha-Sánchez, S. C. (2013). ¿Determinación social o determinantes sociales? Diferencias conceptuales e implicaciones praxiológicas. *Revista de Salud Pública, 15*(6), 797–808.

Navarro, V. (2009). What we mean by social determinants of health. *International Journal of Health Services, 39*(3), 423–441.

Paiva, V., Ayres, J. R., & Buchalla, C. M. (2012). *Vulnerabilidade e direitos humanos – Prevenção e Promoção da Saúde*. São Paulo: Juruá Editora.

Piketty, T. (2014). *Capital in the Twenty-First century*. Cambridge: The Belknap Press of Harvard University Press.

Radcliffe, S. A. (2012). Development for a postneoliberal era? Sumak kawsay, living well and the limits to decolonisation in Ecuador. *Geoforum; Journal of Physical, Human, and Regional Geosciences, 43*(2), 240–249.

Samaja, J. (1998). *Epistemologia e epidemiologia. In: Almeida-Filho, N. Teoria epidemiológica hoje*. Rio de Janeiro: Editora Fiocruz.

Sanahuja, J. A. (2013). Las nuevas geografías de la pobreza y la desigualdad y las metas de desarrollo global post-2015. In *Manuela, M. (coord.). El reto de la democracia en un mundo en cambio: Respuestas políticas y sociales* (pp. 61–100). Madrid: CEIPAZ.

Santos, L., & Ayres, J. R. (2017). *Saúde, Sociedade e História: Uma revisita às contribuições de Ricardo Bruno Mendes-Gonçalves*. São Paulo: Hucitec.

Santos, T. (1979). La crisis de la teoría del desarrollo y las relaciones de dependencia en América Latina. In H. F. Jaguaribe, A. H. Jaguaribe, & A. Ferrer (Eds.), *La dependencia político-económica de América Latina (No. 330.98 D4)*. Ciudad de México: Siglo XXI.

Solar, O., & Irwin, A. (2006). Social determinants, political contexts and civil society action: A historical perspective on the Commission on social determinants of health. *Health Promotion Journal of Australia, 17*(3), 180–5185.

Solar, O., & Irwin, A. (2010). *A conceptual framework for action on the social determinants of health. Social determinants of health discussion Paper 2 (policy and practice)*. Geneva: World Health Organization.

Soliz, M. F. (2014). Exposición, vulnerabilidad y perfil epidemiológico de trabajadores informales en el botadero a cielo abierto del cantón Portoviejo, Ecuador. *Maskana, 5*(1), 57–79.

Spiegel, J. M., Breilh, J., & Yassi, A. (2015). Why language matters: Insights and challenges in applying a social determination of health approach in a North-South collaborative research program. *Journal of Global Health, 11*(9), 1–17.

Starfield, B. (2006). State of the art in research on equity in health. *Journal of Health Politics, Policy and Law, 31*(1), 11–32.

Tajer, D. (2003). Latin American social medicine: Roots, development during the 1990s, and current challenges. *American Journal of Public Health, 93*(12), 2023–2027.

Victora, C. G., Aquino, E. M., do Carmo Leal, M., Monteiro, C. A., Barros, F. C., & Szwarcwald, C. L. (2011). Maternal and child health in Brazil: Progress and challenges. *The Lancet, 377*(9780), 1863–1876.

Waitzkin, H., Iriart, C., Estrada, A., & Lamadrid, S. (2001). Social medicine then and now: Lessons from Latin America. *American Journal of Public Health*, 91(10), 1592–1601.

Wallerstein, I. (2011). *The modern world-system I: Capitalist agriculture and the origins of the European world-economy in the sixteenth century*. San Francisco: University of California Press.

Wilkinson, R. G., & Pickett, K. E. (2006). Income inequality and population health: a review and explanation of the evidence. *Social Science & Medicine*, 62(7), 1768–84.

# Theoretical underpinnings of state institutionalisation of inclusion and struggles in collective health in Latin America

Qamar Mahmood and Carles Muntaner

**ABSTRACT**

Community participation as a strategy in health aims to increase the role of citizens in health decision-making which are contextualised within the institutions of democracy. Electoral representation as the dominant model of democracy globally is based on the elite theory of democracy that sees political decision-making a prerogative of political elites. Such political elitism is counter to the idea of democratic participation. Neoliberalism together with elitism in political sphere have worsened social inequities by undermining working class interests. Latin America has seen adverse consequences of these social inequities. In response, social movements representing collective struggles of organised citizens arose in the region. This paper explores the theoretical underpinnings of democratic participation in contemporary Latin American context at the nexus of emerging social movement activism and policy responses. The paper will use empirical examples to highlight how such democratic practices at the societal level evolved while demanding political inclusion. These societal democratic practices in Latin America are redefining democracy, which continues to be seen in the political sphere only. Health reforms promoting participatory democracy in several Latin American countries have demonstrated that establishing institutions and mechanisms of democratic participation facilitate collective participation by the organised citizenry in state affairs.

## Introduction

This paper explores the experiences of health reform movements in Brazil and Venezuela over the last several decades to demonstrate how the idea of health as a social right emerged. This understanding of health emerged simultaneously with the expansion of citizenship of previously excluded population groups. In parallel, the idea of health and other social sector benefits as part of a social contract between citizens and states also evolved. This paper will argue that the reciprocity of democratic changes in the health sector and in the wider socio-political context was mutually reinforcing and how the Latin American Social Medicine (LASM) had a major part to play in this socially progressive orientation of health. The paper then looks at the state–society nexus and analyses citizen participation in the respective health reforms in both countries. The historical evolution of democratic participation in state affairs and the establishment of institutions of participatory democracy over time provides an insight of deepening democracy in Latin America.

We then use an alternative theory of democracy that has been conceived in the particular experiences of societal democratisation in Latin America to challenge the predominant liberal model of democracy. We contend that it is this predominant liberal system of elite competitive representation that has come to define democracy globally in the post-Second World War era and has systematically restricted participation – one of the core notions of democracy. The idea of citizen/community participation has been around in global public health for at least four decades following the passage of the historic Health for All (HfA) declaration but without much success. Our contention is that it is the conceptualisation of community participation within this liberal democratic paradigm that has restricted true democratic participation in health to take root. We explore these Latin American experiences, empirically, theoretically, and in practice. Through this exploration we intend to argue our position that the political nature of citizens participating in state affairs as a process of societal transformation radically changes the nature of the state and expands the surface area of the state at the state–society nexus. Finally, we mention the dilemmas of participation at this state–society nexus given that such dilemmas are inherently political and contentious.

## Health for all and community participation

This year marks the fortieth anniversary of the passage of the historic Alma Ata Declaration to achieve HfA using the Primary health care (PHC) strategy. Community participation, as an operating principle of PHC, was required in planning, organisation, operation, and control of PHC (World Health Organization [WHO], 1978). It also called for social control of health services. In the years following the passage of HfA, community participation became part of many health interventions globally. On the thirtieth anniversary of Alma Ata and PHC, the World Health Organization (WHO) published its 2008 World Health Report. The report, entitled *Primary Health Care: Now More Than Ever,* reemphasised the role of PHC and reaffirmed its relevance to reduce growing inequalities in health and to achieve HfA (WHO, 2008). Four decades later, HfA remains an elusive target and inequalities in health continue to rise. Challenging in part to the achievement of the HfA goal was the international debate on comprehensive versus selective PHC, the former espoused national liberation sentiment of the post-colonial era and aspiration of welfare-state while the latter originated when neoliberalism was taking hold of the global economic order (Cueto, 2004).

Werner, Sanders, Weston, Babb, and Rodriguez (1997) describe that the declaration shifted focus in health from services to the underlying social, economic, and political causes of poor health. However, a cautionary approach was adopted towards community participation so that the status-quo was not challenged since the WHO, like the other United Nations agencies, is comprised of world governments. According to Navarro (1984) ' … the progressive language of Alma Ata was co-opted; expressions such as "people participation," "decision-making by the people," and "empowerment" became part of the new, official jargon.' He challenged that contrary to the way the HfA was being presented as apolitical, the ' … analysis of the variables without reference to their structural determinants … ' was profoundly political as it takes the focus away from the structural relationships among the elements that define a system, society, or community and the powers they reproduce.

### Democratic participation and participatory governance

Community participation in health essentially is about the democratic participation of the citizenry in health affairs. At its core, community participation and, enacting programmes and policies that are participatory in nature as well as the role of the state are questions about the nature of democracy. ' … democracy meaning the set of relations and institutions which permit the citizenry to control their own lives' (Navarro, 1980). Fundamentally, democracy is about the societal distribution of power and denotes a society where power is in the citizenry (Becker, 1999). Popular participation is about citizens participating in and having control and power over decisions that affect their lives. 'Participatory governance – the co-production of decisions and services – demands not only the activation of civil society but also, unexpectedly, the mobilisation of the state' (Abers & Keck, 2009). Of the various models of democracy such as representative democracy, direct democracy, and participatory democracy, the latter encompasses the idea of participation and democracy. In a participatory democracy, political parties which are genuinely participatory, '… operate within a parliamentary or congressional system complemented and checked by fully self-managed organisations in the workplace and local community' (Held, 2006). Participatory democracy, however, does not represent a political order. It is a broader concept of a new kind of society in which public affairs are integrated into the affairs of the ordinary citizen.

An increasing number of countries became democratic in the second half of the twentieth century and adopted the liberal democratic model. Democracy became increasingly identified with the existence of competitive elections and was limited to the act of voting by citizens every few years (Conway, 2002). According to Warren (2002), the participatory ideals of democracy were pushed to the margins of the mainstream liberal democratic theory while representation did not reflect the interests and opinions of individuals but rather procedures that enabled agreements among large organisations and their interests. Consequently, the gulf between citizens and their representatives widened to the point that people in developed democracies have become disaffected with their political institutions.

### Democratic deficits

Supporters of representative democracy cite evidence that its success in the post-Second World War and in post-Cold War eras indicate the robustness of this form of democracy. It is well-developed in Western Europe while countries in Eastern Europe and Latin America are considered to be on their way to adopting it (Raby, 2006). The negative view of the linkages among capitalism, democracy, and development are quelled by citing the reciprocity between state-makers and capitalism in Western Europe – capitalism and democracy reinforcing each other to achieve human welfare (Barkey & Parikh, 1991). Critics of representative democracy attribute the success of this model in Western Europe to the well-developed welfare-state – a result of popular struggles of working classes and grassroots groups rather than the kind of democracy itself. Thus in developed countries, demands from working classes were organised and represented effectively in the State, which might not be the case in developing countries where State responsiveness to citizens demands may be weak due to weak working class politics (Heller, 2001).

Representative democracy, with its system of citizens electing political elites, who would then make decisions on behalf of the citizenry, thus reinforced economic elite interests through neoliberal policies. Diminishing popular participation in State affairs in representative democracies and the implementation of neoliberal policies have resulted in rising inequalities over the last several decades. Such inequalities were relatively muted in developed relative to developing countries because of positive state–society relations permitting organised working class interests to have a voice in the State. Neoliberalism significantly diminished the role of the State vis-à-vis the markets reducing its crucial functions such as regulating labour markets, finance, commerce, and goods. Additionally, rampant privatisation of services and reduction of social public expenditure weakened the working class further by reducing their access to social and health benefits (Navarro, 2007). Thus, the nature of representative democracy by default favoured the neoliberal system. Occasional participation by the masses in the electoral process meant minimal interference by popular interests in state affairs. In fact, representative democracy has been equated as the political aspect of neoliberalism and that has been instrumental in giving legitimacy to the economic aspects of neoliberalism (Raby, 2006).

### Democratic participation versus elite democratic theory

Avritzer (2002) has challenged the applicability of this elite democracy of competitive electoral representation mentioning three seminal assumptions regarding citizen participation that underpin elite democracy. (1) Max Weber's scepticism that collective decision-making cannot address the complex nature of public administration which should, therefore, be left to bureaucratic elites who have technical knowledge while citizenry's role is in choosing among these political elites. (2) Joseph

Schumpeter's labelling of majoritarian decision-making as potentially undemocratic equating mass participation as irrational and therefore, supporting political decision-making by rational political actors. (3) Anthony Down's reformulation of democratic elitist tradition by introducing the idea of apathy of the masses towards democratic decision-making thereby de-emphasising the idea of the irrationality of masses and rationality of the elites and replacing it with the idea that ' ... it is as rational for the elites to participate as it is for the masses not to participate'.

Democratic elitism's ascription of rationality to political elites and irrationality of majoritarian-based political decision-making is problematic especially in cases of democracies undergoing consolidation and this challenge played out in the Latin American democracies that were transitioning from decades of authoritarian rule. The political society in Latin America after gaining power in several countries displayed undemocratic practices reminiscent of the past authoritarian political regimes (Linz & Stepan, 1996). At the same time, there was an emerging social power in the form of numerous civic organisations and neighbourhood associations that arose and blossomed either independently or because of the repression during the authoritarian period and demonstrated democratic practices while demanding accountability, political inclusion, and sovereignty (Petras & Veltmeyer, 2005). Despite these democratisation efforts at the societal level democracy in Latin America is still considered a domain of the political sphere (Melucci & Avritzer, 2000).

It is in this context that Leonardo Avritzer (2002) proposes his 'Public Space' theory of democracy which stands in contrast to the elitist democratic theory. We argue that Avritzer's theory is most relevant to the arguments presented in this paper and in the Latin American context of democratic consolidation after decades of authoritarian rule for several reasons. (1) The core of his theory relates to citizen participation in democracy. (2) His critique of democratic elitism's assumptions that provide a rationale for limiting citizen participation in political decision-making. (3) His expansion of the notion of democracy to the societal realm rather than solely within the domain of the political society. (4) His elaboration of what such deliberative public spaces could look like and how they could operate.

### Public Space theory of democracy

Avritzer's Public Space theory of democracy arises from his contention that the predominant form of democracy in the political realm is limited in its scope when understanding matters of democratic consolidation especially in cases of democracies in Latin America. He argues that electoral competition of political elites with participation by the masses is generally limited to choosing amongst these elites through voting. He identifies democratic practices at the societal level in many Latin American democracies which he then uses to devise an alternative theory of Public Space democracy. Avritzer links the emergence of political democracy to the formation of a public space where citizens can participate as equals and deliberate on collective projects for society with the intent of guiding formal political decision-making. Central to his theory is the concept of the public sphere which he describes by its location between the market and the State and involving face-to-face deliberations by ordinary citizens that involve communicating about various political and collective projects of society. While identifying democratic practices at the public level in various Latin American countries, Avritzer then emphasizes the need to institutionalize these societal practices.

Avritzer in his elaboration of the Public Space theory of democracy elaborates what such a space means for contemporary democracies facing problems of consolidation. His argument for democracies striving to improve their democratic practices is to focus on democratic societal practices rather than those in the political sphere alone. He contends that such public level democratic practices, which he calls participatory publics, are in need of institutionalisation. See Table 1 for elements of 'participatory publics' as conceived by Arvitzer followed by examples from Brazil and Venezuela to theorize their origin and institutionalisation at the state–society interface.

**Table 1:** The four elements of Participatory Publics (Avritzer, 2002).

(1) 'At the public level of mechanisms of face-to-face deliberations, free expression, and association. These mechanisms address specific elements in the dominant culture by making them problematic issues to be politically addressed.

(2) The second element is the idea that social movements and voluntary associations address contentious issues in the political culture by introducing at the public level alternative practices.

(3) The third element involves transformation of informal public opinion into a forum for public deliberation and administrative decision-making.

(4) The fourth element is that they bind their deliberations with the attempt to search for institutional level the issues made contentious at the public level.'

### Democratic practices in Latin America: the case of Brazil and Venezuela

The neoliberal agenda globally took stronger hold during the Raegan and Thatcher eras (Navarro, 2007). Latin America was a foremost region affected by the neoliberal onslaught and the underlying social cleavages based along class lines and the autocratic regimes provided fertile ground for neo-liberalism to prosper on the continent (Goodale & Postero, 2013). The impact of neoliberalism was across all social and economic sectors of the economy and healthcare was not spared resulting in worsening inequalities, social exclusion, and denial of basic social services like healthcare (Silva, 2009). In response to the consequences of neoliberal policies social movements arose throughout the continent that comprised mainly of these socially excluded groups which demanded state pro-vision of social services such as health but also the inclusion of socially excluded population groups and ensure their rights as citizens (Petras & Veltmeyer, 2005). Brazil and Venezuela stand out as countries that embarked on changing their state–society interface with mechanisms to promote citi-zen engagement across the economy including health.

**Brazil** – Cohn (2008) and Elias and Cohn (2003) describe these changes in the health sector in Brazil and how they were linked with the democratic changes that were occurring in Brazil starting in the 1970s. Historically in Brazil, health as a right was limited to paid contributions by workers and was not seen as a universal right. This segmented healthcare system began to change during the 1970s incorporating notions of universality which coincided with the democratic changes taking place against authoritarian regimes. Social mobilisation in health took the shape of a health move-ment comprised of representatives from trade unions, health workers, academics, progressive sectors of the Catholic Church, and many other civic groups. The democratisation of health, theorised and designed in collective health aimed towards democratisation of the state and its apparatus in addition to the society (Paim, 2008). The space for this progressive health movement, in fact, opened up under the autocratic regime in the 1970s which was looking for social legitimacy across society (Paiva & Teixeira, 2014).

In the 1970s, health professionals and those from academia and research institutes comprised the sanitary movement or *sanitaristas* demanded profound reform in health through the production of knowledge that documented inequities in health and linked them to the political struggles of the time (Cordeiro, 2004). This new knowledge in health brought an explicitly Marxist perspective in health studies which was parallel to other political struggles happening in Latin America in that era (Elias & Cohn, 2003). The *sanitaristas* were instrumental in the creation of the *Centro Brasileiro de Estudos de Saude* (CEBES) and the *Associacao Brasileira de Pos-Graduacao em Saude Coletiva* (ABRASCO) which served as dissemination of their intellectual analysis at the national level (Escorel, 1999). CEBES leader Antonio Sergio Arouca played a pivotal role throughout this process as well as others from ABRASCO who additionally showed intellectual leadership to the mobilisation of organised sections of the society for a democratic change in health (Cordeiro, 2004). The main actors of the health movement were

> Progressive public health professors, researchers from the Brazilian Society for the Advancement of Science, and health professionals engaged with grassroots and trade union struggles ... the health reform movement spread and formed an alliance with progressive members of the congress, municipal health, and other social movements. (Paim, Travassos, Almeida, Bahia, & Macinko, 2011)

As a result of these developments mainly due to this progressive health movement, when the new constitution was being framed towards the end of the 1980s, the health sector was at the forefront with alternative proposals for a new health system Avritzer (2009). The new constitution was passed in 1988.

> Article 198 called for a Unified Health System (SUS) that organised a regionalised and decentralised network of health services, with coordinated management at each level of government, community participation, and the prioritising of prevention as part of an integrated approach to health services delivery. Elias and Cohn (2003)

The new health system was characterised by universality, decentralised with local autonomy, and democratic management under 'social control' (Cohn, 2008).

There were two discerning elements for the success in the implementation of the new health system. One was the formation of Health Councils, which were participative-deliberative fora that would institutionalize citizen participation in health decision-making (Avritzer, 2009). The second was that the social movement in health had a political strategy. Describing this political strategy, Cohn (2008) mentions that the Brazilian Communist Party (PCB) and Brazilian workers party *Partido Trabahaldoris* (PT) were both involved in the health movement. Many of the PCB members occupied positions within the state and worked on the inside. PT, on the other hand, had street power as it was a party of the masses and ensured popular mobilisations that worked from outside. Popular support was achieved by PT while the communists worked to bring about institutional changes within the State. It was the affiliation of PT with the democratisation of health that the *sanitaristas* ultimately found support under Lula's government in 2003. The implementation of the SUS right after its passage in 1988 faced tough challenges under the political turmoil and economic crisis of the 1990s under the Collor (1992), Franco (1992–1995), and Cordso (1995–2003) regimes.

Participation and citizen inclusion in health decision-making were achieved through Health Councils at national, state, and municipal levels and which were composed of representatives from both the state and the civil society (Avritzer, 2009). These Health Councils formed the main mechanism of participatory democracy in the health care system in Brazil. The formation, working, and evolution of this particular form of deliberative-participative institution has been described at length by Avritzer (2009) which he used as empirical evidence to coin the term 'participatory publics' (Table 1) and to build his 'Public Space theory of democracy'. Health Councils have been recognised as the most widespread participatory institution that arose out of the struggle of two social movements namely the popular health movement and the *sanitarista* movement (Avritzer, 2009).

**Venezuela** – With the second largest oil reserves in the world, Venezuela's economy faced booms and busts because of this resource curse. From the 1980s onwards economic neoliberalism started to take hold on the national economy which resulted in rising social inequalities. Armada, Muntaner, Chung, Williams-Brennan, and Benach (2009) describe that in the health sector, these policies manifested as a fiscal reduction of public health services and decentralisation to regional authorities. The poorly financed public health system when decentralised led to increasing privatisation of such services with cost recovery mechanism while continuing to be run under regional authorities. Consequently, social mobilisation against neoliberalism and state authorities grew stronger and led to the destabilisation and overthrow of two regimes in the 1990s.

Hugo Chavez led this political struggle against neoliberalism and attempted a failed coup in 1992 (Alvarado, Martinez, Vivas-Martinez, Gutierrez, & Metzger, 2008) but later won the elections in 1998. Responding to this anti-neoliberal sentiment in the nation, he implemented the most radical reforms to transform the Venezuelan State to '21st century socialism' (Wilpert, 2007). The reform in health was initiated in 2003 and called *Barrio Adentro*, or Inside the neighbourhood. Several publications have since highlighted various aspects of the reform. Feo and Siqueira (2004) focused on the constitutional changes relevant to health. Articles by Muntaner, Salazar, Benach, and Armada (2006, Muntaner, Salazar, & Rueda, 2006) highlighted early years of the reform, focusing on the changes in service delivery. A study by the Pan American Health Organization (PAHO) (2006) focused on improvement in organisation of services, budgetary allocation, and distribution of resources, improvement in access to and utilisation of health services, and the early impact on health outcomes. An article by Alvarado et al. (2008) described the impact of these health policies on the quality of life of the population. A mixed-methods study by Briggs and Mantini-Briggs (2009) used interviews, ethnographic observations, document research, and a household survey to conclude that *Barrio Adentro* is mixed or horizontal in nature instead of being a top-down or bottom-up effort. The authors found that decision-making in *Barrio Adentro* resulted from a collaboration between professionals and residents in underserved communities concluding that such reforms could, therefore, creatively address health inequities. An article by Armada et al. (2009) reported epidemiological evidence related to access, utilisation, and impact of *Barrio Adentro* and survey results from patient satisfaction interviews. In 2012 a study on community participation in *Barrio Adentro* (Mahmood, Muntaner, Leon, & Perdomo, 2012) highlighted that despite challenges from traditional stakeholders opposed to democratising decision-making in health, popular arenas of participation created under *Barrio Adentro* had enhanced citizen participation especially of the most disadvantaged *barrio* residents. Relatedly, an article (Mahmood & Muntaner, 2013) analysed these changes in the sociopolitical context suggesting the success of the reform on the political rather than the technical aspects of *Barrio Adentro*. Our current analysis builds on this scholarship on *Barrio Adentro* further using a theory of participatory democracy contextualised in Latin American experiences to explain the reform as an example of contemporary collective health that was also influenced by LASM principles.

Some milestones aiming for these reforms included: naming a cabinet that consisted mostly of those from the political Left and none from the traditional elites; organising a referendum in order to get approval for a constitutional assembly; and the writing of the new 'Bolivarian' constitution that was approved in December 1999 (Feo & Siqueira, 2004). Citizen participation in State affairs featured prominently in Article 62 of the new constitution, 'the participation of people in the formation, execution and control of public matters … as the means of their complete development both as individuals and collectively.' In health, popular participation was established in the Bolivarian constitution as a mechanism to ensure that the state enforces health as a social right. The relevant articles on health in the constitution (Articles 83, 84, and 85) have the conceptual underpinning of a ' … co-responsibility of the triad of state-individual-society in social participation, which enables citizens and individuals to become the main actors in the new society' (Feo & Siqueira, 2004).

During the initial years of Chavez, efforts to reform the healthcare system in Venezuela prior to *Barrio Adentro* were based on the LASM principles. LASM has long endorsed an approach in health that is collective rather than individual in nature, focused on the political, economic, and social determinants of health, and emphasised attention to factors that produce health inequities (Briggs & Mantini-Briggs, 2009). Corresponding with his initial cabinet appointment of people from the Left (Wilpert, 2007), Chavez appointed two past presidents of the LASM Giberto Rodriguez Ochoa in 1999 and Maria Lopez Urbaneja in 2001 in health who tried to implement a healthcare system based on the principles of LASM through policies and practices. Briggs and Mantini-Briggs (2009) describe that they faced stiff opposition from the Venezuelan Medical Federation that had aligned itself with the traditional political parties that had lost power in the 1990s and the private medical sector that was strongly opposed to Chavez's attempts to reinvent the healthcare system based on his progressive political ideology that advocated a strong public health approach for the healthcare system.

Armada et al. (2009) describe that until 2002, Chavez's efforts in the health sector focused on reversing the effects of neoliberalisation. These efforts included: halting the privatisation of health services and eliminating barriers to access to care; implementation of integrated healthcare with a focus on PHC and prevention; and most significantly, transforming the idea of health as a commodity to be exchanged in the market to that of a fundamental right to be provided by the State. While these changes were significant in their own right, popular demand for improved health services required that more needed to be done (Armada et al., 2009). Implementation of the new 'Bolivarian' constitution required that new and efficient mechanisms are developed that would run parallel to and then replace the existing policy implementation structures. The intent was to avoid undue hurdles within the bureaucracy from those ministries that remained opposed to many of the changes that were being proposed (Muntaner, Salazar, Benach, et al., 2006). One such major change was the creation of 'social missions' which were social programmes that would serve to increase community participation in national programmes and policies (Muntaner, Salazar, Rueda, et al., 2006). The 'health mission' was known as *Barrio Adentro* and it was at the forefront of social missions in terms of its achievements especially in terms of citizen participation in health decision-making (Alvarado et al., 2008).

Reporting on popular participation in *Barrio Adentro*, Muntaner, Salazar, Benach, et al. (2006) mention that it is achieved through the formation of Health Committees through which communities exercise PHC delivery and management. Operation of Health Committees is regulated by the Community Councils Law of April 2006. Coordination of these committees occurs within Communal Councils which are participatory governance structures for public administration within municipalities. Wilpert (007) explains further that the communal councils are modelled on the local participatory budgeting process in Porto Alegre, Brazil and operate at a sub-municipal (*comunidad*) level. Activities of communal councils include gathering and evaluating community projects, working on development plans, mapping community needs, and integrating committees of various social missions. Besides committees for social missions and communal councils, several other institutions and mechanisms for participatory democracy have been put in place. These include referenda, social audit/*Contraloria*, citizen assemblies, and worker cooperatives. All these efforts reflected the government's commitment to ensure popular participation in all spheres of life.

### Challenges of participation

Over the preceding decades, several countries in Latin America experimented with societal transformation to create more participatory societies, which is not without challenges. The literature on participatory experiments identifies several dilemmas of participation (Figure 1) at the state–society interface (Abers, 2000). The framework was developed using empirical evidence from Latin American experiences in participatory democracy and particularly the experience of participatory budgeting in Porto Algre. 'Participatory governance can either result from bottom-up political mobilisation or from committed political leadership … ' (Schonleitner, 2006), however, both can be challenging. State efforts to promote popular participation in state affairs pose questions regarding

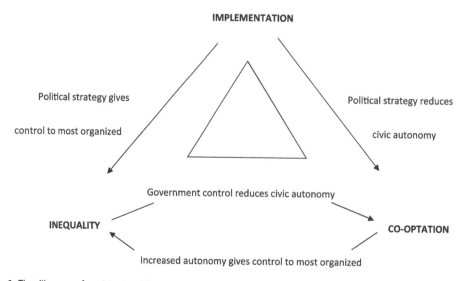

**Figure 1:** The dilemmas of participation (Abers, 2000).

the authenticity of such efforts given its influence over resources and power to structure relations among civic groups and itself (Barkey & Parikh, 1991). Even genuine policy intentions can pose implementation challenges as there could be players in the society that may have a stake in maintaining the status-quo. Conversely, popular participation in state affairs as a bottom-up effort may also be challenging (discussed in the section on inequality). Participatory efforts whether top-down or bottom-up are at the interface of state and society. Brazil and Venezuela's experiences of participatory democracy occurred in times of political and economic neoliberalism, which presented ideological challenges both from outside and inside the national boundaries. The figure depicts three main dilemmas of participatory efforts at the state–society nexus namely implementation, inequality, and co-optation.

**Implementation** – Abers' framework identifies mainly three implementation challenges while implementing participatory policies.

(1) The *ideology* of the ruling party and how it intends to formulate participatory policies would delineate the nature of the reform and how it is implemented. The experience of implementing participatory efforts in the context of decentralisation to local level in Kerala, Porto Alegre, and South Africa are revealing given that all were done by centre-left political parties in power that had strong social movement characteristics. However, South Africa adopted a technocratic approach imbued in neoliberalism which worsened democratic participation as opposed to Kerala and Porto Alegre which opted for progressive and broadly inclusive processes that resulted in deepening of democracy (Heller, 2001). Broadly, the health reform experiences in both Venezuela and Brazil were aligned with the LASM principles of focusing on the collective as opposed to individualised health approach that emphasised democratic participation of citizenry (Paim et al., 2011) (Cohn, 2008) (Elias & Cohn, 2003) (Briggs & Mantini-Briggs, 2009).

(2) The *legal* basis for the implementation of participatory policies may require changes in the constitution and enactment of laws. Laws, for example, can be used for constructing democratic processes by setting the rules and equalising the powers of participants. In Brazil, it took five years after the 1988 constitution for infraconstitutional legislation to pass in 1993 mostly because the conservative sectors of the society confronted the health movement for their defeat over the progressive nature of health articles in the constitution (Mahmood et al., 2012). Abers mentions that despite covering the legal basis of policies that encourage participation, implementation of such policies requires political maneuverability with state bureaucracy. Bureaucracy may create hurdles because there may be those who may not fully agree with the ruling party's policies. Also, the slow pace at which participatory efforts move may be in conflict with the bureaucratic necessities of reaching policy goals rapidly (Abers, 2000). The creation of 'social missions' in Venezuela was specifically to overcome bureaucratic procedures within the ministries (Armada et al., 2009).

(3) On the *administrative* side, whereas there may be a commitment from top-level officials to implement participatory policies, the lower levels may not fully agree or understand the nature of such policies as well as be unwilling to relinquish power to citizen groups and create hurdles in implementation (Abers, 2000). The experience in Brazil was challenging for several local governing units as municipalities and local level officials were reluctant to transfer decision-making authority to them (Abers & Keck, 2009). There may be other groups/businesses whose interest may be to maintain the status-quo that may stall the reform process such as: medical and/or other health associations and pharmaceutical companies if their interest is hurt; service providers may threaten to boycott, relocate, or try other stalling tactics; and media may also side with industry interests and give biased reports to thwart the reform process (Abers, 2000). In Brazil 'The elite supported the proposals for conservative health reforms as these conservative reforms were in their economic interests ... ' (Cohn, 2008). Similarly, the Venezuelan Medical Federation, private media, and big business opposed the reform process (Mahmood et al., 2012).

**Inequality** – The problem of inequality refers to forums of participation dominated by groups that are relatively well-off or enjoy certain prestige or power in communities. Thus, participatory systems can simply reproduce the elitism and inequality, which they aim to eliminate (Abers, 2000). This is one of the biggest threats to effective deliberations in institutions of participations with less representations by the marginalised relative to the well-off due to: the cost of participation may be high for the poor; and the poor may be less organised (Schonleitner, 2006). In addition, they may not be as vocal, lack information to reach decisions or lack formal education. To be genuinely participatory, such efforts should empower and build capacity especially of those that are marginalised. Harnecker (2007) notes that the Ministry of Communal Economy was in Venezuela was created '...to offer professional training and encourage the creation of these socioeconomic organisations by offering access to preferential credit, technical and administrative support.'

**Co-optation** – Abers' (2000) contends that State-initiated participatory policies may only create a façade of public legitimacy by co-opting the poor and marginalised while continuing to pursue a top-down agenda in policymaking. She suggests that a way to explore the quality of participation is by assessing communities are involved in planning and execution of activities, if there are control and delegation, and not simply implementation of pre-designed programmes. Broadly speaking, participatory budgeting fulfils the definition of empowering participatory policy which involves discussion of government policy goals and agendas rather than merely the implementation of pre-designed programmes. Similarly, communal councils were designed on the participatory budgeting experience in Brazil and Venezuela during the reform process in various social sectors including health (Wilpert, 2007) that were participatory-deliberative in nature (Avritzer, 2009).

## Conclusion

This paper has elaborated that while the idea of community participation that has been promoted for decades in global health and development, it has been politically conceived to appear as apolitical. Our contention is that in order to conceive participation of the citizenry in health and other development interventions it needs to be understood in terms of the broader context of democracy. Globally, the dominance of the liberal model of democracy has restricted genuine participation by the citizenry in any areas of the social sectors and broadly in the society as a whole. Capitalism and economic neoliberalism have in fact gained from this exclusionary liberal democratic model. Liberal democracy in Latin America as a system of political elitism has sometimes served to mutually reinforce economic neoliberalism resulting in drastically increasing social inequalities and worsening health and well-being of large swathes of the population. Consequently, the continent has also been leading grassroots forms of societal democracy that organically arose in response to their rejection by the political society. Several Latin American thinkers, scholars, and activists have been documenting and learning from these empirical experiences to build alternative theoretical frameworks that have challenged the long-standing assumptions of the models of democracy that have shunned majoritarian political decision-making.

In this paper we have argued that the social and political context determines the ideological direction and the design of reforms in social sectors. Our focus on the health sector in this paper and in choosing the two country examples was because their respective health sectors were at the forefront of the societal transition to participatory forms of democracy. Knowledge and evidence from a progressive orientation of the health sectors in Brazil and Venezuela fed into the design of reforms in other sectors of the economy. However, social transformation to participatory democracy is not without its challenges. The final part of the paper describes these dilemmas of participation using a framework that was also developed using empirical evidence from participatory democracy experiences in Latin America. These challenges in both Brazil and Venezuela were by no means trivial but commitment from state and engagement from social movements ensured that the historically restricted state–society interface in Latin America progressively expanded and increasingly became inclusive. However, the turn of events on the continent with the political right regaining strength post global recession shows the vulnerability of Latin America to global economic and political pressures.

## Disclosure statement

No potential conflict of interest was reported by the author(s).

## References

Abers, R. N. (2000). *Inventing local democracy: Grassroots politics in Brazil*. Boulder: Lynne Rienner.
Abers, R. N., & Keck, M. E. (2009). Mobilizing the state: The erratic partner in Brazil's participatory water policy. *Politics & Society, 37*(2), 389–314.
Alvarado, C. H., Martinez, M. E., Vivas-Martinez, S., Gutierrez, N. J., & Metzger, W. (2008). Social change and health policy in Venezuela. *Social Medicine, 3*(2), 95–109.
Armada, F., Muntaner, C., Chung, H., Williams-Brennan, L., & Benach, J. (2009). Barrio Adentro and the reduction of health inequalities in Venezuela: An appraisal of the first years. *International Journal of Health Services, 39*(1), 161–187.
Avritzer, L. (2002). *Democracy and the public sphere in Latin America*. Princeton, NJ: Princeton University Press.
Avritzer, L. (2009). *Participatory institutions in democratic Brazil*. Baltimore, MD: The Johns Hopkins University Press.
Barkey, K., & Parikh, S. (1991). Comparative perspectives on the state. *Annual Review of Sociology, 17*, 523–549.
Becker, D. G. (1999). Latin. *America: Beyond 'Democratic Consolidation', Journal of Democracy, 10*(2), 138–151.
Briggs, C. L., & Mantini-Briggs, C. (2009). Confronting health disparities: Latin American social medicine in Venezuela. *American Journal of Public Health, 99*(3), 549–555.
Cohn, A. (2008). The Brazilian health reform: A victory over the neoliberal model. *Social Medicine, 3*(2), 71–81.
Conway, M. (2002). Democracy in postwar Western Europe: The triumph of a political model. *European History Quarterly, 32*(1), 59–84.
Cordeiro, H. (2004). O Instituto de Medicina Social e a luta pela reforma sanitária: contribuição à história do SUS. *Physis (rio De Janeiro, Brazil), 14*(2), 343–362.
Cueto, M. (2004). The origins of primary health care and selective primary health care. *American Journal of Public Health, 94*(11), 1864–1874.
Elias, P. E., & Cohn, A. (2003). Health reform in Brazil: Lessons to consider. *American Journal of Public Health, 93*(1), 44–48.
Escorel, S. (1999). *Reviravolta na saúde: Origem e articulação do movimento sanitário*. Rio de Janeiro: Editora Fiocruz.
Feo, O., & Siqueira, C. E. (2004). An alternative to the neoliberal model in health: The case of Venezuela. *International Journal of Health Services, 34*(2), 365–375.
Goodale, M., & Postero, N. (2013). *Neoliberalism, interrupted: Social change and contested governance in contemporary Latin America*. Stanford: Stanford University Press.
Harnecker, C. P. (2007). Workplace democracy and collective consciousness: An empirical study of Venezuelan cooperatives. *Monthly Review, 59*(6), 27–40.
Held, D. (2006). *Models of democracy* (3rd ed.). Stanford: Stanford University Press.
Heller, P. (2001). Moving the state: The politics of democratic decentralization in Kerala, South Africa, and Porto Alegre. *Politics & Society, 29*(1), 131–163.
Linz, J. J., & Stepan, A. (1996). Toward consolidated democracies. *Journal of Democracy, 7*(2), 14–33.
Mahmood, Q., & Muntaner, C. (2013). Politics, class actors, and health sector reform in Brazil and Venezuela. *Global Health Promotion, 20*(1), 59–67.
Mahmood, Q., Muntaner, C., Leon, R. d. V. M., & Perdomo, R. M. (2012). Popular participation in Venezuela's *Barrio Adentro* health reform. *Globalizations, 9*(6), 815–833.
Melucci, A., & Avritzer, L. (2000). Complexity, cultural pluralism and democracy: Collective action in the public space. *Social Science Information, 39*(4), 507–527.
Muntaner, C., Salazar, R. M., Benach, J., & Armada, F. (2006). Venezuela's Barrio Adentro: An alternative to neoliberalism in health care. *International Journal of Health Services, 36*(4), 803–811.
Muntaner, C., Salazar, R. M., Rueda, S., & Armada, F. (2006). Challenging the neoliberal trend: The Venezuelan health care reform alternative. *Canadian Journal of Public Health. Revue Canadienne de Sante Publique, 97*(6), I19–24.
Navarro, V. (1980). Workers' and community participation and democratic control in Cuba. *International Journal of Health Services, 10*(2), 197–216.
Navarro, V. (1984). A critique of the ideological and political positions of the Willy Brandt report and the WHO Alma Ata declaration. *Social Science & Medicine, 18*(6), 467–474.
Navarro, V. (2007). Neoliberalism as a class ideology; or, the political causes of the growth of inequalities. *International Journal of Health Services, 37*(1), 47–62.

Paim, J. (2008). *Reforma sanitária brasileira: contribuição para a compreensão e crítica*. Salvador: Edufba; Rio de Janeiro: Editora Fiocruz.

Paim, J., Travassos, C., Almeida, C., Bahia, L., & Macinko, J. (2011). The Brazilian health system: History, advances, and challenges. *The Lancet, 377*, 1778–1797.

Paiva, C. H. A., & Teixeira, L. A. (2014). Reforma sanitária e a criação do Sistema Único de Saúde: notas sobre contextos e autores. *História, Ciências, Saúde-Manguinhos, 21*(1), 15–36.

Pan American Health Organization. (2006). *Mission Barrio Adentro: The right to health and social inclusion in Venezuela*. Caracas: Author.

Petras, J. F., & Veltmeyer, H. (2005). *Social movements and state power: Argentina, Brazil, Bolivia, Ecuador*. London: Pluto Press.

Raby, D. L. (2006). *Democracy and revolution: Latin America and socialism today*. Toronto: Between the Lines.

Schonleitner, G. (2006). Between liberal and participatory democracy: Tensions and dilemmas of leftist politics in Brazil. *Journal of Latin American Studies, 38*(1), 35–63.

Silva, E. (2009). *Challenging neoliberalism in Latin America*. New York, NY: Cambridge University Press.

Warren, M. E. (2002). What can democratic participation mean today? *Political Theory, 30*(5), 677–701.

Werner, D., Sanders, D., Weston, J., Babb, S. & Rodriguez, S. (1997). *Questioning the solution: The politics of primary health care and child survival*. Paolo Alto, CA: HealthWrights.

Wilpert, G. (2007). *Changing Venezuela by taking power: The history and policies of the Chavez government*. New York, NY: Verso.

World Health Organization. (1978). *Declaration of Alma Ata*. Retrieved from http://www.who.int/publications/almaata_declaration_en.pdf

World Health Organization. (2008). *The world health report 2008 – primary health care: Now more than ever*. Geneva: Author.

# History and challenges of Brazilian social movements for the achievement of the right to adequate food

Ana Carolina Feldenheimer da Silva, Elisabetta Recine, Paula Johns, Fabio da Silva Gomes, Mariana de Araújo Ferraz and Eduardo Faerstein

**ABSTRACT**
The historical struggles that Brazil faced to overcome malnutrition coincided with the empowerment of civil society and social movements which played a crucial role in the affirmation of health and food as social rights. After two decades under military dictatorship, Brazil went through a redemocratization process in the 1980s when activism emerged to demand spaces to participate in policy-making regarding the social agenda, including food and nutrition security (FNS). From 1988 onward institutional structures were established: the National Council of FNS (CONSEA) convenes government and civil society sectors to develop and monitor the implementation of policies, systems and actions. Social participation has been at the heart of structural changes achieved since then. Nevertheless, the country faces multiple challenges regarding FNS such as the double burden of disease, increasing use of pesticides and genetically modified seeds, weak regulation of ultra-processed products, and marketing practices that affect the environment, population health, and food sovereignty. This article aims at examining the development of the participatory political system and the role played by Brazilian social movements in the country's policies on FNS, in addition to outlining challenges faced by those policies.

During the last few decades the process of political redemocratization in Brazil included the strengthening of civil society organisations and the achievement of institutional spaces for social control of public policies. In parallel with the construction of the Brazilian Unified Health System (UHS, or SUS in Portuguese), Food and Nutrition Security (FNS) became a field of outstanding activism.

Public policies and activism in FNS in Brazil have to deal with complex population health patterns and trends. Comparisons between the 1970s/1980s and the 2010s reveal a reduction in malnutrition among children and adults in all social strata and geographic regions (Monteiro, 2009), which parallels an increase in obesity. However, among the poorest sectors of society, malnutrition coexists with overweight (Monteiro, Mondini, De Souza, & Popkin, 1995). Nationwide survey data for 1974–5 and 2008–9 indicates that overweight nearly tripled among men (from 19% to 50%) and almost doubled among women (from 29% to 48%). As a result, the prevalence of overweight became at least three times higher than that of malnutrition (Conde & Monteiro, 2014).

Disability-Adjusted Life Year (DALY) data reveal that Brazil faces a double burden of diseases: on the one hand, the presence of nutritional deficiencies, infectious diseases, maternal and perinatal conditions and external causes (responsible for approximately 25% of DALYs); on the other hand, high rates of non-communicable chronic diseases (about 75% of DALYs) for most of which overweight is an important risk factor (Leite et al., 2015).

Throughout the second half of the last century, initiatives aimed on tackling malnutrition and macro- and/or micronutrient deficiencies as well as aiming to prevent overweight were mostly focused on health education and communication approaches. In relation to overweight, consisting of recommendations to reduce the intake of calories, fat and carbohydrates and increase energy expenditure through physical activity. However, the effectiveness of these strategies has proven to be limited. Actions taken at national level have not shown effective results in Brazil (as in no other country) in ensuring energy balance at appropriate levels (Curioni & Lourenço, 2005).

The United Nations 2030 Agenda for Sustainable Development (Sustainable Development Goals/ SDGs), and more specifically, the United Nations Decade of Action on Nutrition (2016–2025) call for national and international efforts for the adoption of participatory, structural, and sustainable solutions that can correct failures, prevent the sabotage of food systems and link sustainable and coherent food production, distribution and consumption methods with health and nutrition. In both agendas, the concept of sustainability goes beyond the environmental dimension and includes social and economic sustainability and equity promotion, in addition to the strengthening of local production and distribution processes. (Dangour, Mace, & Shankar, 2017). It is also important to engage people in expanding their concerns from the individual benefits of foods to a broader recognition of the systemic effects of their eating practices on planetary health, and of other dimensions of eating such as its socio-political transformative act.

This article aims at examining the development of the participatory political system and the role played by Brazilian social movements in the country's policies on FNS, in addition to outlining challenges faced by those policies.

## Development of the FNS concept

The concept of FNS in Brazil is the result of a process of historical construction strongly influenced by social participation. In Brazil and worldwide, during the 1950s food security had a narrow focus on increasing food availability through the expansion of agricultural production; thus, food insecurity was defined as resulting from insufficient food production. This premise was used to justify the productivity increase in the 'Green Revolution' model – i.e. investments concentrated in agricultural technology, monocultures, mechanisation and pesticide use. However, this model failed to address the problem of hunger and resulted in adverse social and environmental impacts such as rural flight, threats to biodiversity, soil and food contamination and increased dependence on large corporations (Burity et al., 2010, p. 11). At that time, the Brazilian population had an epidemiological scenario with low life expectancy at birth, high infant mortality rates, malnutrition and micronutrient deficiencies, especially among children and women of childbearing age (Batista Filho & Rissin, 2003).

By the 1980s, an international social movement[1] had gained strength to broaden the concept of food security, incorporating other dimensions such as sufficiency (protection against hunger and malnutrition), access to safe food (biologically or chemically uncontaminated), quality (nutritional, biological, sanitary and technological) and food appropriateness – i.e. food produced and consumed in an environmentally sustainable, socially just, culturally acceptable manner, incorporating the idea of access to information. (Burity et al., 2010, p. 12; Maluf, 2007, p. 20).

A milestone in this process was the Food Security Treaty, which resulted from civil society's demands and was achieved at the World Civil Society Conference during the United Nations Conference on Environment and Development (UNCED), or Eco '92. The 3rd item of the Food Security Treaty emphasises that the world food insecurity problem is a result of an undemocratic and inequitable distribution of and access to resources (such as land, credit, information and incentive), rather than a problem of global food production. As a result, there is a concentration of production in certain regions and in the hands of fewer and fewer intensive producers, to the detriment of the other regions, small scale farmers and local food security (Food Security Treaty, 1992).

The Brazilian concept of FNS considers the dimensions of food security, food safety and the result in terms of the human process of eating (i.e. nutrition and health) to be inextricably linked. Integrating the human process into the concept includes the socioeconomic and cultural aspects expressed by culture and food heritage. There is also a dialogue with another concept – that of food sovereignty – in order to assert the right of peoples to define their own policies and sustainable food production, distribution and consumption strategies. It seeks to protect and promote food production based on small and medium producers, respecting cultures and the diversity of peasant, fishing and indigenous modes of agricultural production.

The concept of FNS approved at the Brazilian 2nd National FNS Conference (2004) was influenced by contributions from both social movements and governmental agencies:

> Food and Nutrition Security is the fulfilment of the right of everyone to regular and permanent access to quality food in sufficient amounts without compromising access to other essential needs, based on health-promoting dietary practices that respect cultural diversity and are socially, economically and environmentally sustainable.

Thus, the Brazilian concept of FNS considers the dimensions of food security, food safety and the result in terms of the human process of eating (i.e. nutrition and health) to be inextricably linked. Integrating the human process into the concept includes the socioeconomic and cultural aspects expressed by culture and food heritage. There is also a dialogue with a more recent concept – that of food sovereignty – in order to assert the right of peoples to define their own policies and sustainable food production, distribution and consumption strategies. It seeks to protect and promote food production based on small and medium producers, respecting cultures and the diversity of peasant, fishing and indigenous modes of agricultural production.

This understanding of what FNS means gave rise to the concept of appropriate and healthy food:

> Healthy and appropriate eating is the fulfilment of a basic human right, with the guarantee of permanent and regular access, in a socially just manner, to a dietary practice that is appropriate to the biological and social aspects of individuals, according to their life cycle and special dietary needs, based on traditional local references. It must meet the principles of variety, balance, moderation and pleasure (taste), the dimensions of gender and ethnicity, and environmentally sustainable means of production, free of physical, chemical and biological contaminants and genetically modified organisms (CONSEA, 2007).

The concept adopted by the Ministry of Health in 2013 incorporates additional aspects:

> Adequate and healthy eating is understood as the dietary practice that is appropriate to the biological and socio-cultural aspects of individuals as well as to a sustainable use of the environment. Thus, it must be in accordance with the needs of each phase of life and with special dietary needs; referenced by food culture and by gender, race and ethnicity; accessible from a physical and financial standpoint; harmonious in quantity and quality; based on adequate and sustainable production practices; and with minimal quantities of physical, chemical and biological contaminants (Brazil, 2013).

## History of social movements linked to FNS in Brazil

Over time, the FNS concept has been refined as the involvement of civil society in formulating public policy increased. Brazil has been under long periods of dictatorship (1937–45 and 1964–85) during which decision-making processes and the management of the social welfare systems were restricted to large federal bureaucracies.

Societal aspiration for democracy, coupled with a social security financing crisis and the economic recession of the 1980s drove social demands, bringing together public health academics and professionals, labour unions, and grassroots movements (Paim, Travassos, Almeida, Bahia, & Macinko,

2011). In 1986, the 8th National Health Conference outlined the principles for the construction of Brazil's Universal Health System (UHS, SUS in Portuguese). Subsequently, the National Constituent Assembly (1987–8) defined the legal basis for the UHS, detailed by Organic Health Laws 8.080 and 8.142 of 1990): health as a fundamental human right, and food as a determinant of health (Brasil, 1990a, 1990b); the UHS national directorate was given the role of formulating, evaluating and supporting food and nutrition policies.

In the mid-1990s, driven by popular support for the impeachment of President Collor (due to corruption charges) and for the Ethics in Politics Movement, the Citizenship Action against Hunger and Poverty and for Life (CAHPL) was organised through local committees that developed grassroots actions. The decentralised committees included varied sectors of Brazilian society, and their degree of capillarity at the organisation's peak period was unprecedented at that time. CAHPL's main impact was to broaden the agenda of the fight against hunger in Brazilian society and to mobilise many thousands of people in actions to donate food to vulnerable groups (CONSEA, 1994; Silva & Gomes da Silva, 1991). During the same period, the Institute of Applied Economic Research (IPEA) launched the Hunger Map (Peliano, 1993).

The political effervescence resulting from the presidential impeachment process helped supporting the proposal for a national FNS policy, and led to the creation of the National Food and Nutrition Security Council (CONSEA) in 1994 (Decree 807). The CONSEA's objectives were: a) to develop guidelines for the Plan to Combat Hunger and Poverty; b) to design an appropriate strategy for its execution; c) to mobilise necessary resources to meet these objectives; d) to encourage partnership and integration among public, private, national and international agencies in order to ensure the mobilisation and streamlining of resource use as well as the complementarity of the actions developed; e) to coordinate public awareness campaigns to combat hunger and poverty in order to coordinate government and civil society efforts; and f) to encourage and support the creation of state and municipal committees to combat hunger and poverty (Maluf, 2007).

In 1994, the 1st National Food Security Conference (NFSC) was held. Its theme was 'Hunger – a National Issue'. The NFSC had specific objectives: a) to discuss the concept of food security as a component of a national project to transform the reality that produces and reproduces hunger, poverty and exclusion; b) to reach a consensus on priorities and guidelines for policy formulation and the proposal of intervention instruments; c) to discuss the process of citizenship building; d) to identify alternatives and promote the exchange of experiences in development in civil society; and e) to identify new forms and mechanisms of partnership and coordination between governmental and non-governmental actions with a view to building a new relationship between the government and civil society (CONSEA, 1994, 1995).

In this NFSC, a broader concept of food security was adopted as a set of principles, policies, measures and instruments to permanently ensure that all Brazilians have access to food at affordable prices, with the quantity and quality necessary to meet the nutritional requirements for a dignified and healthy life as well as other rights of citizenship. In addition, he final report mentions the need the need for sustainable economic and social development that should include the consolidation of the agrarian reform process (CONSEA, 1995).

However, President Cardoso abolished CONSEA and established the Community Solidarity Program (CSP), which focused on actions to combat poverty in municipalities (Decree 1.366, 1995). The CSP's objective was to 'coordinate government actions aimed at serving the portion of the population that does not have the means to meet its basic needs, and especially to fight hunger and poverty' (Silva, 2001).

The CSP priorities were: a) reducing infant mortality; b) food; c) supporting elementary education; d) urban development; e) generating employment and income; and f) professional training. According to critics, CSP transferred the responsibility for social policies to civil society (e.g. NGOs) on the grounds of solidarity, which resulted in fragmented, selective and narrowly-focused actions (Silva, 2001, pp. 76–77). weakening actions' alignment actions and delaying public policies.

The CSP was not structured as a traditional governmental programme but rather as a strategic proposal to combat poverty, 'a multi-purpose program' that encompassed emergency and structural programmes, inserting itself into social policy without exhausting it (Burlandy & Labra, 2003, p. 124). Its guiding axes were: a) the articulation, coordination and convergence of government social actions for municipalities and the poorest population groups, with the simultaneous implementation of the greatest possible number of actions in these localities, seeking complementarity and synergy; b) decentralisation; c) the restructuring of the administrative apparatus to avoid overlapping actions; d) the allocation of resources with transparent criteria; and e) the promotion of solidarity as a value capable of mobilising government partnerships with civil society in order to raise resources for tackling poverty. (Burlandy & Labra, 2003; IPEA, 1996).

This structure introduced civil society into the management of policies and programmes in a unique way. Montaño (2002) claimed that this kind of civil society protagonism is linked to the 'third sector' concept, derived from the fragmentation of society into three spheres: the state ('first sector', the political sphere), the market ('second sector', the economic sphere) and civil society ('third sector', the social sphere).

In 1998, the federal government established the Active Community Program within the CSP framework. This programme was based on the principles of Integrated and Sustainable Local Development and aimed to maximise the resources of communities themselves in the fight against poverty, thus making municipalities self-sufficient (IPEA, 1996). In the area of food and nutrition, programmes were selected such as the Programme to Combat Maternal and Child Malnutrition, and Food Stock Distribution.

As noted by Valente (2002), the CSP gradually distanced itself from civil society, and its main limitations were: (1) its different institutional format and lack of managerial support: it lacked the tools and adequate institutional space to implement its proposed actions; and (2) representativeness: it lacked the legitimacy of the broader civil society. It was not possible to advance the understanding and institutional fulfilment of the social demands of population segments that were not organised to put pressure on the government. Therefore, the CSP objectively failed to achieve social impact and change local realities (Burlandy & Labra, 2003).

In 2003, President Lula instituted the Zero Hunger Program and reinstalled CONSEA: its presidency must be exercised by a representative of civil society and the secretariat exercised by the Minister for Food Security and Fight against Hunger. Since then, CONSEA has been a key player in the process of institutionalising FNS in Brazil. It operates through permanent commissions, that is, micro-structures organised around strategic issues, in charge of elaborating ideas and proposals to be presented at CONSEA plenary sessions. Four national conferences held to date generated a political process leading to the approval of the FNS Organic Law (2006), the National FNS Policy (2010); a constitutional amendment that included food as a social right; and two national FNS plans (2012–15 and 2016–19). In addition to actively participating in restructuring the National School Meal Program, it has promoted debates about the enforceability of the right to food, pesticide use and genetically modified seeds, and the nutritional needs of indigenous and traditional communities, among other issues.

## National achievements in the FNS field

The process of specifying the human right to adequate food in the international sphere gave momentum to movements seeking to legally recognise this right at the national level. In 1966, the International Covenant on Economic, Social and Cultural Rights (ICESCR), adopted by UN General Assembly Resolution No. 2200-A (XXI) had affirmed the right to food in its broadest sense (Article 11). Brazil is a party to the ICESCR and in 1992 was incorporated into national law by Decree No. 591. The country is also involved in the recognition of this right by means of the 1969 American Convention on Human Rights (Pact of San José), ratified by Brazil in 1992, and the Additional Protocol to the American Convention on Human Rights in the Area of Economic, Social and Cultural

Rights of 1988 (San Salvador Protocol) which refers to the right to food in its Article 12 (internally promulgated by Decree 3.321 of 1999).

The concept of the human right to adequate and healthy food is gaining momentum as a result of national and international social movements' demands. For example, the non-governmental organisations FoodFirst Information and Action Network International, the World Alliance on Nutrition and Human Rights and the Institut Jacques Maritain coordinated the development of the Code of Conduct on the Human Right to Adequate Food in 1997, to be included in the United Nations and the Food and Agriculture Organization agendas. In 1999, the United Nations Committee on Economic, Social and Cultural Rights drafted General Comment 12 on the Right to Adequate Food, which emphasises the broadest concept of FNS.

With the resumption of CONSEA in 2003, the creation of a legal and institutional framework to protect and promote the Human Right to the Adequate Food was advocated. In 2006. the Organic Law of Food and Nutrition Security (Law No. 11.236), established the National Food and Nutrition Security System (NFNSS) and defined universality, equity, autonomy, social participation and transparency as its principles.

The NFNSS brings together various government sectors to coordinate FNS policies (Leão & Maluf, 2012, p. 30). The following are the main bodies that manage the NFNSS at the federal level:

- The National Conference on FNS: 2/3 of its participants are from civil society and 1/3 are from the government; It occurs every four years to recommend guidelines and priorities to CONSEA for the national FNS Policy and Plan and to evaluate the NFNSS;
- CONSEA: 2/3 of its advisors are from civil society and 1/3 is from the government; it is a direct advisory body for the presidency of the republic. It proposes guidelines and priorities and suggests the budget required to implement the FNS Policy and Plan;
- The Inter-ministerial Chamber of Food and Nutrition Security (ICFNS): composed of Ministers of State and Special Secretaries; it prepares the FNS Policy and Plan based on CONSEA's guidelines.

Initiatives derived from the work of CONSEA and ICFNS include the 1st and the 2nd National Plan of FNS (2012–2015 and 2016–2019).Of utmost importance has been the interaction between the National School Meal Program and the National Program to Strengthen Family Agriculture: legislation passed in 2009 (Law 11,947) established that at least 30% of food purchased for the school meal programme (in natura or minimally processed) must come from small family farmers.

Of no less importance was the publication of the Food and Nutritional Education Reference Framework for Public Policies (Brasil, 2012) and the new Food Guide for the Brazilian Population (Brasil, 2014) based on FNS principles, which achieved international recognition.

### Challenges for the FNS agenda: political context, regulation, public-private relations

In the current political context of Brazil, similarly to the prevailing context of an increasing number of countries worldwide, public policies have been strongly influenced by private interests of large corporations (Stuckler and Nestle, 2012).

This situation is no different in the FNS field, where an example of such conflicts between public and private interests in Brazil has been observed in relation to the National Technical Biosafety Commission (NTBC). Academics and civil society organisations have pointed out the NTBC tendency to echo arguments made by the marketing teams of companies that produce pesticides and genetically modified organisms (Zanoni et al., 2011). This situation has turned Brazil into the largest consumer of pesticides in the world (ASP-TA, 2010), in addition to approving the use of pesticides that are banned in other parts of the world, such as Europe.

The political strategy of large economic conglomerates dealing with unhealthy products (e.g. tobacco, alcohol and ultra-processed foods and beverages) to avoid regulations that would reduce their profits have been widely documented in the case of the tobacco industry (Ulucanlar, Fooks, & Gilmore, 2016) and have been also increasingly documented in the food and nutrition field (Brownell & Warner, 2009; Gomes, 2015). These companies, as well as the organisations related to them (Gomes, 2015), act not only at the national level, but also in the sphere of the United Nations by funding activities and playing a role that sometimes can compete with the role of Member States (Mialon, Swinburn, Allender, & Sacks, 2017).

A frequent strategy of such corporations and related actors to distort, weaken or avoid regulatory policies is to propose public-private interactions so called 'partnerships' with regulatory authorities (Burlandy et al., 2016; Gomes & Lobstein, 2011; Richter, 2004), such as the voluntary agreement between the Brazilian federal government and the Brazilian Food Industry Association to reduce sodium content in processed and ultra-processed food and drink products (Martins, 2014). In addition to its dubious effectiveness, this agreement has several potentially negative side effects. While explicitly attacking government policies aimed at promoting adequate and healthy food, the industry can guarantee a seat at the table in negotiating regulatory policies (Kearns, Schmidt, & Glantz, 2016). Thus, an ambiguous message is conveyed to the public that ultra-processed products should be avoided (according to the recommendations of the Dietary Guidelines for the Brazilian Population), yet the public may perceive such products as recommended for consumption, since they see government and manufacturers negotiating voluntary reformulations of such products, when government's recommendation is for their avoidance (Monteiro and Cannon, 2012).

In 2016, several soft drink industry trade associations opposed the adoption of the Bill 430/2016 which would tax soft drink, claiming that it will lead to job and income losses ("ALIANZA LATINOAMERICANA," 2015). Through this discursive strategy, the industry tries to represent legitimate interests of various sectors of society (Ulucanlar et al., 2016).

Therefore, it is necessary to adopt mechanisms to identify and analyse conflicts of interest in order to safeguard public health (Mialon, Swinburn, & Sacks, 2015; Pralle, 2006) In 2013, several Brazilian scientific societies, professional associations, researchers, and health professionals gathered at the 'Front for Regulation of the Public-Private Relationship in Food and Nutrition', aimed at increasing awareness about conflict of interests related to the Brazilian FNS agenda (Frente pela Regulação, 2013).

While Brazil stands out as a reference in social participation and control in relation to FNS actions, the established participatory bodies have not been sufficient to avoid the deleterious political influence of agribusiness and big food companies. For example, in the 2014 general elections, the financing of electoral campaigns by large ultra-processed food companies outpaced that of all other business sectors (Abramo, 2014).

In order to face such challenges, it is needed a constant dialogue and coordination among social movements, through the actions of structured national councils and by strengthening civil society organisations truly engaged with the FNS agenda. Active social control coupled with partners such as universities are also needed to defend FNS.

Initial steps towards the implementation of intersectoral public policies need to be strengthened, in line with the spirit of the United Nations SDGs. This 2030 Agenda states as its Goal 2: 'End hunger, achieve food security and improved nutrition and promote sustainable agriculture (...)' Also, that 'it is time to rethink how we grow, share and consume our food. If done right, agriculture, forestry and fisheries can provide nutritious food for all and generate decent incomes, while supporting people-centred rural development and protecting the environment.' (http://www.un.org/sustainabledevelopment/hunger/).

In comparison with the previous Millenium Development Goals , the process leading to the SDGs involved more consultations to governments, academia and civil society. The achievement of theses objectives requires efforts aimed at deepening their discussion and implementation under democratic principles. The structural causes underlying the set of challenges expressed in SDGs require paradigm shifts in the development models of most countries, including Brazil.

## Note

1. According to Blumer (1939),

> Social movements can be viewed as collective enterprises to establish a new order of life. They have their inception in the condition of unrest, and derive their motive power on one hand from dissatisfaction with the current form of life, and on the other hand, from wishes and hopes for a new scheme or system of living

## Disclosure statement

No potential conflict of interest was reported by the author.

## References

Abramo, C. W. (2014). Poder econômico e financiamento eleitoral no Brasil. Parte 2: Concentração e efetividade das doações privadas. ONG Transparencia Brasil. Retrieved from https://www.transparencia.org.br/downloads/publicacoes/Concentracao.pdf

ALIANZA LATINOAMERICANA DE ASOCIACIONES DE LA INDUSTRIA DE ALIMENTOS Y BEBIDAS. DECLARACION DE QUITO. 10 y 11 de marzo de 2015. Retrieved from http://copal.org.ar/wp-content/uploads/2015/07/declaracion_quito.pdf

AS-PTA Assessoria e Serviços a Projetos em Agricultura Alternativa. "Com mais transgênicos, Brasil supera recorde de consumo de agrotóxicos". Em pratos limpos, 13 maio 2010. Retrieved from http://pratoslimpos.org.br/2010/05/13/com-mais-transgenicos-brasil-supera-recorde-de-consumo-de-agrotoxicos/

Batista Filho, M., & Rissin, A. (2003). Nutritional transition in Brazil: Geographic and temporal trends. *Cadernos de Saúde Publica*, 19, S181–S191.

Blumer, H. (1939). Collective behavior. In Robert E. Park (Ed.), *An outline of the principles of sociology* (pp. 60–61). New York: Barnes and Noble.

Brasil, C. C. (1990a). Lei n° 8.080, de 19de setembro de 1990: Dispõe sobre as condições para a promoção, proteção e recuperação da saúde, a organização eo funcionamento dos serviços correspondentes e dá outras providências. *Diário Oficial da União*, 128(182), 18055.

Brasil, C. C. (1990b). Lei n°: 8.142, de 28de dezembro de 1990. Dispõe sobre a participação da comunidade na gestão do Sistema Único de Saúde (SUS) e sobre as transferências intergovernamentais de recursos financeiros na área da saúde e dá outras providências. *Diário Oficial da União*, 28, 25694.

Brasil. Ministério da Saúde (MS). Secretaria de Atenção à Saúde. Departamento de Atenção Básica. (2014). *Guia alimentar para a população brasileira*. Brasília: Ministério da Saúde.

Brasil. Ministério do Desenvolvimento Social e Combate à Fome. (2012). *Marco de referência de educação alimentar e nutricional para as políticas públicas*. Brasília: MDS. Retrieved from http://www.ideiasnamesa.unb.br/files/marco_EAN_visualizacao.pdf

Brazil. Ministry of Health of Brazil. Secretariat of Health Care. Department of Primary Health Care. (2013). *National food and nutrition policy/ Ministry of health of Brazil, secretariat of health care, department of primary health care*. Brasilia: Ministry of Health of Brazil.

Brownell, K. D., & Warner, K. E. (2009). The perils of ignoring history: Big Tobacco played dirty and millions died. How similar is Big Food? *Milbank Quarterly*, 87(1), 259–294.

Burity, V., Franceschini, T., Valente, F., Recine, E., Leão, M., & Carvalho, M. D. F. (2010). *Direito humano à alimentação adequada no contexto da segurança alimentar e nutricional*. Brasília, DF: Abrandh.

Burlandy, L., Alexandre, V. P., Gomes, F. D. S., Castro, I. R. R. D., Dias, P. C., Henriques, P., … Castro Júnior, P. C. P. D. (2016). Health promotion policies and potential conflicts of interest involving the commercial private sector. *Ciencia & saude coletiva*, 21(6), 1809–1818.

Burlandy, L., & Labra, M. E. (2003). Comunidade Solidaria: engenharia institucional, focalização e parcerias no combate à fome, à pobreza e à desnutrição. *Ciência & Saúde Coletiva, Rio de Janeiro*, 8(1), 176–196.

Conde, W. L., & Monteiro, C. A. (2014). Nutrition transition and double burden of undernutrition and excess of weight in Brazil. *The American Journal of Clinical Nutrition*, 100(6), 1617S–1622S.

CONSEA. (2007). *III conferência Nacional de Segurança Alimentar e Nutricional. Documento Base*. Brasília: Author.

CONSEA. Conselho Nacional de Segurança Alimentar e Nutricional. (1994). *I Conferência Nacional de Segurança Alimentar – Relatório Final*. Brasília: Author.

CONSEA. Conselho Nacional de Segurança Alimentar e Nutricional. Secretaria Executiva Nacional da Ação da Cidadania. (1995). *I Conferência Nacional de Segurança Alimentar e Nutricional*. Brasília: Author.

Curioni, C. C., & Lourenço, P. M. (2005). Long-term weight loss after diet and exercise: A systematic review. *International Journal of Obesity, 29*(10), 1168–1174.

Dangour, A. D., Mace, G., & Shankar, B. (2017). Food systems, nutrition, health and the environment. *The Lancet Planetary Health, 1*(1), e8–e9.

Frente pela Regulação da Relação Público-Privado em Alimentação e Nutrição. Manifesto de criação da Frente pela Regulação da Relação Público-Privado em Alimentação e Nutrição. Novembro de 2013. Retrieved from http://regulacaopublicoprivado.blogspot.com.br/p/manifesto.html

Global Forum at Rio de Janeiro. The NGO Alternative Treaties. 19 - Food Security Treaty. June 1–15, 1992.

Gomes, F. D. S. (2015). Conflicts of interest in food and nutrition. *Cadernos de saude publica, 31*(10), 2039–2046.

Gomes, F. S., & Lobstein, T. (2011). Food and beverage transnational corporations and nutrition policy. *SCN News,* (39), 57–65. Retrieved from http://citeseerx.ist.psu.edu/viewdoc/download?doi=10.1.1.466.1285&rep=rep1&type=pdf#page=57

IPEA. Instituto de Pesquisa Econômica Aplicada. (1996). Cadernos Comunidade Solidária: Segurança Alimentar e Nutricional no Brasil, 2.

Kearns, C. E., Schmidt, L. A., & Glantz, S. A. (2016). Sugar industry and coronary heart disease research: A historical analysis of internal industry documents. *JAMA Internal Medicine, 176*(11), 1680–1685.

Leão, M., & Maluf, R. S. (2012). A construção social de um sistema público de segurança alimentar e nutricional: a experiência brasileira. *ABRANDH, Brasília, BRA.*

Leite, I. D. C., Valente, J. G., Schramm, J. M. D. A., Daumas, R. P., Rodrigues, R. D. N., Santos, M. D. F., ... Mota, J. C. D. (2015). Burden of disease in Brazil and its regions, 2008. *Cadernos de Saúde Pública, 31*(7), 1551–1564.

Maluf, R. S. J. (2007). *Segurança alimentar e nutricional.* Petrópolis: Vozes.

Martins, A. P. B. (2014). Redução de sódio em alimentos: uma análise dos acordos voluntários no Brasil. *Série Alimentos, Instituto Brasileiro De Defesa Do Consumidor (IDEC), São Paulo,* 1–90.

Mialon, M., Swinburn, B., Allender, S., & Sacks, G. (2017). 'Maximising shareholder value': A detailed insight into the corporate political activity of the Australian food industry. *Australian and New Zealand Journal of Public Health, 41* (2), 165–171.

Mialon, M., Swinburn, B., & Sacks, G. (2015). A proposed approach to systematically identify and monitor the corporate political activity of the food industry with respect to public health using publicly available information. *Obesity Reviews, 16*(7), 519–530.

Montano, C. (2002). *Terceiro setor e questão social: crítica ao padrão emergente de intervenção social.* São Paulo: Cortez Editora.

Monteiro, C. A. (2009). A queda da desnutrição infantil no Brasil. *Cadernos de Saúde Pública, 25*(5), 950–950.

Monteiro, C. A., & Cannon, G. (2012). The impact of transnational "big food" companies on the south: A view from Brazil. *PLoS Medicine, 9*(7), e1001252. doi:10.1371/journal.pmed.1001252

Monteiro, C. A., Mondini, L., De Souza, A. L., & Popkin, B. M. (1995). The nutrition transition in Brazil. *European Journal of Clinical Nutrition, 49*(2), 105–113.

Paim, J., Travassos, C., Almeida, C., Bahia, L., & Macinko, J. (2011). The Brazilian health system: History, advances, and challenges. *The Lancet, 377*(9779), 1778–1797.

Peliano, A. M. (1993). O mapa da fome: subsídios à formulação de uma política de segurança alimentar. In *IPEA. Documento de Política* (No. 14). Ipea.

Pralle, S. B. (2006). *Branching out, digging in: Environmental advocacy and agenda setting.* Washington, DC: Georgetown University Press.

Richter, J. (2004). Public–private partnerships for health: A trend with no alternatives? *Development, 47*(2), 43–48.

Silva, L. I. L, & Gomes da Silva, J. (1991). *Política Nacional de Segurança Alimentar.* São Paulo: Governo Paralelo.

Silva, M. O. (2001). *O Comunidade Solidária: o não-enfrentamento da pobreza no Brasil.* São Paulo: Cortez Editora.

Stuckler, D, & Nestle, M. (2012). Big food, food systems, and global health. *PLoS Medicine, 9*(6), e1001242. doi:10.1371/journal.pmed.1001242

Ulucanlar, S., Fooks, G. J., & Gilmore, A. B. (2016). The policy dystopia model: An interpretive analysis of tobacco industry political activity. *PLoS Medicine, 13*(9), e1002125. doi:10.1371/journal.pmed.1002125

Valente, F. L. S. (2002). *Direito Humano à Alimentação – desafios e conquistas.* São Paulo: Cortez Editora.

Zanoni, M, Melgarejo, L, Nodari, R, Dal'Saglio, F., Kessler, K. P., Ferraz, J. M., ... Deffune, G. (2011). O biorrisco e a Comissão Técnica de Biossegurança: lições de uma experiência. In M. Zanoni & G. Ferment (org) (Eds.), *Transgênicos para quem? Agricultura, Ciência e Sociedade* (pp. 244–276). Brasília: MDA.

# La Revolución Ciudadana and social medicine: Undermining community in the state provision of health care in Ecuador

Karin Friederic and Brian J. Burke

**ABSTRACT**

Under President Rafael Correa (2007–2017), Ecuador's Ministry of Health established a state-centred health care regime that incorporates elements of Latin American social medicine into post-neoliberalism. These initiatives – which are part of 'The National Plan for Good Living (*Buen Vivir*)' – include free healthcare, greater attention to social determinants of health, a focus on equity and inclusion, and increased coordination across welfare, health, and development sectors. However, the reforms also use health services to build a sense of inclusive, participatory citizenship, with the Ecuadorean state as the central figure in service provision. In this paper, we demonstrate that state-centred health care reforms have paradoxically weakened community organising for collective health. Drawing on seventeen years of ethnographic research and health solidarity work in rural Northwest Ecuador, we illustrate how Ecuador's health reforms have reconfigured relations among local civil society, transnational NGOs, and the state. Established modes of community participation and international collaboration have been undermined largely because these reforms ignore community sovereignty and self-organisation and overemphasise the threat of neoliberalism. The lessons about balancing the state-based fulfilment of rights with community power are relevant to social medicine advocates, particularly those working in rural communities that are already organising creatively for their own health and well-being.

## Social medicine and *La Revolución Ciudadana*

The Latin American social medicine (LASM) movement, which draws on over a century of primarily Marxist social thought in Europe and the Americas (Arango Panesso, 2008; Laurell, 1989; Tajer, 2003), foregrounds the social determination of health and promotes well-being via community-controlled health care and social transformation.[1] The movement is built on a way of understanding illness and health centred on the following referents, some of which have become commonplace in global public health more broadly: (a) analysing disease not as a purely biological phenomenon but also as a result of capitalist development, socio-economic inequality and related working and living conditions, and national policy; (b) considering the subjects of health care to be not only individuals or a national population of homogeneous individuals but rather a stratified population comprised of classes (defined according to economic status, race/ethnicity, gender differences, urban/rural residency, etc.); and (c) responding to disease via preventative measures, policies for universal and equitable health care, the broader elimination of social inequities that lead to unequal health outcomes, the reduction of environmental and workplace hazards, and the promotion of empowered communities able to manage and advance their own health and healing (Arango Panesso, 2008; Granda Ugalde, 2009; Laurell, 1989; Tajer, 2003; Waitzkin, Iriart, Estrada, & Lamadrid, 2001). In some cases, LASM also adopted an anti-colonial attitude toward health economics and technology development (Breilh, 1995).

Under President Rafael Correa's administration (2007–2017), the Ecuadorean Ministry of Health (MoH) has established a state-centred, populist health care regime that incorporates elements of Latin American social medicine into a post-neoliberal platform (see, for example, Ministerio de Salud Pública, 2013). Correa's policies thus represent a backlash against nearly two decades of neoliberal policies that aimed to radically marketise society, minimise the welfare and regulatory arms of the state, and convert basic social services into commodities (North, 2013). Neoliberals hoped that commoditising or marketising social services would prompt the more 'efficient' provision of services while fuelling growth through capital accumulation among national and global elite (Harvey, 2005). Unfortunately, the flip side of market efficiency is surrendering democratic decision-making to impersonal market logics of supply, effective demand, exclusion, and profitability. Ecuador never implemented a formal package of neoliberal reforms in the health sector – as it had in other sectors – but 'the health sector in Ecuador suffered a "silent" neoliberal reform' through piece-meal initiatives to reduce public health budgets, restrict government health insurance, increase private contracting, and decentralise decision-making (De Paepe, Tapia, Santacruz, & Unger, 2012, p. 219). As Navarro (2008) and Rasch and Bywater (2014) point out, a privatised health care system is particularly conducive to narrowly conceived biomedical approaches that ignore the social determination of health, diverse measures of well-being, and community decision-making.

The post-neoliberal reforms initiated by Correa's administration entailed the reversal of this silent revolution. Launched primarily via 'The National Plan for Good Living (*Buen Vivir*)' (SENPLADES, 2010) as part of Ecuador's 'Citizens' Revolution,' the reforms included the introduction of free healthcare, greater attention to social determinants of health, and better coordination across welfare, health, and development sectors. Ecuadoreans have seen significantly increased health funding, movements toward a unified national health system, the establishment of primary and preventative health care as a universal right and a responsibility of the state, and an intersectoral approach through which multiple ministries consider health-related aspects of their work. The Citizens' Revolution seems to have had a positive impact on health and equity. Between 2006 and 2016, the poverty rate decreased by 38%, inequality dropped,[2] and social spending doubled as a percentage of GDP (Ray & Kozameh, 2012; Weisbrot, Johnston, & Merling, 2017). The Ministry of Health (MoH) saw a 70% increase in its budget during Correa's first year, a significant increase in consultations, and a doubling of the use of diagnostic tools, such as x-rays and mammography (De Paepe et al., 2012). The Correa administration also improved access to medical services by mandating higher salaries and a (longer) 40-h workweek for doctors, establishing mobile clinics, and partnering with the Cuban government to benefit from Cuban doctors, medications, and expertise (Ministerio de Salud Pública, 2014). While it is difficult to directly attribute improved health outcomes to these policy changes, during the same period Ecuador saw improvements in infant and child mortality (Pan-American Health Organization, 2017; World Health Organization, 2017), which often outpaced 'similar countries' (Ray & Kozameh, 2012), and significant declines in the number of reported malaria cases and deaths, tuberculosis cases and deaths, and deaths due to HIV/AIDS (World Health Organization, 2017).

Ecuador's vision of *Buen Vivir* includes strong socialist principles consistent with the LASM socio-political vision of health – such as redistribution, democratisation of the means of production, and a guarantee of dignified work – as well as a commitment to 'citizen power' and decentralised, democratic participation (SENPLADES, 2010, p. 7). In many ways, however, *Buen Vivir* remains aspirational. Hartmann (2016, p. e1) convincingly argues that the so-called 'postneoliberal public health care models' implemented in Ecuador, Bolivia, and Venezuela 'neither fully incorporate social medicine nor completely reject neoliberal models.' They adopt the LASM tenets that health is a right of all citizens and must be seen as a socio-political issue, and they go beyond LASM by emphasising interculturalism or pluriculturalism. However, they depend on neoliberal policies favouring export-oriented primary commodity extraction (especially mining) and the partial privatisation of health care and health insurance. From the perspective of LASM's structural analysis, these macroeconomic and institutional deficiencies must be seen as serious contradictions, even if Ecuador's improved health outcomes have been welcome.

In this article, we shift to a more local scale to examine how the Citizens' Revolution has been experienced by historically marginalised people and communities; how ideals of decentralisation, community participation, and citizen power have been put into practice; and how this has transformed community health activism. Our long-term perspective illustrates that, despite the rhetoric of inclusion and equity, state-centred health care reforms have weakened community organising for collective health and turned rural people into increasingly passive recipients of state services. More specifically, these reforms have replaced community–NGO–state collaborations that were planned and evaluated largely in terms of community goals with state-led medical services based on abstract, quantified, and centralised metrics of 'production.' While these paradoxical impacts may not be generalisable across the country, they provide important insights into a state–community tension that must be negotiated effectively for either LASM or postneoliberalism to have genuinely liberatory effects.

Methodologically, this article draws from seventeen years of ethnographic research and health-related solidarity work in rural northwest Ecuador. Since 2001, Friederic has conducted both ethnographic and historical research alongside applied work with a community health centre and microeconomic projects, all established through collaborations between the local village council and a transnational NGO that she helped form (see Friederic, 2011, 2015 for discussion of the author's positionality as a scholar-activist). From 2001 to 2006, she conducted focus groups, interviews, demographic surveys, and participant observation about gender relations, common household illnesses and treatments, health care services and utilisation, and community health education and promotion. From 2007 to 2008, Friederic conducted long-term ethnographic fieldwork on gender violence and family well-being in the context of broader cultural politics of development in the region. Since then, co-authors Friederic and Burke have returned every year or two to assess the effects of the Correa administration policies on health care delivery, utilisation, and community organising through focus groups, participant-observation, and interviews with health care staff and community members.

## Participation, community sovereignty, and the reconsolidation of the Ecuadorean state

Before turning to our case study, it is worth examining what is required for meaningful community participation in health care, as well as how exactly the Correa administration envisions state and community power. As Vázquez, Siqueira, Kruze, Da Silva, and Leite (2002) note, although participation is a nearly universal principle of health reform, it takes extremely varied forms in practice. Achieving deep forms of participation requires basic civil and political rights and access to health information (Backman et al., 2008), traditions of community organising, and institutional mechanisms for soliciting, hearing, and responding to citizen input and ensuring accountability (Cornwall & Coelho, 2007; Hickey & Mohan, 2004; Vázquez et al., 2002).

Correa's platform appears to value deep participation. The five branches of the Citizens' Revolution – democratic, ethical, economic, social, and international revolutions – all suggest increased individual and community influence over a state committed to people's rights and wellbeing. The National Plan for Good Living provides the guiding framework for how these revolutions should be understood and achieved. The Plan was ostensibly built upon the indigenous notion of *sumak kawsay*, a Kichwa term most often translated as *buen vivir* in Spanish and *living well* or *good living* in English. However, many scholars have critiqued the technocratic appropriation of this dynamic concept that, at root, implies a transformative and alternative vision of development (Acosta, 2008, 2013; Fernández, Pardo, & Salamanca, 2014; Bretón, Cortez, & Garcia, 2014; Macas, 2010; Whitten & Whitten, 2015). Though the meaning of *sumak kawsay* varies across indigenous groups, Whitten and Whitten (2015) note that in Canelos Quichua of Amazonia, it 'means something like "beautiful life" or "beautiful life force"' and it incorporates related concepts such as deep knowledge, community, conviviality, kinship, and integration with nature and the supernatural (193). Thus, in its original sense, *sumak kawsay* is embedded in an indigenous ontology, ethical paradigm, and way of living that envisions 'human beings with respect and in harmony with each other, nature, and the spiritual world' (Sieder & Barrera Vivero, 2017, p. 5). This constellation of meanings contrasts sharply with the interpretations of *Buen Vivir* that appear in the National Plan, which are 'based on capitalist wealth accumulation, albeit for a common good' (Whitten & Whitten, 2015, p. 193), raising questions about the extent to which revolutionary changes and indigenous ontologies can be pursued through state frameworks (Becker, 2011, 2012). So, while *Buen Vivir* retains echoes of its original meaning (e.g. community participation, the rights of nature, and collective rights), it loses its dynamism when taken up as a project by the state, one that must be planned, implemented, measured, and incorporated into the current socio-economic context. Intellectually, the Ecuadorean state's vision of Buen Vivir is framed not in terms of indigenous cosmovision but rather in terms of a historical critique of neoliberal policies that marketized public services, neo-colonial foreign relations that increased Ecuadorean dependency, and the exclusion of ethnic minorities within Ecuador. The linchpin to all three problems, according to the Plan, is to reconsolidate state power primarily by increasing public services. Returning social services to the government will reduce foreign influence and increase citizens' engagement with and esteem for the central state. Doing this within a 'plurinational' framework ensures that even ethnic minorities are included. And strengthening government control over key resource sectors (e.g. oil) while decreasing foreign financial influence (via loans) will provide the capital for public services.

Rebuilding the state – and earning popular trust in the state – was extremely important in Ecuador, which had had seven presidents in ten years (1997–2007) and nine health ministers in five years (2001–2005). Neoliberal policies, natural resource dependency, and high levels of corruption had severely weakened social programmes. However, a close examination of the intellectual framing of *Buen Vivir* raises concerns about how communities would fare in this new political landscape. First, the historical justification for *Buen Vivir* is a highly simplified story consisting of only two actors: the state and the market. This history ignores the actual dynamics of power and action that Ecuadorean communities have engaged in, including non-state/non-market interventions in health. As a result, the Plan repeatedly portrays communities and individuals as blank slates that need to be formed into citizens in order to have any agency beyond their market demand. Second, the Plan oversimplifies imperialism. It collapses all forms of North–South interaction into neoliberal empire and thus ignores the fact that communities within Ecuador have often gained power in the face of marketisation via transnational links of solidarity (for examples, see Alvarez, Faria, & Nobre, 2004; Cole & Phillips, 2008; Radcliffe, 2001; Sawyer, 2007). Such international alliances could be harnessed to support both citizen power and the state, but only if they were visible. Overall, then, the Citizens' Revolution appears to be driven by an extreme fixation on the neoliberal enemy and the need for state-building, with paranoia obscuring nuance. The result is that historically marginalised groups are interpellated as participants in *Buen Vivir* exclusively as citizens of the state and not in terms of other ways that they have pursued wellbeing.

Indigenous experiences negotiating community autonomy illustrate that our concerns with the discourse of *Buen Vivir* are warranted. Constitutional reforms in 1998 and 2008 declared Ecuador a pluricultural and plurinational state and recognised a broad range of indigenous rights, including the rights to their own judicial systems. However, a 'lack of clarity around diverse national, regional, and local sovereignties' over mineral resources and cultural patrimony (Hill & Fernández-Salvador, 2017, pp. 119–120), and the absence of 'coordinating rules that would define the relationship between customary law and national law' (Thomas, 2017, p. 46), have left many questions of community self-governance open to executive or judicial interpretation. In a state whose legitimacy depends on development programmes financed by resource exploitation, 'local sovereignty is overwhelmingly overridden by national forms of sovereignty and control, despite state discourses of decentralisation' (Hill & Fernández-Salvador, 2017, pp. 132–133). As a result, the Correa administration has repeatedly eroded indigenous autonomy via regulations on mining, water, education, and the meaning of 'legitimate' indigeneity, and by increasing systems of resource exploitation that undermine 'the material conditions for the reproduction of indigenous communities' (Becker, 2013; Sieder & Barrera Vivero, 2017, p. 16).

The statist worldview of *Buen Vivir* and the Citizens' Revolution may work well in places where neoliberal policies, state weakness, and the lack of public services were accepted passively. Prior to the Citizens' Revolution, however, the people of Las Colinas[3] had already self-organized as an active citizenry engaged in substantial self-governance. They had claimed their 'citizen's power' by mobilising to get what they needed from the central government and from other actors via patronage, citizenship demands, and transnational alliances, but according to their own desires rather than the vision from Quito. These efforts can be thought of as 'vernacular statecraft' (Colloredo-Mansfeld, 2009) or the construction of 'state-ness' (Martínez, 2017). What follows, then, is a description of what happens when the state-led revolution is enacted upon already active communities. How do vernacular states respond to the reconstitution of the national state?

## Grassroots health activism in rural northwest Ecuador

Las Colinas – a rural, cloudforest region in the northwestern coastal province of Esmeraldas – has a long history of community self-organisation dating to the first *mestizo* colonists of the 1960s and 1970s (Friederic, 2014a, 2014b). Accustomed to political instability, the people of Las Colinas have tended to privilege autonomy and self-reliance in their negotiations with outsiders. These negotiations have become prominent in the last twenty years, as community leaders, transnational NGOs, and state agencies have initiated various development programmes in the region. Shifts in community organising for health care in Las Colinas reveal how relations between local civil society, transnational NGOs, and the state have been reconfigured during the Correa administration (2007–2017).

Since the 1960s and 1970s, most of the region's inhabitants have emigrated from the neighbouring province of Manabí, where agrarian reform, inheritance laws, overpopulation, and climatic conditions made cultivable land scarce. These *mestizo* colonists used cooperatives and patronage networks to carve homesteads, villages, and road networks into the cloudforest. To some degree, they fit national stereotypes of people from Manabí, which is seen as a lawless frontier where fiercely independent men lead self-reliant families and order is kept through internal justice (DeWalt, 2004; Hidrovo Quiñonez, 2003; Friederic, 2014b; Striffler & de La Torre, 2008). Now as then, Las Colinas' inhabitants live in a precarious state of poverty. They survive on minimal income and, as squatters without formal land rights, they suffer from an insecure relationship to the land that sustains them. Despite this, they have typically appreciated their distance from '*la mirada del estado*' (the view of the state).[4] For many years, visible state presence in Las Colinas consisted of brief police forays into the region in pursuit of fugitives and sporadic visits by the Ministry of the Environment. Even today, government infrastructure is limited to intermittent, short-term road improvements and inconsistent electricity; the government has yet to provide water or sanitation services, which are managed by households and communities themselves (Comité de Gestión, 2007; Friederic, 2014b).

In the 1990s, government agencies and NGOs became interested in the rich biodiversity of this region's virgin cloudforest which was threatened by colonisation. In 1996, the region was declared a national biological reserve, and most *campesinos* lost their land rights. Not surprisingly, Las Colinas' residents grew increasingly distrustful of the state over the next two decades. On the one hand, they criticise the state's failure to provide basic services – and yet, they often reframe their position by celebrating their own self-reliance. Don Marcelo, one of the first settlers in this area, described these processes in the following way:

The people who first arrived in this region came with very few possessions, just those they carried on their backs. Then from one moment to the next, the state comes in and says 'this is my property and we are no longer going to give you any land title because this is mine, this is protected area now, it is primary forest.' So, how do the people feel? They feel cheated, tricked, betrayed. Most of them had sold whatever little property they had in Manabí, or wherever they came from, and they wanted to resettle here and buy land and security for their children; but then they couldn't. Some just returned to Manabí, but for those of us who have stayed, the lack of trust has only increased. Nobody knows what is going to happen. Most people hope for change, but we have lots of doubt because we have lived through so many government deceptions. (Interview, 2008)

During the early 2000s, local leaders increasingly collaborated with transnational NGOs to access goods and services; however, they also used these collaborations to maintain their own autonomy and leverage attention from the Ecuadorean state (Friederic, 2015). At that time, there were low rates of coverage, especially for rural populations, and the health sector suffered from a severe lack of coordination (De Paepe et al., 2012). Las Colinas' residents had to travel to the district capital of Quinindé to access health services – a trip that could take up to two or three days depending on which village one came from, the state of the roads, and the season – and they often arrived to find the hospital with insufficient medication and staff.

Las Colinas' health difficulties came to a head in 2001, when cerebral malaria ravaged many of the region's villages. Local leaders from all 26 villages assembled to discuss how to fill the health service gap. They agreed to construct a small health post, asking a German doctor volunteering in the region to raise money to complement community contributions of labour and supplies. The doctor returned home to establish a German NGO and, over the next couple of years, Friederic and others formed sister organisations in the U.S., the UK, and Canada. A Quito-based NGO was established to receive donations from the Global North to assist with construction and administrative expenses of the health centre. In the remainder of this paper, we refer to this network of organisations as the NGO.

At a community assembly in April 2002, NGO funds were disbursed to a democratically elected, community health committee. The Campesino Health Committee, consisting of four men and two women, directed construction efforts, managed funds with oversight from the Quito based NGO, and solicited further assistance from Ecuador's central and municipal governments. The Campesino Health Committee and the NGOs agreed that the health centre should be fully owned by the community and built on legally recognised land. Propelled by surprisingly strong support from international donors, the municipality, and Las Colinas communities, the plan quickly grew from a basic health post to a full-service health centre. To support this expansion, NGO volunteers conducted research across the region to assess local people's health status according to conventional metrics and to gather data on how they conceptualised good health. This input led to a broader definition of health in line with LASM's social determination model; as focus group discussions progressed, definitions of health expanded from 'no illnesses' to healthy families, mutually respectful communities, clean environments, and the ability to meet basic needs. The health project therefore developed a new set of objectives focused on primary and preventative health care as well as improving the quality of life through community health education, environmental health, women's health, microeconomic initiatives, and capacity building.

After several months of feeling each other out, the NGO, health committee, MoH, and the Quinindé municipal hospital formalised a unique four-way partnership. This was the only partnership of its kind in Esmeraldas and one of only a few nationally. According to the *Convenio* (the formal agreement), the health centre remained under community ownership but was designated an official MoH '*subcentro de salud*' (or primary care subcentre). This made the MoH responsible for providing a rural doctor (or *médico rural*, a required post-graduate residency programme in rural areas), nurse, dentist, some equipment, and access to free medicine and nationwide health programmes (such as *Maternidad Gratuita*, or Free Maternity), though these obligations were rarely fulfilled in the first five years of the project.[5] The NGO was responsible for coordinating international medical volunteers, providing medical supplies and equipment, and raising funds to support the Campesino

Health Committee. The Health Committee worked with the NGO to supervise health centre staff and volunteers, to design community development programming and capacity building, and to plan, manage, and evaluate health centre operations.

During these early years, donations from the global North covered most health centre expenses (including medications and a laboratory technician, administrator, cooking/cleaning person, and nurse, all of whom were from Las Colinas and were supervised by the Campesino Health Committee), as well as two employees and an office in the Quito-based branch of the NGO. In addition, the NGO coordinated dozens of volunteer doctors and nurses for stays ranging from 3 to 12 months to complement MoH staff but with a focus on community outreach. The NGO's main goal, however, was not to finance the health centre but to enhance the health committee's management capacity and ability to negotiate with the MoH, so that the Campesino Health Committee could guarantee sustainable access to quality healthcare and support community autonomy moving forward. In fact, we initially expected that the NGO could cease its involvement in the region within five to ten years. However, this was compromised when the MoH implemented free universal health care in 2006, eliminating a one-dollar-per-consultation fee that was central to the health centre's plans for financial sustainability (Eckhardt, Forsberg, Wolf, & Crespo-Burgos, 2011).

Another significant aspect of the health project was the establishment of a network of community health workers (CHWs) and direct-to-village medical brigades. The CHWs met monthly to discuss local health needs and participate in workshops on skills including first aid, emergency medicine, family planning, nutrition, malaria prevention, community organising, public speaking, leadership, and basic accounting. The curriculum for CHWs was based on a combination of CHW input, medical volunteer and staff expertise, and input from the Health Committee and NGO staff (many of whom were well-versed in the principles of social medicine and primary health care). In their own communities, CHWs represented the health centre by promoting and providing information about health centre services, holding health education workshops, administering first aid, and attending emergencies using supplies from NGO-provided kits. Their most visible role in their communities was as organisers for health centre medical brigades, when doctors, nurses, dentists, and others visited distant communities to provide consultations and health education. In these early years, brigades were also intentionally designed to build trust and share knowledge through community meetings, focus groups, and interviews, as well as team building activities and informal conversations. At least twice a year, the medical team (accompanied by one member of the Campesino Health Committee and a CHW) would visit multiple communities, often taking a week or more for each brigade.

Throughout the 2000s, health services in Las Colinas remained imperfect. The resources gathered by Northern volunteers and the MoH were never adequate to meet all of the region's health needs (Ordóñez Llanos, 2005). Some volunteers were still medical students, placing us in the ethically tricky position of providing staff who had not finished their training, a practice that was abandoned once MoH staff were provided on a constant basis. And the CHWs' work was a significant responsibility that only partially compensated for a lack of government resources. As unpaid volunteers whose work was not always recognised by their fellow community members, CHWs' commitment and participation waxed and waned; yet nearly all communities had a CHW representative who offered their services with pride (Ordóñez Llanos, 2005). One CHW from that period described his experience in the following way,

> First of all, we come here to participate in workshops, and then we take that knowledge back to our communities and inform people about the themes, for example, how to prevent certain diseases. But we know that we can't do everything, we are not doctors who can diagnose, but we can offer what we have learned, orient people, or give them first aid. (Interview, 2005)

Many described this work as empowering both individually and for their communities. As another CHW remarked,

I've been very content with my participation over these years, even when people in my community don't recognize how much I've spent of my time and money to participate in this project. But it feels good, good to serve others, good to fulfil this role, almost as if it lifts the soul. (Interview, 2005)

Through the 2000s, the NGO built significant community-owned health assets, including the health centre, an ambulance, and a multi-use building to house volunteers, MoH medical staff, and special events. The Campesino Health Committee took a leadership role with regards to health and other forms of community development, providing substantial direction to volunteer and government medical staff. Also, NGO staff in Quito and the health centre administrator served as representatives from the community to the state and transnational partners. The health administrator, for example, regularly lobbied (and continues to lobby) the municipal hospital for required medications, health centre equipment and supplies, and the best *médicos rurales*. This built-in intermediation was meant to ensure a key goal of social medicine: the 'redistribution of power and resources among the distinct groups implicated in healthcare decisions,' (Vázquez et al., 2002, p. 33).

The health impacts were impressive. Depending on the season and staffing, the health centre treated anywhere from 40 (in 2001–2002) to 300 patients per month (2006). Through extensive distribution of bed nets during health brigades and via CHWs, malaria transmission in the region was eliminated, despite the fact that malaria was one of the most prevalent and deadly illnesses when the project was initiated. Though reliable data are still difficult to access, childhood vaccination rates have increased at least five-fold since 2001.

The *Convenio de Integración* was important for fostering and sustaining this deep participation. Community members take great pride in the fact of their ownership, in keeping with their ideal of self-reliance and mistrust of both the state and other potential partners. In interviews and meetings, they repeatedly emphasise their ownership and management of the health centre as evidence of their success in community organising and their capacity for self-governance. The NGO has viewed the *Convenio* as an important indication that they are not merely creating a relationship of dependency but instead they are supporting participatory governance by local institutions (in this case, both the state and the community). And the national and municipal governments saw the *Convenio* as a convenient way to provide services to a population in need without investing many resources, since most of the work and funding fell to the NGO and management fell to the community. As we will see, though, this perspective changed in the late 2000s. The history of state–community–NGO relations in Las Colinas contradicts assertions that NGOs are unambiguously part of neoliberal projects; while NGOs have sometimes substituted for state service provision, local inhabitants have also used NGO partners to struggle with and against the state and to expand both the state presence and community autonomy (see also Friederic, 2015; Biermann, Eckhardt, Carlfjord, Falk, & Forsberg, 2016).

## *La Revolución* in practice: post-neoliberal health care and changes in grassroots health activism

One measure of the partnership's success was increased state commitment to fulfilling basic health rights. Though bolstered by national increases in health funding authorised by Correa as minister of economy and then as president, Las Colinas received a particularly large increase in government support due to community activism. By constructing a high-quality health centre, the community and NGO laid the groundwork for significant MoH involvement. By 2008, the MoH was providing full-time staffing for the health centre and all major medications at no cost. However, as MoH capacity grew, and as MoH staff grew tired of hearing demands from the community and NGO, they began to ignore and sometimes actively resist the *Convenio*, often treating the health centre as if it were their own. One particularly comedic example of this came in 2009, when we returned from a medical brigade to learn that two MoH administrators had visited the health centre and volunteer house in our absence to inventory 'their' equipment, including a dental chair, exam beds, coffee pots, and toaster ovens that belonged to the community and even international volunteers. Aside from the question of fictitious ownership, increased government involvement led to professionalisation and 'seeing like a state' rather than community input, planning, and evaluation (Scott, 1998). This critique of Correa's administration extends to other sectors, with Ecuadorean activists remarking that 'after the Constitution in 2008, people disengaged from politics because that's when people got incorporated into the bureaucratic system,' which also 'weakened social organising' more broadly (Miranda, 2017). In Las Colinas, in particular, the strengthening of the state deeply affected both community participation and basic health service delivery.

From 2008 on, the role and participation of CHWs declined overall, despite punctuated bursts of activity due to short term programmes that garnered their interest (for example, a NOKIA-funded mobile communications and data collection project and the implementation of malaria rapid tests). The MoH explicitly encouraged the participation of CHWs in its planning, yet workshops with CHWs led by MoH medical staff were often characterised as 'boring' or 'too technical.' CHWs still valued the learning, but they complained that they did not feel like their input or work was being appreciated. As one long-time CHW characterised the shift:

> It's just not like it was before, when we participated, and we laughed so much. We were welcome to sleep at the health centre when we couldn't get back to our communities after full day workshops. We were tired but we enjoyed it because we felt it was our home, it was another family…. We were all in the work together. Now we just sit and listen to the experts tell us things. They are nice and they know a lot, but it's not like it was. (Interview, 2014)

CHWs no longer felt essential to the project, instead seeing their responsibilities reduced to 'bringing letters' to their community about health centre services and events, but 'that's it.'

The NGO and Campesino Health Committee initially celebrated the fact that the MoH was taking more responsibility for service provision and, as governance of the health project evolved, the NGO shifted its focus to outreach in distant communities. By 2012, however, CHWs were significantly less active and the frequency of brigades had declined to one to two per year. Perhaps most importantly, the Campesino Health Committee had substantially less influence over health centre programming, primarily because bureaucratic demands on medical staff allowed them less flexibility to adapt to community needs.

While outreach is still important on paper to the MoH, staff complain that the need to show 'high production,' or a high quantity of patients, disincentivises outreach in distant communities. Amid isolated homesteads, they see fewer patients than they would at the health centre located in the region's most densely populated village. As doctors tried to compensate for the 'unproductivity' of brigades, they increased formal workshops and talks and decreased the amount of time dedicated to building trust and soliciting community input. Furthermore, brigades now required complex and onerous planning, coordination, and paperwork. Medical staff regularly complained about needing to solicit permission to be absent from the clinic, put in requests for extra medication, and wait for those to arrive (which they often did not). After brigades, they then had to produce official reports verifying that they saw enough patients and dispensed enough medications to justify the brigade.

The emphasis on metrics and documentation has changed the way health education is provided, as evidence in the following excerpt from Friederic's field notes:

> Last night, the young rural doctor was up until 11 pm creating a poster for today's talk on breastfeeding. The perfectionist that he is, he was up for three hours tracing drawings from books of maternal figures with babies. In the morning, he asked me to take pictures of him with his precise, intricate drawings. When I asked why he needed the photographs, he said, 'The Ministry [MoH] wants to see what we are doing for the community. I have to have documentation of meetings with community members so I need to get a photo of the meeting today and a photo of the attendance sheet. But they always want to see if I am making a good poster. It's important that we do this. But I tell you, it is a shame that I can't do a talk on dengue, considering the outbreak we're in the midst of!' When I asked why not, he replied, 'Well, because it's international breastfeeding week, and it's part of the planning we were given for the month, so we have to give at least one talk about that theme in the community with at least 20 participants. They have a set calendar and schedule of the important themes throughout the year.'

At the talk later that day, the doctor, who was quite shy when it came to public speaking, explained the important nutrients that mothers passed on to their babies through breastmilk. He was meticulous, but he used difficult medical language and failed to connect with his audience. The crowd was uncomfortable and a bit confused, though certainly appreciative of his efforts. After the talk, I asked a friend what she thought, and she said, 'it was good, he was very knowledgeable.' When I urged her to explain to another friend what it was all about, she said, 'I don't remember the details, but he told us it is very important to breastfeed.' (Fieldnotes, 2014)

Outreach, or increased contact with people outside the clinical setting, is certainly valued by the MoH and health centre staff. However, outreach is prioritised (at least in part) because deeper penetration into the communities allows for greater surveillance and coverage, two concepts that are central to the MoH's national health care plan. Outreach is also planned at national and municipal levels, disallowing the type of flexible and adaptive work that the Campesino Health Committee once promoted. Whereas health education was once community driven, with health promoters choosing the themes, shaping the content of workshops, and often participating in the delivery of workshops, they (like the rest of the population) have become passive beneficiaries. So, while MoH health centre staff characterise recent shifts in national health care as increasingly oriented towards community outreach, there have been major changes in what counts as outreach, which activities are prioritised, and what form of participation they provoke. In order to fulfil the community outreach requirement, it is well-known that most staff prefer giving educational talks in the central village (and counting the number of heads present, or that walk by), or visiting households in the nearest communities, which can be accessed by car and visited in one day so that staff can sleep in their own apartments.

Audit culture and the fetishisation of 'production' has transformed the provision of health care in Ecuador, much like it has in the field of global health more broadly (Adams, 2016; Brotherton, 2012). In recent years, teams of vaccinators have been hired and trained by the MOH on a short-term basis. They travel out to remote areas with low rates of vaccination coverage, like Las Colinas. In 2014, we travelled with one of the medical brigades to a community six hours from the health centre. Even before the doctors began to see patients, the vaccinator walked up to every adult present, including those participating in the soccer game beside the school, and began administering vaccines with little to no explanation. He barely mumbled which vaccine he was giving, he did not ask adults if they had received the vaccination before, and he failed to notify people if they needed follow-up booster shots. In most cases, they did. The vaccinator even pressured two of our students into getting yellow fever and tetanus vaccinations, diligently logging them into his notebook, despite the fact that these non-Ecuadorean students had already been immunised. The vaccinator was getting paid and evaluated per dose administered. If he did not administer all of the doses, he would be chastised, as valuable doses would have to be thrown out. Plus, as with medications in the health centre, the quantity used during this brigade would determine how many we would be given for future brigades. As the dentist noted when jumping onto her mule to leave the community, 'the only thing the Ministry cares about is production, production, production, it's all about the numbers.'

This was a common sentiment among MoH medical staff and the long-term health centre staff hired by the Campesino Health Committee. In 2014, Friederic asked a community staff member (who had been with the health project since 2002) about the increased role of the MoH in health care in Las Colinas:

Yes, there have been good changes. For example in terms of medications, we're better stocked … . But it all depends … on 'production,' or on all of the work that the doctor does. Because everything begins from there. And also the people who come, the patients. For example we can look at the patients with chronic illnesses, like the diabetics. This is an established program and it's already in the hospital but [resources] all depend on whether the patient comes from month to month, does their check-up, is taking their medications, is having their exams, and is controlling things. Then the doctor takes his report [about patient compliance] and passes it on. Here we have 20 diabetics and this month all showed up, so this means that for the next month, all of the medicine will come for those patients. But if the patient doesn't come, the doctor doesn't have to report [that they exist], and then we don't get the medications. Sometimes we don't have medicine for diabetics, or we don't have the strips to do the exams. [Also], the things that have to do with family planning sometimes don't come. It all depends on the production, on the [patients] who come, because one isn't going to ask [for resources] on behalf of patients who aren't doing their controls. It's just not possible.

On the other hand, for example, right now we've been asking for lab supplies for more than a month. So in this case it's the hospital's problem. I was asking for them and they don't give them … . Sometimes there's a delay in purchasing or uploading requests … when there are administrative changes in the region. And sometimes this has happened and we don't have medicine here. Sometimes patients come and there's no medicine. Then it's no longer our fault. Maybe it's the region's fault. But yes, things have gotten a lot better in this respect.

This focus on numbers, coverage, and statistical surveillance reveals that the 'revolución ciudadana' (insofar as it concerns healthcare) is successfully reaching most populations, but it encourages token forms of inclusion while discouraging deeper types of participation. This system is not currently designed to respond to needs but to provide coverage, which is broadly and shallowly construed, and to be highly visible in the performance of providing coverage.

People in the village seem quite content. Like the woman at the breastfeeding workshop and the long-term health centre staff we cited above, they remark on the performance of coverage (informative talks, increased house visits, vaccination campaigns, etc.) and downplay questions about effectiveness. The health centre doctor is enthusiastic about his role 'serving the pueblo' with an increased emphasis on prevention, but he acknowledges that the medication is always running out, and the demands of data collection are completely out-of-touch with reality. 'But,' he says, 'if we had money and good infrastructure (like technology, roads, medication), then this would be another story.' In response, the dentist (who was trained in Cuba) responded, 'no, this is all a farce. I mean, it looks good on paper, but that's it,' later implying that the entire emphasis of the new programmes was on metrics and shallow participation.

## Conclusions

The health activism we describe here was only one facet of Las Colinas' self-organisation. From 2000 to 2008, the community also lobbied the government and NGOs for other initiatives, including clean water, road improvements, police presence, economic cooperatives, and ecotourism. At the time, it seemed that new community organisations were forming at every turn, and both NGO staff and community members would marvel at the unified organising that seemed to be at the heart of community life in Las Colinas. Of course there were factions and most of the workload fell on an 'elite' group of leaders, but all would agree that this was a period of growth, excitement, and possibility. The hopeful rhetoric of the Citizens' Revolution really captured this spirit – and in fact, the majority is still Correísta. However, the last several years have left people struggling to explain the splintering and de-activation of so many local organisations. People in Las Colinas often attribute the current 'apathy' or 'lack of organisation' to 'the youth of today who don't know what it means to really suffer' or a culture of 'handouts' that has made people lazy. Others point out that a generation of community leaders has moved, died, or directed their efforts to improving life for their own families rather than the community. While contributors to the slowdown in organising are diverse, we posit that the state-centred and context-blind approach of the Citizens' Revolution and Buen Vivir are also a major cause of community de-mobilization. Interestingly, post-neoliberalism promotes state-based decentralisation as an antidote to neoliberalism's market-based decentralisation, but both approaches ignore a third option of community-based decentralisation.

Our case study makes an important contribution to research on the Latin American Pink Tide by illustrating that the Ecuadorean state's contradictory approach to decentralisation and participation is governed not only by a desire to appropriate extractivist revenues for reinvestment in social programmes, but also by a broader state-building project. In our case, the state is undermining local sovereignty and communal institutions because they need to accomplish the identity work of the cultural/citizens' revolution. Instead of autonomy, it offers a new model of citizenship that incorporates rural people as beneficiaries of the Citizens' Revolution, but in a way that reinscribes their marginality and poverty – 'receiving' is key to the performative symbolism of citizenship, just as 'providing' is key to the state's performances. To bring everyone into their roles, the state has to undo competing sovereignties in order to re-incorporate community members as citizens. In short, the Citizens' Revolution is inclusive not through invitation but through the erosion of alternative sovereignties.

Ultimately, however, to avoid the romanticisation of community we must evaluate the trade-offs between state and community. Advocates of post-neoliberalism and LASM, which hope for strong and generous states, cannot automatically opt for community power. As Atun, et al. argue, decentralised health systems like the one in Las Colinas circa 2004 can democratise health services and empower communities, but they have also 'generated more complex environments for governance and performance management' and raise the possibility for new forms of inequality and health system fragmentation (2015, p. 1235). Furthermore, states in the process of re-consolidation may fear that community power and vernacular statecraft will yield counterhegemonic movements that are not only anti-neoliberal but also anti-state. As Martínez (2017) notes, communities succeed in taking control over resources and governance – even in the face of corporate and state opposition – primarily when they have strong organising traditions, are able to use rights discourses effectively in official spheres, and build a strong web of translocal allies. The Ecuadorean state's position is, most likely, that it is far better to surrender community power to an ostensibly democratic and well-intentioned state than to risk transnational alliances that may support communities but may also be backdoors for neoliberal and neocolonial resurgences.

While we continue to welcome the strengthening of the Ecuadorean state and increased funding and reform in the MoH, we believe there are both normative and pragmatic reasons to be concerned about the erosion of community self-organising. Among the latter, we would like to underscore four. First, as we have shown here, and Rasch and Bywater (2014) have argued regarding urban Ecuador, top-down, state-administered health systems are often insufficiently responsive to local needs and demands. Second, states in countries as diverse as Ecuador rarely represent local interests adequately, but this can be addressed in large part by creating mechanisms for real community influence. Third, democratic and progressive governance is further undermined in Ecuador by the central contradiction of post-neoliberalism – that the anti-neoliberal state and its public services are dependent upon transnational capital and precarious petrodollars. And finally, the erosion of community organising leaves communities vulnerable in the event that the Ecuadorean state is destabilised in the future.

Crucially, the cautionary tale of Las Colinas' health activism also applies to LASM itself. As critical public health activists promote basic rights to health and combat political and economic determinants of disease, state policy and state services will be among the most valuable levers for change. Engaging the state with oversimplified understandings of local context, however, will often be counter-productive, especially in traditionally marginalised communities that are already organising creatively for their own health and well-being. A more sound approach might include strengthening transnational solidarities, establishing *convenios* between official and vernacular states, and encouraging empowered communities to create alternatives to standardised metrics so they can establish health priorities and health professionals can be flexible enough to meet local needs. We hope that a more mature Citizens' Revolution will encourage state- and citizen-building through state–community–NGO partnerships, even when those partnerships magnify contradictions in the national project.

## Notes

1. In this article, we use the term 'social determination of health' when referring to LASM and Marxist approaches to health, and we use 'social determinants' as a broader term referring to the more proximate social factors that influence health and illness, as it is used by the World Health Organization. As Morales-Borrero, Borde, Eslava-Castañeda, and Concha-Sánchez (2013) note, these terms are not synonymous; instead, they reflect different conceptual understandings of causation and prevention, as well as distinct ethical-political entry points.

Whereas 'social determination of health' invokes a critique of capitalist development, 'social determinant' approaches identify risk factors and propose improvements 'within an inherently unjust system' (Eslava, Borde, Morales, & Torres-Tovar, 2015; Morales-Borrero et al., 2013).

2. Inequality declined as measured by the GINI coefficient and as the ratio between the top and bottom deciles of the income distribution (Ray & Kozameh, 2012; Weisbrot et al., 2017).

3. In keeping with anthropological convention, we use a pseudonym, Las Colinas, to refer to the region discussed in this article.

4. To be clear, we are not arguing that the state is irrelevant even in this 'out-of-the-way' place (Tsing, 1993; McCullough, Brunson, & Friederic, 2014; Friederic, 2014b). 'Vernacular statecraft' through seemingly autonomous practices (e.g. communal labour organising, self-organized land colonisation, and the use of local judicial councils) is nonetheless shaped by Quito's selective presence and absence (Colloredo-Mansfeld, 2009).

5. Later, the MoH would provide an OB-GYN, additional staff, and other programmes.

## Acknowledgements

This article is dedicated to our dear friend, Guido. Thank you to staff and volunteers at the health clinic in Las Colinas (a pseudonym) and the NGO for your collaboration. At various stages, Karin Friederic's fieldwork was supported by the National Science Foundation, the Wenner-Gren Foundation, the P.E.O. Foundation, the Harry Frank Guggenheim Foundation, the Feminist Review Trust, the University of Arizona, and Wake Forest University. IRB Approval was attained through the University of Arizona and Wake Forest University, and a research permit attained through the Ministry of the Environment in Ecuador (2007). Brian Burke's fieldwork in Ecuador was supported by the Goodnight Family Sustainable Development Department at Appalachian State University.

## Disclosure statement

In accordance with Taylor & Francis policy and my ethical obligation as a researcher, I, Karin Friederic, am reporting that I have served as a co-founder and volunteer board member of a non-profit organisation that has developed projects in this region of Ecuador, as noted in the article. I have no reason to believe that my organisation will benefit from publication of this article or that any other conflicts of interest may arise from this affiliation.

## Funding

At various stages, Karin Friederic's fieldwork was supported by the National Science Foundation, the Wenner-Gren Foundation, the P.E.O. Foundation, the Harry Frank Guggenheim Foundation, the Feminist Review Trust, the University of Arizona, and Wake Forest University. Brian Burke's fieldwork in Ecuador was supported by the Goodnight Family Sustainable Development Department at Appalachian State University.

## References

Acosta, A. (2008). El buen vivir, una oportunidad por construir. *Ecuador Debate, 75* (December), 33–47.

Acosta, A. (2013). *El buen vivir: Sumak kawsay, una oportunidad para imaginar otros mundos.* Barcelona: Icaria.

Adams, V. (2016). *Metrics: What counts in global health.* Durham: Duke University Press.

Alvarez, S., Faria, N., & Nobre, M. (2004). Another (also feminist) world is possible: Constructing transnational spaces and global alternatives from the movements. In J. Sen, A. Anand, A. Escobar, & P. Waterman (Eds.), *World social forum: Challenging empires* (pp. 199–206). New Delhi: Viveka Foundation.

Arango Panesso, Y. (2008). Referentes socio-históricos latinoamericanos: Contribución a los fundamentos políticos de la promoción de salud. *Revista Cubana de Salud Pública, 34*(1), Retrieved from http://ref.scielo.org/y6s34f

Atun, R., Monteiro de Andrade, L. O., Almeida, G., Cotlear, D., Dmytraczenko, T., Frenz, P., … Wagstaff, A. (2015). Health-system reform and universal health coverage in Latin America. *The Lancet, 385*, 1230–1247.

Backman, G., Hunt, P., Khosla, R., Jaramillo-Strouss, C., Fikre, B. M., Rumble, C., … Vladescu, C. (2008). Health systems and the right to health: An assessment of 194 countries. *The Lancet, 372*(9655), 2047–2085.

Becker, M. (2011). Correa, indigenous movements, and the writing of a new constitution in Ecuador. *Latin American Perspectives, 38*(1), 47–62.

Becker, M. (2012). Building a plurinational Ecuador: Complications and contradictions. *Socialism and Democracy, 26* (3), 72–92.

Becker, M. (2013). The stormy relations between Rafael Correa and social movements in Ecuador. *Latin American Perspectives, 40*(3), 43–62.

Biermann, O., Eckhardt, M., Carlfjord, S., Falk, M., & Forsberg, B. C. (2016). Collaboration between non-governmental organizations and public services in health – a qualitative case study from rural ecuador. *Global Health Action, 9*, 32237.

Breilh, J. (1995, November). *La medicina social ecuatoriana; promesas y falencias en 50 años de producción: avances y problemas conceptuales, metodológicos y técnicos.* Paper presented at the Congreso Ecuatoriano de Biopatología Andina y Tropical.

Bretón, V., Cortez, D., & Garcia, F. (2014). En busca del sumak kawsay: Presentación del dossier. *Íconos Revista de Ciencias Sociales, 48*, 9–24.

Brotherton, P. S. (2012). *Revolutionary medicine: Health and the body in post-soviet Cuba.* Durham, NC: Duke University Press.

Cole, S., & Phillips, L. (2008). The violence against women campaigns in Latin America: New feminist alliances. *Feminist Criminology, 3*(2), 145–168.

Colloredo-Mansfeld, R. (2009). *Fighting like a community: Andean civil society in an era of Indian uprisings.* Chicago: University of Chicago Press.

Comité de Gestión. (2007). *Propuesta: Resolución de conflictos de tenencia de la tierra dentro de la Reserva Ecológica.* Unpublished document. Comité de Gestión de 'El Páramo,' Esmeraldas, Ecuador.

Cornwall, A., & Coelho, V. S. P. (2007). Spaces for change? The politics of participation in new democratic arenas. In A. Cornwall & V. S. P. Coelho (Eds.), *Spaces for change? The politics of participation in new democratic spaces* (pp. 1–32). London: Zed Books.

De Paepe, P., Tapia, R. E., Santacruz, E. A., & Unger, J.-P. (2012). Ecuador's silent health reform. *International Journal of Health Services, 42*(2), 219–233.

DeWalt, K. M. (2004). *Women's work and domestic violence in Manabí, Ecuador.* Paper presented at the annual meeting of the society for applied anthropology, Dallas, TX.

Eckhardt, M., Forsberg, B., Wolf, D., & Crespo-Burgos, A. (2011). Feasibility of community-based health insurance in rural tropical Ecuador. *Revista Panamericana de Salud Pública, 29*(3), 177–184.

Eslava, J. C., Borde, E., Morales, C., & Torres-Tovar, M. (2015, November 20). Social determination of the health-disease process: a new insertion to the lexicon. IHP: Switching the Poles in International Health Policy. Retrieved from http://www.internationalhealthpolicies.org/social-determination-of-the-health-disease-process-a-new-insertion-to-the-lexicon/

Fernández, B. S., Pardo, L., & Salamanca, K. (2014). El buen vivir en Ecuador: ¿marketing político o proyecto en disputa? Un diálogo con Alberto Acosta. *Íconos Revista de Ciencias Sociales, 48*, 9–24.

Friederic, K. (2011). The challenges of advocacy in anthropological research on intimate partner violence. *Practicing Anthropology, 33*(3), 27–31.

Friederic, K. (2014a). Violence against women and the contradictions of rights-in-practice in rural Ecuador. *Latin American Perspectives, 41*(1), 19–38.

Friederic, K. (2014b). The 'SONY Nightclub': Rural brothels, gender violence, and development in coastal Ecuador. *Ethnos, 79*(5), 650–676.

Friederic, K. (2015). Gender violence, social change, and applied anthropology in coastal Ecuador. In J. R. Wies & H. H. Haldane (Eds.), *Applying anthropology to gender-based violence: Global responses, local practices.* (pp. 167–182). Lanham, MD: Lexington Books.

Granda Ugalde, E. (2009). *La salud y la vida. Vol. 1.* Quito: Imprenta Noción.

Hartmann, C. (2016). Postneoliberal public health care reforms: Neoliberalism, social medicine, and persistent health inequalities in Latin America. *American Journal of Public Health, 106*(12), 2145–2151. Advance online publication. doi:10.2105/AJPH.2016.303470.

Harvey, D. (2005). *A brief history of neoliberalism.* Oxford: Oxford University Press.

Hickey, S., & Mohan, G. (2004). *Participation: From tyranny to transformation? Exploring new approaches to participation in development.* London: Zed Books.

Hidrovo Quiñonez, T. (2003). *Manabí histórico: Del conocimiento a la "comprensión".* Portoviejo: Editorial Mar Abierto.

Hill, M. D., & Fernández-Salvador, C. (2017). When cultural and natural patrimony collide: Sovereignty, state power, and political strategy among the picapedreros (stonemasons) of San Pablo, Ecuador. *The Journal of Latin American and Caribbean Anthropology, 22*(1), 116–136.

Laurell, A. C. (1989). Social analysis of collective health in Latin America. *Social Science and Medicine, 28*(11), 1183–1191.

Macas, L. (2010). Sumak Kawsay: La vida en plenitud. *América Latina en Movimiento, 452*, n.p.

Martínez, J. C. (2017). The state in waiting: State-ness disputes in indigenous territories. *The Journal of Latin American and Caribbean Anthropology, 22*(1), 62–84.

McCullough, M. B., Brunson, J., & Friederic, K. (2014). Introduction: Intimacies and sexualities in out-of-the-way places. *Ethnos, 79*(5), 577–584.

Ministerio de Salud Pública. (2013). *Manual del Modelo de Atención Integral de Salud – MAIS.* Quito: Ministerio de Salud Pública del Ecuador.

Ministerio de Salud Pública. (2014). Ecuador firma cinco convenios de salud con Cuba. Retrieved from http://www. salud.gob.ec/ecuador-firma-cinco-convenios-de-salud-con-cuba/#

Miranda, B. (2017, April 3). As Correa's historic presidency ends, 6 Ecuadorian activists reflect on the results of La Revolución Ciudadana. REMEZCLA. Retrieved from http://remezcla.com/lists/culture/six-ecuadorian-activists-reflect-correa-presidency/

Morales-Borrero, C., Borde, E., Eslava-Castañeda, J. C., & Concha-Sánchez, S. C. (2013). Conceptual differences and praxiological implications concerning social determination or social determinants. Revista Salud Pública (Bogota), 15(16), 797–808.

Navarro, V. (2008). Neoliberalism and its consequences: The world health situation since Alma Ata. Global Social Policy: An Interdisciplinary Journal of Public Policy and Social Development, 8, 152–155. doi:10.1177/ 14680181080080020203

North, L. L. (2013). New left regimes in the Andes? Ecuador in comparative perspective. Studies in Political Economy, 91(1), 113–136.

Ordóñez Llanos, G. (2005). Inequities and effective coverage: Review of a community health programme in Esmeraldas – Ecuador. (MA), KIT (Royal Tropical Institute), Amsterdam, Netherlands.

Pan American Health Organization (PAHO). (2017). Country profile: Ecuador. Infant and maternal morality. In Perfiles de Salud, Core health indicators initiative, health information platform for the americas (PLISA). Washington, DC: Pan American Health Organization. Retrieved May 30, 2018, from http://www.paho.org/data/ index.php/es/analisis/perfiles-de-salud/275-perfiles-nacional-mortalidad-infantil-materna.html

Radcliffe, S. A. (2001). Development, the state, and transnational political connections: State and subject formations in Latin America. Global Networks, 1(1), 19–36.

Rasch, D., & Bywater, K. (2014). Health promotion in Ecuador: A solution for a failing system. Health, 06(10), 916– 925. doi:10.4236/health.2014.610115

Ray, R., & Kozameh, S. (2012). Ecuador's economy since 2007. Washington, DC: Center for Economic and Policy Research.

Sawyer, S. (2007). Empire/multitude—state/civil society: Rethinking topographies of power through transnational connectivity in Ecuador and beyond. Social Analysis, 51(2), 64–85.

Scott, J. C. (1998). Seeing like a state: How certain schemes to improve the human condition have failed. New Haven, CT: Yale University Press.

Secretaría Nacional de Planificación y Desarrollo (SENPLADES). (2010). Republic of Ecuador national development plan. National plan for good living 2009–2013: Building a plurinational and intercultural state. Quito: SENPLADES.

Sieder, R., & Barrera Vivero, A. (2017). Legalizing indigenous self-determination: Autonomy and buen vivir in Latin America. The Journal of Latin American and Caribbean Anthropology, 22(1), 9–26.

Striffler, S., & de La Torre, C. (2008). Introduction. In S. Striffler & C. de La Torre (Eds.), The Ecuador reader: The history, culture, politics (pp. 1–7). Durham: Duke University Press.

Tajer, D. (2003). Latin American social medicine: Roots, development during the 1990s, and current challenges. American Journal of Public Health, 93(12), 2023–2027.

Thomas, M. S. (2017). The effects of formal legal pluralism on indigenous authorities in the Ecuadorian highlands. The Journal of Latin American and Caribbean Anthropology, 22(1), 46–61.

Tsing, A. L. (1993). In the realm of the diamond queen: Marginality in an out-of-the-way place. Princeton, NJ: Princeton University Press.

Vázquez, M. L., Siqueira, E., Kruze, I., Da Silva, A., & Leite, I. C. (2002). Los procesos de reforma y la participación social en salud en América Latina. Gaceta Sanitaria, 16(1), 30–38. doi:10.1016/S0213-9111(02)71630-0

Waitzkin, H., Iriart, C., Estrada, A., & Lamadrid, S. (2001). Social medicine in Latin America: Productivity and dangers facing the major national groups. The Lancet, 358, 315–323.

Weisbrot, M., Johnston, J., & Merling, L. (2017). Decade of reform: Ecuador's macroeconomic policies, institutional changes, and results. Washington, DC: Center for Economic and Policy Research.

Whitten, Jr., N. E., & Whitten, D. S. (2015). Clashing concepts of the 'good life': Beauty, knowledge, and vision versus national wealth in Amazonian Ecuador. In F. Santos-Granero (Ed.), Images of public wealth or the anatomy of well-being in indigenous Amazonia (pp. 191–215). Tucson: University of Arizona Press.

World Health Organization. (2017). Ecuador statistics summary (2002 – present). Quito: World Health Organization Country Office. Retrieved from http://www.who.int/countries/ecu/en/

# Social transformation, collective health and community-based arts: 'Buen Vivir' and Ecuador's social circus programme

J. B. Spiegel, B. Ortiz Choukroun, A. Campaña, K. M. Boydell, J. Breilh and A. Yassi

**ABSTRACT**
Worldwide, interest is increasing in community-based arts to promote social transformation. This study analyzes one such case. Ecuador's government, elected in 2006 after decades of neoliberalism, introduced *Buen Vivir* ('good living' derived from the Kichwan *sumak kawsay*), to guide development. Plans included launching a countrywide programme using circus arts as a sociocultural intervention for street-involved youth and other marginalised groups. To examine the complex ways by which such interventions intercede in 'ways of being' at the individual and collective level, we integrated qualitative and quantitative methods to document relationships between programme policies over a 5-year period and transformations in personal growth, social inclusion, social engagement and health-related lifestyles of social circus participants. We also conducted comparisons across programmes and with youth in other community arts. While programmes emphasising social, collective and inclusive pedagogy generated significantly better wellbeing outcomes, economic pressures led to prioritising productive skill-building and performing. Critiques of the government's operationalisation of *Buen Vivir*, including its ambitious technical goals and pragmatic economic compromising, were mirrored in social circus programmes. However, the programme seeded a grassroots social circus movement. Our study suggests that creative programmes introduced to promote social transformation can indeed contribute significantly to nurturing a culture of collective wellbeing.

## Introduction

The election of a national government in Ecuador in 2006 that dubbed itself the 'Citizens' Revolution' responded to the demand for social change that was sweeping Latin America. The new Ecuadorian Constitution enacted in 2008 proposed *Buen Vivir* as the guiding principle for government policies (Government of Ecuador, 2008), with national development plans (Secretaria Nacional de Planificación y Desarrollo [SENPLADES], 2009, 2013), emphasising wellbeing beyond conventional economic indicators. *Buen Vivir* translates roughly to 'good living' derived from the Kichwa *Sumak Kawsay*, albeit not without considerable controversy (Macas, 2010). The *Buen Vivir* Plan set the stage for one of the world's largest government-sponsored programmes using circus arts as a sociocultural intervention with communities in precarious situations.

Popularised in the later decades of the twentieth century, there are now over 350 'social circus' programmes around the world (Cirque du Soleil home page) -using a combination of juggling, clowning, acrobatics, aerials, and balancing disciplines amongst others, to promote inclusivity, trust, and creative expression (Spiegel, 2014). While many programmes approach circus as a means of promoting psychological and social transformation of participants, some programs focus on artistic training for economically marginalised groups, with the professionalisation of its participants – or at least labor and economic inclusion – increasingly constituting 'success', others some programs focus particularly on artistic training for economically marginalised groups.

Building from grassroots circus and theatrical initiatives already underway, *Circo Social Ecuador* materialised in April 2011 through an agreement between the then Vice-President, Lenin Moreno (now President) and several municipalities in Ecuador, followed a month later by an accord with the giant Montreal-based transnational circus company, *Cirque du Soleil* (Spiegel, in press-b; Spiegel, Breilh, Campana, Marcuse, & Yassi, 2015).[1] While *Cirque du Soleil's* branding as well as the 'services' it offers communities have been frequently problematised (Hurley & Léger, 2008; Leroux, 2012; Leslie & Rantisi, 2016), it remains the world's largest diffuser of social circus pedagogy. Drawing on the social circus model developed by this transnational entertainment corporation, the extensive Ecuadorian State support for this national community arts programme was remarkable for the ways in which it explicitly aims to promote a transformation in social and cultural logic. According to Mr. Moreno, *Circo Social Ecuador* was designed to: (1) create a cultural alternative for empowering vulnerable communities; (2) support protection of children and adolescents at-risk; (3) bring together young people to promote social movements and strengthen their sense of national cultural identity in a manner appropriate to each locality; (4) facilitate integrative activities with other national social projects as well as public and private initiatives; and (5) develop values of solidarity, participation, discipline, concentration, cooperation, self-esteem, personal and collective development, and a sense of belonging. Importantly, the goal was also explicitly to 'achieve a multiplier effect throughout the country' (Programa Circo Social Ecuador, 2012).

As practices are appropriated and re-appropriated, disbursed through global networks of 'development programmes', the 'beneficiaries', and indeed, even the 'practitioners' of such circulating practices are caught in the nexus of the institutional cultures through which they encounter and diffuse the arts deemed 'transformative'. As Homi Bhabha (Bhabha, 2012) famously theorised, this practice of engaging with new images and visions can involve cultural submission, cultural resistance, or sometimes both simultaneously, particularly within the context of colonial practices and cultural hierarchies. Commenting on the new social vision of the Ecuadorian government, cultural theorist Catherine Walsh queried:

> It is a project that entails, and demands, the creation of radically different conditions of existence and of knowledge, power, and life, conditions that could contribute to construct really intercultural societies, where the values of complementarity, relationality, reciprocity, and solidarity get to prevail …. [But] Are they willing to think and act with the historically subordinated and marginalized peoples; to unlearn their uninational, colonial, and monocultural learning; and to relearn to learn so as to be able to complement each other, and co-exist and co-live ethically? (Walsh, 2009, p. 235, 212)

This vision – and the social, cultural and epistemological politics and challenges toward which it points – was the context of our inquiry. In light of the post-colonial ambitions that characterised the launching of *Circo Social Ecuador*, it became crucial for us to develop a lens of inquiry in keeping with the stated aims, and constructed through dialogue concerning these goals, in order to assess how the social and cultural policies of social circus enacted under the new rubric were affecting individuals and communities.

The extent to which various visions of social circus are being actualised worldwide, under what conditions, and with what challenges has only begun to be examined. Gains have been found in helping participants to 'reconnect to their bodies' and increase their physical expression and mobility (Kelaher

& Dunt, 2009; Loiselle, 2015; Spiegel & Parent, 2017), 'feel empowered' or 'self-confident' (Archambault, 2014; Kelaher & Dunt, 2009; Loiselle, 2015; McCaffery, 2011; Savolainen & Suoniemi, 2015; Spiegel & Parent, 2017; Trotman, 2012), as well as increase their general 'sense of happiness', wellbeing or 'fun' (Cadwell & Rooney, 2013; Kinnunen, Lidman, Kakko, & Kekäläinen, 2013; Trotman, 2012). Improvements in interpersonal skills, intercultural relations, and 'social participation' or 'engagement' are also being reported and analysed (Kelaher & Dunt, 2009; Kinnunen et al., 2013; Loiselle, 2015; Savolainen & Suoniemi, 2015; Spiegel, 2016b; Spiegel & Parent, 2017; Trotman, 2012). In studying the role of the *Machincuepa* social circus in Las Aguilas, Mexico (McCauley, 2011) – a community described as struggling with the impacts of poverty, including open drug use in the streets – McCauley stressed that social circus offered an otherwise non-existent 'safe' gathering place, thus providing youth with an essential space to combat alienation and share experiences and resources.

To examine the impacts of Ecuador's social circus programme, we begin by discussing the Ecuadorian context followed by a description of our methodology and research techniques. We then proceed to (1) analyze how political ideologies and social discourses affected the operationalisation of social circus in the various municipalities; (2) assess how these policies and programmes shaped the ways in which participants were able to access and control the conditions of their own lives and that of their communities; and (3) examine how the implementation of this sociocultural initiative influenced personal growth as well as individually and collectively constructed behaviours that impact how health and well-being are experienced and transformed. We conclude by analysing the significance of our study for deepening understandings of the relationships amongst politics, social policy and the ways in which community arts programmes impact collective health, drawing parallels between the operationalisation of *Buen Vivir* and Ecuador's social circus programme itself.

## Toward a post-colonial methodology: a community-based transdisciplinary approach

The neoliberal economic model that dominated Ecuador from the 1990s and into the twenty-first century led to poverty rates exceeding 60% (Weisbrot, Johnston, & Merling, 2017). Despite the new government's considerable investment in infrastructure and social services including health and education (Instituto Nacional de Estadística y Censos (INEC), 2011), and despite greater attention to the rights of children and youth (UNICEF, 2002), 70% of youths were still living in poverty by 2011 (Carriel Mancilla, 2012). In this socioeconomic context, Moreno saw the potential of social circus to improve health and social outcomes.by:

> Creating a cultural alternative for empowering vulnerable communities … and developing values of solidarity, participation, discipline, concentration, cooperation, self-esteem, personal and collective development, and a sense of belonging.

*Circo Social Ecuador* was thus launched as part of broader social policies of *Buen Vivir*, reflecting the convergence of left intellectual discourse on wellbeing and the emergence of an organised Ecuadorian indigenous movement, promoting recovering indigenous communal values, cultural empowerment and identity. The extent to which policies and programmes have actually respected any of these principles has been hotly debated, with critics contesting that *Buen Vivir* was not a vision of a new civilisation but rather a cosmetic instrument for renewed governance of modernised capitalism (Alonso González & Vázquez, 2015; Becker, 2011; Walsh, 2010; Yates & Bakker, 2013).

Amidst these debates, our study sought to investigate how Ecuador's social circus programme has been altering ways of interacting, creating, realising potential and accessing collective resources needed for health and wellbeing. Our analysis adopts the notion of 'social *determination* of health' whereby health is conceptualised as a complex multidimensional dialectic deeply rooted in social and political processes in which socia*l groups* have 'ways of living' defined by their position in class/gender/ethno-cultural relations, in turn expressed in *individual* lifestyles and bio-psychological embodiments (Breilh, 2010, 2013; Krieger, 2011). The social *determination* of health approach, in contrast to the more traditional social *determinants* of health analytic framing, focuses attention not merely on the discrete factors or conditions that impact health and wellbeing (e.g. nutrition, housing, education, income, etc.), but rather on the structural processes at the societal level that lead to these social inequities, and the interrelationships among these (Breilh, 2008). The overall research objective of the study was thus to better understand how social policies, as well as their associated social interventions employing the arts (sociocultural interventions), intercede in the dominant modes of constructing ways of being and lifestyles at the individual and collective level.

Building on a longstanding collaboration between Ecuadorian and Canadian researchers, the study was conducted over an almost 5-year period beginning in 2013, drawing in researchers from the arts, humanities, health and social sciences. The metaphor of the rhizome (Deleuze & Guattari, 1987) characterises the way in which we merged disciplines (Boydell, Spiegel, & Yassi, in press); dissimilar from the root of a tree, a rhizome has no beginning and ending, only points connecting to other points with multiple points of entry. This metaphor of the rhizome reflects how our study blended epistemologies; its *relational* focus (Fox & Alldred, 2015) allowed for creativity, connection, experimentation and multiplicity in thinking to flourish (Fornssler, McKenzie, Dell, Laliberte, & Hopkins, 2014). Drawing from the lead author's previous studies of social circus in Quebec (Spiegel, 2015, 2016b; Spiegel & Parent, 2017), we also combined our interdisciplinary methods with the potentialities of community artists, including Ecuadorian author BO who trained instructors for *Circo Social Ecuador* [CSE]) in 2012 and had been the pedagogical director of CSE for 5 months in 2013, to analyze how transformations in 'ways of living' and lifestyles of youth were being effected by their participation in social circus. By interacting extensively and sharing data from one source to inform the others, we also sought to analyze the extent to which the processes operationalised embodied the vision and/or constraints associated with *Buen Vivir* in Ecuador and/or surfaced new potential for social transformation.

Our qualitative data gathering methods included participant observation in which lead author JBS observed social circus training, participating in the workshops where she could, and interacted with participants and instructors to understand their experiences, their concerns, their joys, and the challenges they faced. Other team members also visited the programmes in the various municipalities. Discussions were held with personnel from *Cirque du Soleil*, Ecuador's Vice Presidency and Ministry of Culture, as well as municipal programme directors, social workers, coordinators and instructors. JBS also conducted 16 confidential interviews to supplement the group discussions that involved well over 100 participants in these various sessions.

We analysed documents, training materials, programme plans and a myriad of information that helped us understand how and the extent to which the programmes were meeting goals. The considerable expertise of co-author BOC regarding the history of the programmes, the pedagogy and the challenges, facilitated appreciation of the nuances of each situation, always conscious of positionality. Indeed, we adopted a high degree of reflexivity (Rice & Ezzy, 1999), well aware that research perspectives are continuously bound up not only with academic biographies but also with the 'interpersonal, political and institutional contexts in which researchers are embedded' (Mauthner & Doucet, 2003).

The quantitative component of the study consisted of a large retrospective-prospective longitudinal survey, with comparison group, specifically including 254 youth or young adults who were participating – or had participated – in social circus across the country, and 167 youths enrolled in various other art and cultural activities in the *Casa Metro* youth centres in Quito's metropolitan area, including 63 involved in collective creative practices generally more physically demanding – such as personal defense, dance, break dancing, capoeira, and parkour – as well as 104 participating in other pursuits – including music, guitar, percussion, art, language studies and other activities. We adapted questionnaires that had been used in other studies by JBS and included questions focused specifically on understanding the impact of community-based creative practice on the emotional and physical wellbeing of participants. We asked respondents to compare how they remember feeling, or what their situations were, before they began social circus or their other arts-related activities, compared to afterwards, using a retrospective post-then-pre questionnaire design (Rockwell &

Kohn, 1989), to avoid 'loss to follow-up' that characterises many studies of street-involved youth (Hampshire & Matthijsse, 2010). The questionnaire included constructs of personal growth (Robitschek, 1998) and social inclusion, understood as 'the means, material or otherwise, to partici-pate in social, economic, political and cultural life' (Huxley et al., 2012). In addition, it comprised questions that probed social engagement and health-related outcome (nutrition, fitness, substance use, housing, income, etc.), as well as an index of social class (Breilh, Campaña, Felicita, & al., 2009).[2]

The analysis presented here is drawn from the larger study[1] that further incorporated arts-based research methods (Marcuse, Fels, Boydell, & Spiegel, in press), as well as analysis of the pedagogical philosophy and practices (Fels & Ortiz Choukroun, in press). Several workshops served as sites of encounter at once providing a space for sharing and problematising research techniques, modes of study and ways of developing and experiencing praxis. The institutional hierarchies of knowledge, the ways in which they continue to stratify social and professional participation, and the complexity of overcoming colonial dynamics were, however, omnipresent; in our data collection and analysis across methods we sought to mitigate and transforms these dynamics as much as possible.

## Ecuador's national social circus programme: operationalisation of new social policy

> In history we were conquered, we also had bad governments that suppressed communities. ... By revitalizing the spiritual part of a person, as with social circus, we can start to work to improve self-esteem ... have an Ecua-dorian point of view not from a submissive stance but from a position of being able and capable of creating and proposing new ideas and change. ... Depending on who is in charge of the social circus [program] it can just be a local spectacle and the essence of social change could be completely lost. We [the central government] must look after preventing that. Official from the Ecuadorian Ministry of Culture and Heritage, November 2014

In his article 'New Models of Cultural Policy in Latin America', Cecchi noted that in the first decade of the twenty-first century the cultural field took on much more prominence in Latin America in the countries that had 'reconstructed' themselves by recognising their multiethnic and pluricultural identities (Cecchi, 2015). He observed that political decisions about how cultural policies are implemented open possibilities 'for social inclusion and mutual recognition, and finally also extend-ing the margins of citizenship' (pg.15). Ecuador, alongside countries like Venezuela and Bolivia, saw culture elevated to a constitutional right, with corresponding large increases in government spend-ing; much of the transformation was focused on who participates in cultural production.

A social circus programme driven so strongly by a national government was unprecedented, as was the level of investment of public funds.[3] This provided an opportunity to promote values con-sistent with the 2013–2017 Plan Nacional Buen Vivir, such as 'social inclusion, self-esteem and pro-found collective confidence in the country' (SENPLADES, 2013), with government documents suggesting that social circus could act 'as a powerful lever of social transformation'. The emphasis on social principles contrasts with goals in social circus programmes elsewhere; for example, the partnership of La Tarumba in Perú, Circo del Mundo in Chile, and Circo Social del Sur in Argentina, with the Inter-American Development Bank and Cirque du Soleil, describes itself as 'an alternative to improve the employability ... . training of entrepreneurship and ... a model to help lower the rate of youth unemployment in the region' (MIF, 2013). While CSE also offers participants the opportunity for professionalisation and decent work, the declared focus is on promoting personal and social development as a form of social transformation.

There are four main activities in CSE: First, instructor training (Photos 1–3) to prepare instructors with the social pedagogy needed to be effective mentors. Secondly, réplicas – workshops offered to groups of usually up to 20 participants in sessions once to three times per week, lasting about 3–4 months conducted either at the location of a partner civil society organisation or onsite at a munici-pal venue (Photos 4 and 5); these workshop sessions are the backbone of the programme. Third are the 'open circus' sessions where instructors and volunteers (usually youth with advanced training) work with children and other members of the public using circus arts (Photos 6 and 7), often invol-ving hundreds of participants; and fourthly performances/demonstrations (Photos 8 and 9).

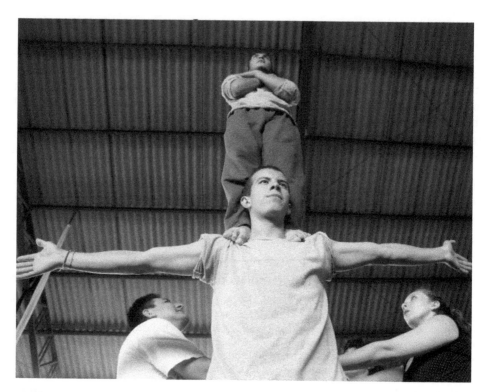

**Photo 1.** Volunteers in Cuenca learning a group confidence-building exercise, reflecting the social pedagogy (2013). Photo credit: B. Ortiz Choukroun.

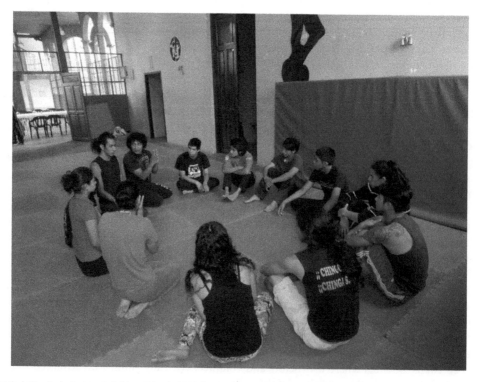

**Photo 2.** Instructor/volunteer training session in Loja discussing pedagogical approaches (2014); the social theory behind each exercise is taken quite seriously. Photo credit: A Campaña

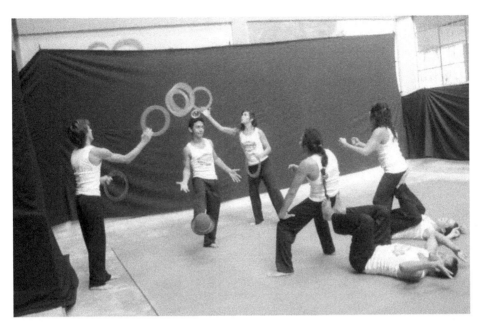

**Photo 3.** Demonstration by instructors/volunteers in Tena at the culmination of a training session (2012). Photo courtesy of Circo Social Tena.

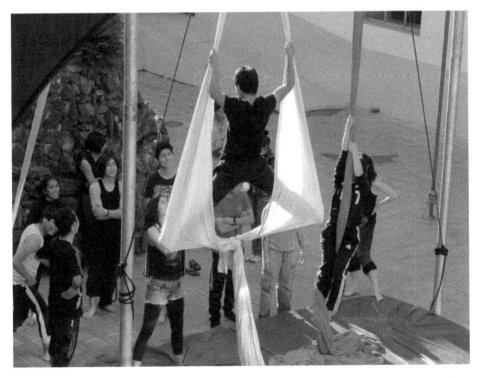

**Photo 4.** Réplica with youth in Loja; the instructor adapts the exercise on silks to the level of the participants (2015). Photo credit: B. Ortiz Choukroun.

However, the relative importance of each of these activities varies by programme site, as do the target populations prioritised and the pedagogical structure, in turn influenced by the political stances of the various governmental authorities (see Table 1). Notably, misperceptions of the objectives of

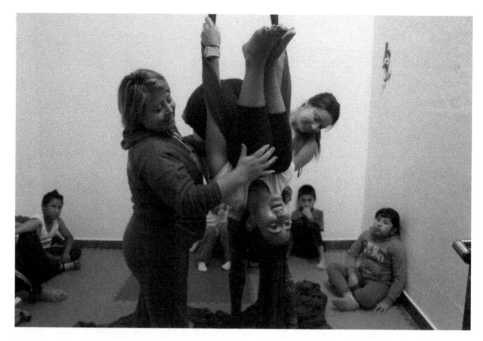

**Photo 5.** Social worker and volunteer in replica in Cuenca. (2013); Cirque du Monde pedagogy emphasises the importance of direct involvement of social workers in all the workshops. Photo credit: B. Ortiz Choukroun.

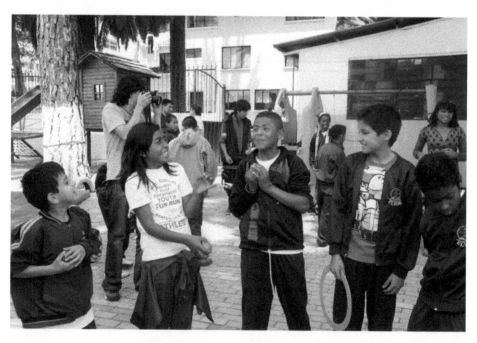

**Photo 6.** Children from la Fundación REMAR Ecuador enjoying an Open Circus event by Circo Social Quito 2013; an estimated well over 50,000 children have attended Open Circus or social circus performance events across Ecuador. Photo credit: B. Ortiz Choukroun.

social circus were exacerbated by the influence of *Cirque du Soleil* imagery (Fricker, 2016; Hurley & Léger, 2008) creating inappropriate expectations of marginalised groups performing in large cos-tume-clad majestic productions. Moreover, the grandiose (never-achieved) government plan to

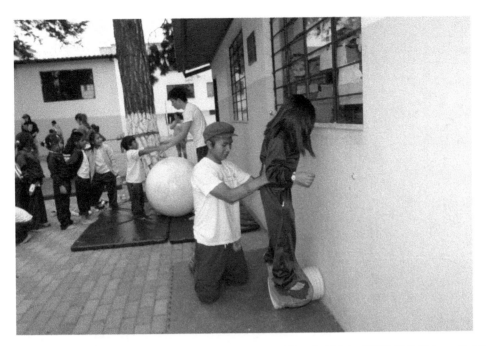

**Photo 7.** Youth volunteers working with children in an Open Circus event of Circo Social Quito, REMAR, 2013. Photo credit: B. Ortiz Choukroun.

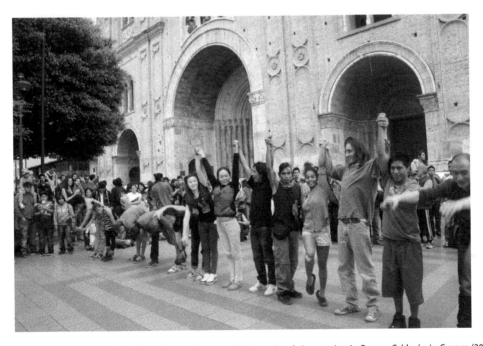

**Photo 8.** Volunteers from Circo Social Ecuador performing with international circus artists in Parque Calderón in Cuenca (2013). Photo credit: B. Ortiz Choukroun.

mount a 'big tent' in each city (against the advice of its social circus pedagogy advisors) distracted considerably from the programme's social objectives (Spiegel, Ortiz Choukroun, Campaña, & Yassi, in press). In light of these discrepancies, we ask, was social circus indeed encouraging broader

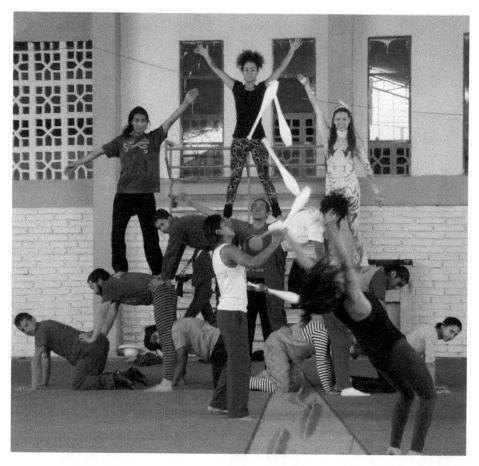

**Photo 9.** Juggling, clowning, acrobatics, and collective acrobatics (pyramid) by Circo Social Quito and Circo Social Cuenca volunteers in 2013 rehearsing for a show at the inauguration of the big tent in Cuenca (2013). Photo credit: B. Ortiz Choukroun.

co-construction of the cultural life of the country across ethnic and class divisions? And if so, what were the broader well-being implications of the shift?

## Social reach, cultural participation, and collective wellbeing

The driving force behind dominant theories of change related to social circus is the conviction that embodying collective creation, collective risk-taking and collective trust builds solidarity and propels positive socially transformative actions. It is hoped that when those who have been marginalised from social, cultural and economic access create together in this way, social inclusion will improve, thereby increasing social equity and improving collective living conditions (Spiegel & Parent, 2017). This desire is not unique to Ecuador's programme, but rather anchored in the very vision for social circus disseminated by *Cirque du Soleil's* social citizenship programme, *Cirque du Monde*, operating in over 80 communities globally (Cirque du Monde, 2014). However, brought to Ecuador, where disparity propelled by decades of neoliberalism is stark, and adapted to a new paradigm that aimed to trigger transformative mobilisation to redress social inequities, these objectives take on a particular tenor.

Our survey showed significant transformations in educational goals and career prospects amongst social circus participants, as well as in softer indicators of social inclusion such as '*satisfied with social life*' and '*sense of group-community belonging*' (Figure 1). However, living conditions and food

**Table 1.** Socioeconomic and political profile, social policies and pedagogy, programme metrics and observations/outcome overall and by city.

| | Socio-economic & political context | Social circus policy decisions/pedagogy | Programme metrics | Observations/impacts |
|---|---|---|---|---|
| National (Circo Social Ecuador-CSE) | High rates of poverty and inadequate social programmes due to neoliberal structural adjustment policies were replaced by some redistributive policies with the election of *Alianza País (AP)* in 2006. In 2017, Lenín Moreno (former AP vice-president) was elected President. | CSE began in 2011, as part of the *Buen Vivir* development plan, with a national pedagogical director and local counterparts (until mid-2013) who trained instructors in social pedagogy, along with two one-week trainings by *Cirque du Monde* yearly. By 2013, CSE was completely decentralised, with the Ministry of Culture and Heritage playing a much-reduced role. | CSE had served over 100,000 people by the end of 2016 – 15,000–30,000 individuals annually – since its inception. For example, in 2016 there were 1384 participants registered in replicas and training; ~30 volunteers, ~18,000 Open Circus participants and ~10,000 members of the general public who participated in the audiences. | Overall, the programme achieved excellent results with respect to personal growth (PG): 17.5% increase from baseline; social inclusion (SI): 12.3% increase; and social engagement (SE): 15.4% increase. Improvements with respect to fitness, nutrition and drug use were also noted; best results were in those with lowest baselines and in age group 14–25, but all benefited. Interviews and focus groups illustrated that participants developed a strong sense of community, but also revealed tensions. |
| Circo Social Quito | Capital city and second largest in the country, Quito, located in the Sierra (Andean) region, had a progressive mayor (from the AP party) until 2014, when a right-wing mayor was elected. Quito has a history of social awareness, but inequitable urban development. | Even before CSE, there was grassroots circus activity in youth centres and streets of Quito. Early on (from 2012) the CSE programme thrived with a strong sense of community among marginalised youth; gradually the inclusion of more people from diverse backgrounds led to dual camps – the technical and the social. By the end of 2017, the programme was actively serving diverse needs, encouraging small enterprises related to circus; instructors and volunteers often performed at city events. | The largest programme in CSE, the numbers of 'beneficiaries' increased over time, but with less intensive focus. In 2013, there were 525 participants in replicas and 1750 Open Circus attendees; 2016 had 293 participants in replicas and trainings, with 15,000 Open Circus attendees and ~3600 general public audience. | With no circus school in Ecuador, this programme provided social circus as well as circus arts 'professional' training, diluting the social focus. Survey data showed gains in measures of PG (18.0%), SI (12.8%) and SE (13.3%), but less impressive than in Loja. Qualitative research revealed strong sense of community, but also tensions between the 'social' and 'technical' camps. |
| Circo Social Cuenca | Medium size city in the Sierra. Cuenca had a progressive mayor (AP) until 2014 followed by a centre-left mayor. There was much activity demanding social and health rights related to mining and environmental concerns. | This was the first programme to launch (2011); the original focus was street-involved youth but in 2014 shifted to children from marginalised communities and the elderly; interviewees attributed this partly to avoiding difficulties with (seen as unruly) youth. This programme was the only one to retain social workers throughout its history. | The programme grew steadily until 2016 (40–331 replica participants), although Open Circus attendees fluctuated, and target age groups changed. Higher participation was not always matched by increased numbers of instructors. | Youth participation was limited, which may explain less impressive results than elsewhere; adjusting for age the programme was no less successful than the others. Interviewees noted difficulties in finding social workers with the right profile, however partnering with universities helped. |
| Circo Social Guayaquil | Located on the coast, the country's largest city and main economic driver, Guayaquil has profound social inequity with high rates of poverty and crime. With strong | The programme in Guayaquil, from the beginning in 2012, rejected social circus pedagogy as proposed by the Vice Presidency with its focus on social | Updated information on CS Guayaquil participants is unavailable. In 2012, an estimated 300 people participated in this programme, including 18 workshop | Too few completed surveys precluded conclusions. Interviews with former participants and volunteers confirmed the lack of 'social' focus. However, |

*(Continued)*

**Table 1.** Continued.

| | Socio-economic & political context | Social circus policy decisions/pedagogy | Programme metrics | Observations/impacts |
|---|---|---|---|---|
| | populism and right-wing governments almost since 1992, this region was the source of major opposition to the previous AP government. | objectives; instead it strived to build professional skills, modelling, TV, and obtaining employment. Nevertheless, the programme recently (2017) joined the network of social circus so a more socially-oriented approach is now expected. | beneficiaries. (Permission to study this programme with surveys and interviews was not granted.) | interviewees suggested that recently hired instructors, who were part of the first training process, could make a positive change. |
| Circo Social Tena | This small city in the Amazon, near oil extraction and agro-industrial areas, has a large indigenous population. In 2014, a right-wing major was again elected, focused on economic development, and at odds with the AP government. | The programme, which began in 2012, had outreach to indigenous communities deep into the jungle, as well as serving diverse populations in Tena (people with disabilities and the elderly as well as youth and children). The programme closed in December 2014 at the end of the first year of the new municipal government. | Workshop participants reached 200 in 2014 while number of volunteers fluctuated across years. Open Circus and general public participation peaked in 2013 with 1400 participants. | Too few surveys were completed to allow quantitative conclusion due to the programme having closed by the time the survey was completed. Interviews indicated that the programme had been very well received prior to the change in government. |
| Circo Social Loja | A small city located in the Sierra, Loja had centr-left governments since the project began in 2013; however, the mayor, elected in 2014 holds conservative views regarding social programmes, marginalised youth and the role of the arts. | The programme started operations later than other CS programmes; hired more instructors and provided more instructor and volunteer training than any other programme, targeting marginalised youth as well as children. In December 2016, a disagreement between the instructors and the mayor regarding performing at a city event led to the restructuring of the programme. | In 2016, Loja's CS programme served over 7000 individuals: 360 participants in replicas and trainings, ~5 volunteers, ~2000 Open Circus attendees, and ~5000 audience members at demonstrations. | This programme provided the most impressive results in the survey: 20.2% increase in PG; 15.2% increase in SI, 26.0% increase in SE; significantly better than some of the other programmes, even controlling for age and social class. However, the results were obtained before the changes at the end of 2016, after which the number of social circus workshops was decreased considerably. |

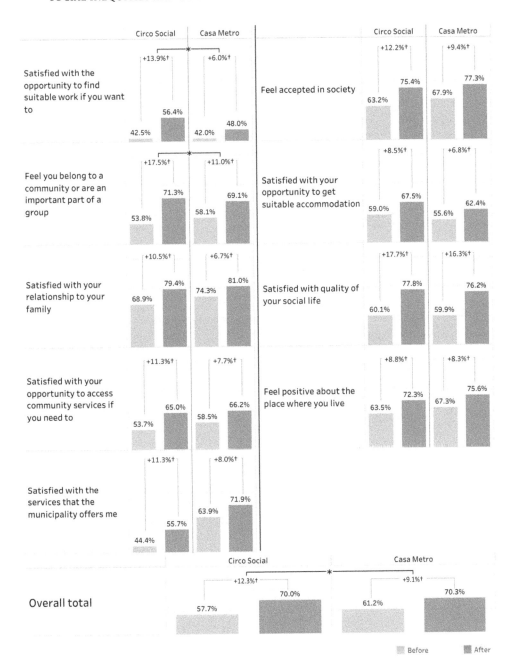

**Figure 1.** Changes in social inclusion pre versus post beginning social circus, ages 12–39, comparing respondents from *Circo Social* with respondents from *Casa Metro* programmes. † Paired t-test shows the average participant response improved significantly with 95% confidence; * T-test shows that the average change between programmes is significantly different, with 95% confidence.

security were only slightly improved (8% increase in '*satisfaction with housing*'; 39% still reporting inadequate *diet*), understandable given that such changes require longer-term effort at the macro societal level. Participants in other community arts (*Casa Metro*) also showed significant improvements, however social circus participants reported significantly more impact than their counterparts in other arts and cultural activities for both social inclusion and personal growth (Figure 2). Social circus participants also significantly increased their social engagement while those from *Casa Metro* did not. Indeed social circus respondents scored higher on all four social engagement questions after

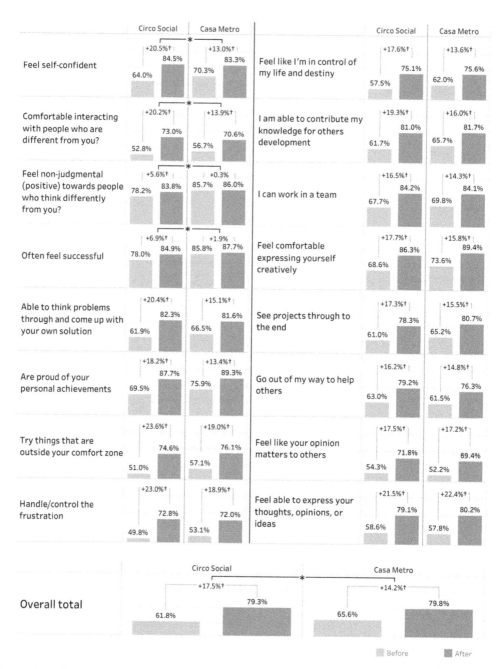

**Figure 2.** Personal growth mean comparison pre versus post participation and between *Circo Social Ecuador* and *Casa Metro* (ages 12–39). †,* -see legend for Figure 1.

participation in social circus, with a significant upsurge in '*participate in organizations, community projects or social activism*' (Figure 3), suggesting this programme may indeed be spurring activism needed for macro-level social transformation.

Interestingly, parkour and capoeira had results that were similar to social circus for personal growth and social inclusion, and less consistent with findings for the other *Casa Metro* programmes (Figure 4), an observation likely explained by similarities in the activities and profile of youth they tend to draw. Our interviews with the *Casa Metro* director suggested that, like social circus, parkour

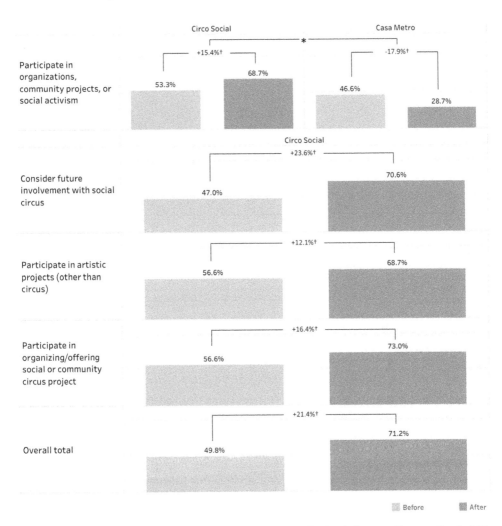

**Figure 3.** Social engagement mean comparison pre versus post participation of various indictors, and between *Circo Social Ecuador* and *Casa Metro* (ages 12–39) overall. †,* -see legend for Figure 1.

and capoeira attracted youth from lower socio-economic backgrounds, and/or who are interested in collective counter-cultural activities, consistent with the literature on youth involvement in these art forms (Ugolotti & Moyer, 2016), including youth attraction to social circus (Hurtubise, Roy, & Bellot, 2003). Scholars discuss youth engagement with capoeira and parkour as the medium through which struggles about belonging and citizenship take place (Ugolotti & Moyer, 2016), describing how participants 'challenge dominant regimes of representation, while also attempting to improve their life conditions and reach their personal goals'.

It is important to note that the socio-cultural and political conditions varied substantially between the Ecuadorian cities that hosted social circus programmes, manifesting in marked differences between their programmes, and thus the impacts achieved varied, as shown in Table 1. The target population for *Circo Social Quito*, which we studied most intensively, fluctuated considerably over the years. In November 2014, the coordinator described their participants as follows:

> It is diverse. Many of them come because they don't have a place to go and then they stay because they like it; others like circus arts a lot and come to exercise and learn techniques. People are from different social classes […] including street children who were [performing] at the traffic lights or kids in school who like arts and want to spend the evening, or kids who have decided to become circus artists and want to become professional.

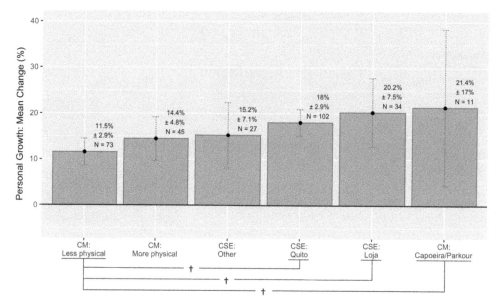

**Figure 4.** Social inclusion change, comparison by physical level, ages 18–39. † T-test shows a significant different between groups, each individual t-test having 95% confidence; none of the differences reach statistical significance for age-group 12–39, nor using the more rigorous Tukey test, nor when controlling for differences in baseline values within the groups. (It is noteworthy that CS Loja had significantly lower baselines compared to all other groups except the Capoeria/Parkour group).

Partly for pragmatic reasons to serve this diverse population that had grown to over 200 regular participants by 2017, the social pedagogical content was reduced, focusing more on technical and artistic content. The tensions within the operationalisation of social circus thus played out most transparently in Quito's programme, largely as there were no circus schools in Ecuador, militating for catering to those who want to professionalise in circus arts as well as those who come mainly for social engagement. In addition to supporting professionalisation, the programme encourages the creation of enterprises, bringing *Circo Social Quito* closer to the 'employability' objective characterising the Peruvian-Chilean-Argentinian programmes financed by the Inter-American Development Bank (MIF, 2013).

As explained by a former social worker with *Circo Social Quito* interviewed in October 2015, the changes since the programme began in 2011 had far reaching implications on programme demographics:

> Most of the young people [recruited in the early years] were living in the streets, and did not want to study or improve their quality of life . .... They consumed drugs, alcohol,[and were] involved in that world. So that's what the initial project was about, trying to help them out of those high-risk situations . .... The new kids, from what I have seen, come from a different background . .... It's no longer because they are in a vulnerable situation ... I think that reflects the current vision of the program ... , Before it felt like a family, I am not sure what they [the participants] think now ... Maybe it's just like another program.

*Circo Social Loja* outperformed all the other social circus programmes. This appears to be due to stronger adherence to the original focus and envisioned pedagogy both in terms of target participants (in Loja, the focus remained on youth in precarious conditions, whereas other programmes served a wider range of communities) as well as better staff-to-participant ratio and instructor training in social pedagogy. Across programmes, those with lower starting scores had significantly greater improvements than those with higher baselines in personal growth, social inclusion, and social engagement indicators.[4] Also, our data suggested that those aged 14–25 benefitted significantly more than younger or older participants. However, even adjusting for age, sex and social class differences, the Loja group showed significantly greater improvement than other social circus participants, suggesting that the pedagogy adopted does matter (Table 1).

## Relationships between individual and collective wellbeing

> The impact of the social circus in my life is integral. It made me a more humanitarian, empathetic and proactive person. Female participant, Loja

Social circus, like most community-arts, is inherently a social activity. Grounded in collective embodied creation, well-being impacts are linked to how individuals engage with larger social and collective activities and conditions (Spiegel & Parent, 2017). Nevertheless, we found that the collective processes had profound but variable effects on individuals' personal development and lifestyles. The overall substantial improvement in all the indicators of personal growth (Figure 2) especially in *'trying things outside my comfort zone', 'feeling comfortable to express my thoughts'*, and *'feeling self-confident'* was indeed associated with changes in lifestyles (*diet, substance use, fitness* – Figure 5). And there was a clear relationship between ways of creating collectivity and lifestyles that youth are able to adopt based on their economic and social conditions. Our interviews indicated that this was due in large part to a sense of opening horizons offered through the learning of collective embodied expression, and taught with a sense of openness to others.

> I don't even want to remember what it was like before. It was very bad. I had no future – [I was an] enemy of my own family and myself. … It [social circus] made me love myself and my family. It was a time to re-evaluate. I became a better human being, more sensible. Because we are circus artists we can express our feelings when we perform, this enables us to communicate our deepest emotions, sadness, happiness, crying … . All the things that have happened to you as a child and throughout our lives, I really like that. It's almost like falling into an unconscious state and in that state you are able to let go of those deep feelings, no matter what those are. Male participant, Quito

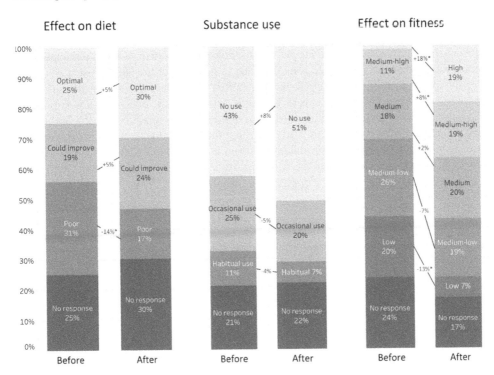

**Figure 5.** Attitudes and practices related to diet, substance use and physical fitness at baseline and after participation, for participants in a *Circo Social Ecuador* programme (ages 12–39). * Chi-squared tests show proportions before and after are significantly different with 95% confidence.

For many, social circus became at once a lifestyle and a desired way of living. 'Our expectation from the circus [workshops] is to earn enough money to live and maybe travel and take it with us. Have the right tools to create more', explained one participant. His partner elaborates:

> Travel and be able to have that experience with social circus, go to other places and try with a difference audience /demographics and culture. It's very interesting to see people how they really are and learn to respect that as well.

Those who reaped the greatest gains were youth who also volunteered[5]; they spoke of the importance of sharing and knowledge transfer, leading to a transformation both in how they related to others and to finding their own path. Whether this was because participants who most appreciated the programme were the ones who became volunteers, or conversely, the volunteering gave rise to greater benefits, cannot be determined and likely a dialectical process is at work. Highlighting a theory of change that points to the logic of transition from an 'individual' to a 'collective' mode of production, a participant from Quito noted how delighted they were to work with children:

> The objective is to transform each individual and gradually change society. Learn not to judge others for their condition, appearance or way of thinking. It's a journey … I feel it [social circus] has helped me find other alternatives, roads. I feel a need to communicate with society …. Before I had no interest at all in dealing with society, I wanted to be left aside. Now I am very interested in children. … When you recognize yourself as an individual, then you can be part of society and have some sort of impact. Change starts with oneself.

Here the logic still begins with the individual, in ways that repeat a neoliberal individual-based theory of wellbeing, however one that not only moves toward the collective but is underscored by social policies that facilitate this transition.

## Collective culture, neoproductivism, and the politics of transition

A major critique of the government's operationalisation of its *Buen Vivir* strategy is that it relies too heavily on a neo-productivist logic that prioritises product and performance over respect for the processes and contributions of all (Alonso González & Vázquez, 2015). Much of the tension that emerged in the social circus programme could be linked to the uneasy relationship between the ways in which the well-being of the 'collective' and of 'society' became linked to the extent to which participants, often economically and otherwise vulnerable, were expected to perform for the 'greater good'.

Given the importance of economic resources, we asked why 'volunteers' who work with children in the *réplicas,* or who perform at events at the request of the Municipality, are not provided with financial remuneration. In response, the coordinator of the Quito programme noted that the training provided was their main compensation, also describing the different ways social circus participants can generate income, including a mask-making business, a coffee shop with baked goods, and a shop to build monocycles. Explaining that the Municipality supported such endeavours by providing physical space, promotion and some expertise, she noted:

> Because these are business ventures, they require some level of commitment and additional effort. Throughout this process they learn to share their skills with others … those who are studying different careers can actually use those skills at these new business ventures. For example, one of them is studying business development and management, the group has an expectation that this person will become the future manager of the business venture…. We are planning a big event soon and … masks were going to be very important. So, everyone made a commitment to creating two masks each to sell. So this is what we consider a "Colectivo".

The lack of financial compensation when asked to perform publically was particularly problematic for several young social circus artists who stated that they '*felt exploited*'. A former instructor from Loja explained:

> Once the local government put money into the project, they had the feeling of ownership of the project and the kids. It was like they could 'rent' them and make them perform during the different events the city organized.

A participant from Loja, however, clarified that most participants are grateful for the free space to practice and learn – as well as for the intense sense of community developed; he noted that he

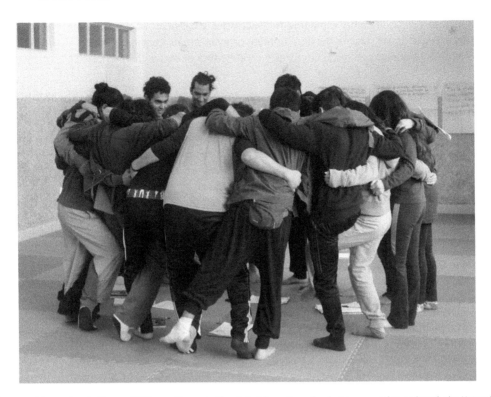

**Photo 10.** Photo taken in Cuenca, 2015 at a Cirque du Monde training where the decision was taken to launch the Network – Tejido de Circo Social. (Photo credit: Alex Grijalva)

liked to volunteer to help others, but he stressed that how they feel about performing for free depends on the audience and the purpose. The tension here mirrors ongoing debates concerning the politics of 'transition', particularly the justification by the *Alianza Pais* government of extractivism on the basis of its generating funds for social investment – a rationale that critics refer to as a populist neo-productivist model antithetical to *Buen Vivir* (Acosta, 2011; Alberto, 2016; Breilh, 2017). The term for this practice – (neo)extractivism – was coined by Gudynas (Gudynas, 2009) to refer to post-neoliberal policies of progressive governments to control the extraction of resources through renegotiating contracts, increasing taxes and export duties, and even nationalising companies, so as to generate surplus revenue to reduce poverty, diversify local economies, enhance social inclusion and maintain political stability. In light of such concerns, other scholars have advocated for an expansion of the concept of extractivism 'beyond its sectorialization in raw materials' to the very concept of 'development' itself (Gago, 2017; Mezzadra & Gago, 2017). Here we offer this notion as a lens through which to understand the tensions now at work in the social and cultural development strategies in the government's social circus programmes. In particular, our study problematises: (1) an emerging focus on technical prowess for performance over social objectives, (2) the expectation of free labour from participants in exchange for the opportunity to 'develop themselves' and their own personal wellbeing, and (3) the aims to produce 'productive' citizens through collective business endeavours. Trajectories for further addressing ongoing inequities are now being actively explored (Spiegel, in press-a). Partly in resistance to the precarity of relying completely on the State, by the end of 2015 the social circus community across the country began to form a network, *Tejido de Circo Social* (Photo 10), with a general objective of:

> promoting and developing social circus in Ecuador ... both in the country and the region as in the rest of the world, aiming to improve society and lead to the construction of a just and creative world through horizontal work with individuals and the community.

The launch of *Tejido*, arguably signalling the successful attainment of the State-envisioned 'multiplier effect', began a new stage in the development of social circus in Ecuador, opening the possibility of new actions to encourage social circus as a creative tool of social change.

### Community arts as a microcosm of the *Buen Vivir* paradox: implications for thinking about the socio-politics of community art and wellbeing

The attempt to actualise the concept of *Buen Vivir* via social circus suggests multiple avenues for rethinking the relationship between individual and collective wellbeing and the role of cultural and artistic practice therein.

Our study highlighted the ways in which personal transformation, social inclusion and collective practice are intrinsically linked and mutually affect one another. Consistent with Bourdieu's theories on the relationships among economic capital, cultural capital and social capital (Bourdieu, 1997 [1986]; Spiegel & Parent, 2017), the study not only reinforced research noting that those from lower social classes had lower starting scores for personal growth and social inclusion indicators (Richman, Clark, & Brown, 1985; Twenge & Campbell, 2002), but that the net benefit was greater where programmes put in place policies to reach out to youth in precarious conditions. It thus supports the call by health promotion scholars for such programmes to provide widespread coverage but pay special attention to those most vulnerable (Frohlich & Potvin, 2008), while also underlining the benefits of encouraging interaction between youth who might not otherwise come in contact with one another, offering exposure to different styles of living and breaking down class and cultural prejudice.

The ongoing challenges in realising the visions of the programme – and in particular, in blending a desire for inclusive collectively-oriented processes with high-performance products as techniques for supporting collective wellbeing – point to a broader tension. Scholars have argued that the declared social aims of *Buen Vivir* programmes were constrained by economic compromising and short-term political considerations, characterising the actions of Ecuador's government as pragmatic (Caria & Dominguez, 2016), aiming to redistribute resources without antagonizing Ecuadorian exporters, or as Becker put it, embracing 'the humaneness of socialism while pursuing the efficiency of capitalism' (Becker, 2014, p. 132). Instructors being drawn away from social pedagogy to prepare performances can be linked to the pragmatic need to 'show' benefit in technical terms. This tension dogged all the programmes, albeit to different extents and at different time periods; the ambitious plans for technical achievement under expensive big circus tents that never did materialise, became a distraction from the main purpose of the social circus programme. Indeed, the contradiction revealed here may be inherent in the social policy of capital-driven societies more broadly, and is linked to the very 'need' to approach sociocultural interventions as forms of building 'capital' for essentially economically-oriented development models.

The pressure and pull away from collective wellbeing toward utilising a collective process for productive ends, advancement of select individuals, and, as such, national cultural and economic 'success' as oriented by market values, is far from unique to Ecuador. It is a trend that has been seen worldwide, in social circus programmes as well as in the repurposing of public programmes more broadly. Indeed, in Quebec, home of *Cirque du Soleil*, official partner of Ecuador's social circus programme, the first venue created for social circus has long since been repurposed as a recreational and professional training centre (Spiegel, 2016a). In Ecuador, however, ongoing commitment to the collective wellbeing goals of the programme particularly by instructors, volunteers and participants themselves, suggests an avenue for rethinking the connection between the promotion of cultural agency and collective wellbeing as a factor not only increasing short-term indicators of health (fitness, nutritious diet, personal growth, etc.), but in acting as a force towards establishing future policy and institutions committed to the principles of inclusivity and social support. As Escobar noted: '*The most interesting cases [of social transformation] might arise at moments when the State/social movement nexus is capable of releasing the potential for imagination and action of autonomous social movements'* (Escobar, 2010). In generating a movement to conjoin artistic processes to the transformation of conditions associated with the social determination of health, our study suggests that such creative programmes can contribute significantly to the development of a global culture of collective wellbeing. As such a culture grows, research must embrace epistemologies able to go beyond the development of positivist markers of individual improvement to also value holistic changes in social dynamics and cultures of transformations themselves.

## Notes

1. As this goes to press, a book written about this project, entitled *'The Art of Collectivity: Social Circus and the Cultural Politics of a Post-Neoliberal Vision'*, edited by Jennifer Beth Spiegel and Benjamin Ortiz Choukroun, is currently under review. We reference chapters from this book, as it is expected to be available in 2019.
2. For cohort definition in each city and programme, data gathering techniques, response rates, measures to mitigate 'survivor bias' as well as the specific statistical tests and statistical programmes employed in each set of analyses, see Yassi and Campaña (in press).
3. In a 2015 *Cirque du Monde's* survey with responses from over 200 social circus organisations, social circus programmes in Ecuador reported that 91% of their funding was from government, compared to only 31% worldwide, where there is much greater dependence on foundations or the private sector – see Spiegel (in press-b), and www.cirquedusoleil.com/en/about/global-citizenship/social-circus/cirque-du-monde.aspx.
4. Circo Social participants with low baselines saw a 54.8% greater improvement in personal growth ($p < 0.0001$), 17.5% greater improvement in social inclusion [$p < 0.0001$], and 35.4% greater improvement in social activism ($p < 0.0001$) compared to those with higher baselines. Other statistical analyses indicated that this was not simply a ceiling effect – see Yassi and Campaña (in press).
5. The 78 volunteers who responded to the survey had an overall 21.6% change in personal growth compared to 15.8% in the 176 non-volunteering participants; $p = 0.03$.

## Acknowledgements

We sincerely thank all the participants, volunteers, current and former staff of the programmes as well as the Ecuadorian government, municipal directors and Cirque du Soleil personnel who generously gave their time. We thank the individuals and participating organisations for giving us permission to use the photos. We are also grateful to our inspiring research collaborators especially Lynn Fels and Judith Marcuse at Simon Fraser University and Patrick Leroux at Concordia University, as well as Karen Lockhart, Steven Barker and the other skilful staff at the University of British Columbia and Universidad Andina Simon Bolivar.

## Disclosure statement

No potential conflict of interest was reported by the authors.

## Funding

This work was supported by the Canadian Institutes of Health Research (CIHR) under grant MOP-133595, *'Social Circus and Health Equity: An interdisciplinary, intercultural, international collaboration'*. Lead author JBS was also supported by grant #895-2012 – 1008, *'Art for Social change: An integrated research program in teaching, evaluation and capacity-building'*, from the Social Sciences and Humanities Research Council (SSHRC) as a research fellow; and senior author AY is supported by the Canadian government under their Canada Research Chairs funding.

## References

Acosta, A. (2011). Extractivism and neoextractism: Two sides of the same curse. In M. Lang & D. Mokrani (Eds.), *'Mas alla del desarrollo'* (pp. 61–85). Quito: Abya Yala Ediciones.

Alberto, A. (2016). Aporte al debate. El extractivsmo como categoría de saqueo y devastación. *FIAR, 9*(2), 24–33.

Alonso González, P., & Vázquez, A. M. (2015). An ontological turn in the debate on Buen Vivir-Sumak Kawsay in Ecuador: Ideology, knowledge, and the common. *Latin American and Caribbean Ethnic Studies*, 1–20. doi:10.1080/17442222.2015.1056070

Archambault, K. (2014). *Évaluation d'un programme novateur de réadaptation par les arts de la scène pour des jeunes présentant un trouble psychiatrique stabilisé: Le programme Espace de Transition.* Montreal: Université de Montréal.

Becker, M. (2011). Correa, indigenous movements, and the writing of a new constitution in Ecuador. *Latin American Perspectives, 38*(1), 47–62. doi:10.1177/0094582×10384209

Becker, M. (2014). Rafael Correa and social movements in Ecuador. In S. Ellner (Ed.), *Latin America's radical left: Challenges and complexities of political power* (pp. 127–148). Lanham, MD: Rowman and Littlefield.

Bhabha, H. K. (2012). *The location of culture.* London: Routledge.

Bourdieu, P. (1997 [1986]). The forms of capital. In A. Halsey, H. Lauder, P. Brown & A. Stuart Wells (Eds.), *Education: Culture, economy, society* (pp. 46–58). Oxford: OUP.

Boydell, K., Spiegel, J. B., & Yassi, A. (in press). Collectivity and the art of transdisciplinary community-based research: A rhizomatic approach. In J. B. Spiegel & B. Ortiz Choukroun (Eds.), *The art of collectivity – Social circus and the cultural politics of a post-neoliberal vision.* Montreal: McGill – Queen's University Press.

Breilh, J. (2008). Latin American critical ('social') epidemiology: New settings for an old dream. *International Journal of Epidemiology, 37,* 745–750. doi:10.1093/ije/dyn135

Breilh, J. (2010). *La epidemiología crítica: una nueva forma de mirar la salud en el espacio urbano.* Quito, Ecuador.

Breilh, J. (2013). La determinación social de la salud como herramienta de transformación hacia una nueva salud pública (salud colectiva). *Revista de la Facultad Nacional de Salud Pública, 31*(suppl 1), S13–S27.

Breilh, J. (2017). *Extractivismo petrolero, crisis múltiple de la vida y los desafíos de la investigación.* Quito: UASB.

Breilh, J., Campaña, A., Felicita, O., & al., e. (2009). *Environmental and health impacts of floriculture in Ecuador.* Quito, Ecuador. Retrieved from Research Report Project IDRC-CRDI (103697-001)

Cadwell, S., & Rooney, B. (2013). *Galway community circus – Community impact survey.* Retrieved from http://www.academia.edu/10219178/Galway_Community_Circus_Impact_Study

Caria, S., & Dominguez, R. (2016). Ecuador' *Buen Vivir:* A new ideology for development. *Latin American Perspectives, 43*(1), 18–33. doi:10.1177/0094582X15611126

Carriel Mancilla, J. (2012). Public expenditure in health in Ecuador [Gasto público en salud en el Ecuador]. *Rev Med FCM-UCSG, 18*(1), 53–60. Retrieved from http://editorial.ucsg.edu.ec/ojs-medicina/index.php/ucsg-medicina/article/view/603/547

Cecchi, L. E. (2015). *New models of cultural policy in Latin America: A comparative analysis (2000–2014).* VIII Congreso Latinoamericano de Ciencia – Política, organizado por la Asociación Latinoamericana de Ciencia Política (ALACIP). Pontificia Universidad Católica del Perú, Lima.

Cirque du Monde, Cirque du Soleil. (2014). *ParticiPant handbook cirque du Monde training – Part 1.* Retrieved from www.educircation.eu/documentation/

Cirque du Soleil home page. Social circus – Cirque du Monde. Retrieved from http://www.cirquedusoleil.com/en/about/global-citizenship/social-circus/cirque-du-monde.aspx

Deleuze, G., & Guattari, F. (1987). *A thousand plateaus: Capitalism and schizophrenia (trans. Brian Massumi).* Minneapolis: University of Minnesota Press.

Escobar, A. (2010). Latin America at a crossroads. *Cultural Studies, 24,* 1–65. doi:10.1080/09502380903424208

Fels, L., & Ortiz Choukroun, B. (in press). Pedagogy of Circo Social Ecuador: Launching the ball. In J. B. Spiegel & B. Ortiz Choukroun (Eds.), *The art of collectivity – Social circus and the cultural politics of a post-neoliberal vision.* Montreal: McGill Queen's University Press.

Fornssler, B., McKenzie, H. A., Dell, C. A., Laliberte, L., & Hopkins, C. (2014). "I got to know them in a new way" Rela (y/t) ing rhizomes and community-based knowledge (brokers') transformation of western and indigenous knowledge. *Cultural Studies? Critical Methodologies, 14*(2), 179–193. doi:10.1177/1532708613516428

Fox, N. J., & Alldred, P. (2015). New materialist social inquiry: Designs, methods and the research-assemblage. *International Journal of Social Research Methodology, 18*(4), 399–414. doi:10.1080/13645579.2014.921458

Fricker, K. (2016). "Somewhere between science and legend": Images of indigeneity in Robert Lepage and Cirque du Soleil's Totem. In L. P. Leroux & C. Batson (Eds.), *Cirque global – Quebec's expanding circus boundaries* (pp. 140–160). Montreal: McGill – Queen's University Press.

Frohlich, K., & Potvin L. (2008). Transcending the known in public health practice. *American Journal of Public Health, 98*(2), 216–221. doi:10.2105/AJPH.2007.114777

Gago, V. (2017). *Neoliberalism from below: Popular pragmatics and baroque economies.* Durham, NC: DUKE University Press.

Government of Ecuador. (2008). *Republic of Ecuador – Constitution of 2008.* Retrieved from http://pdba.georgetown.edu/Constitutions/Ecuador/english08.html

Gudynas, E. (2009). Diez Tesis Urgentes sobre el Nuevo Extractivismo: Contextos y Demandas Bajo el Progresismo Sudamericano Actual. In J. Schuldt, A. Acosta, A. Barandiará, A. Bebbington, M. Folchi, A. Alayza & E. Gudynas (Eds.), *Extractivismo, Política y Sociedad* (pp. 187–225). Quito: caap/claes.

Hampshire, K. R., & Matthijsse, M. (2010). Can arts projects improve young people's wellbeing? A social capital approach. *Social Science and Medicine, 71,* 708–716. doi:10.1016/j.socscimed.2010.05.015

Hurley, E., & Léger, I. (2008). Les corps multiples du Cirque du Soleil, translated by Léger. *Globe: revue internationale d'études québécoises, 11*(2), 135–157.

Hurtubise, R., Roy, S., & Bellot, C. (2003). Youth homelessness: The street and work: From exclusion to integration. In L. Roulleau-Berger (Ed.), *Youth and work in the post-industrial city of North America and Europe* (pp. 395–407). Boston: Brill Leiden.

Huxley, P., Evans, S., Madge, S., Webber, M., Burchardt, T., McDaid, D., & Knapp, M. (2012). Development of a social inclusion index to capture subjective and objective life domains (phase II): Psychometric development study. *Health Technology Assessment, 16*(1), 1–248. doi:10.3310/hta16010

Instituto Nacional de Estadística y Censos (INEC). (2011). *Ultimos resultados de pobreza, desigualdad y mercado laboral en el Ecuador.* Quito, Ecuador.

Kelaher, M., & Dunt, D. (2009). *Evaluation of the community arts development scheme.* Retrieved from https://www.vichealth.vic.gov.au/~/media/ … /arts/cads/cads_final_for_web.pdf?la=en

Kinnunen, R., Lidman, J., Kakko, S., & Kekäläinen, K. (2013). "They're smiling from ear to ear" wellbeing effects from social circus. Retrieved from http://www.uta.fi/cmt/index/wellbeing-effects-from-social-circus.pdf

Krieger, N. (2011). *Epidemiology and the people's health: Theory and context.* New York: Oxford University Press.

Leroux, L. P. (2012). *Cirque in Space! The ethos, ethics, and aesthetics of staging and branding the individual of exception.* Guest talk at the Centre for Canadian Studies, Duke University, Durham North Carolina.

Leslie, D., & Rantisi, N. (2016). Creativity and place in the evolution of a cultural industry: The case of Cirque du Soleil. In L. P. Leroux & C. Batson (Eds.), *Cirque global Quebec's expanding circus boundaries* (pp. 223–239). Montreal: McGill Queen's University Press.

Loiselle, F. (2015). *Retombées du cirque social (Cirque du Soleil) en contexte de réadaptation sur la participation sociale de jeunes adultes avec déficiences physiques en transition vers la vie active – Étude qualitative.* Montreal: University of Montreal.

Macas, L. (2010). Sumak Kawsay. La vida en plenitud. *América Latina en Movimiento, 452,* 14–16. Retrieved from http://icci.nativeweb.org/yachaikuna/Yachaykuna13.pdf

Marcuse, J., Fels, L., Boydell, K., & Spiegel, J. B. (in press). Through their own bodies, eyes and voices: Social circus, social inquiry and the politics of facilitating "collectivity". In J. B. Spiegel & B. Ortiz Choukroun (Eds.), *The art of collectivity – Social circus and the cultural politics of a post-neoliberal vision.* Montreal: McGill – Queen's University Press.

Mauthner, N., & Doucet, A. (2003). Reflexive accounts and accounts of reflexivity in qualitative data analysis. *Sociology, 37*(3), 413–431. doi:10.1177/00380385030373002

McCaffery, N. (2011). *Streetwise Community Circus, Knockavoe School evaluation An evaluation of the impact of teaching circus skills to people with learning disabilities.* Retrieved from www.sccni.co.uk/assets/knockavoe-final-evaluation2.pdf

McCauley, J. (2011). *The circus she calls me: Youth at risk in a social circus.* (International Development MSc.), University of Amsterdam

Mezzadra, S., & Gago, V. (2017). In the wake of the plebeian revolt: Social movements, 'progressive' governments, and the politics of autonomy in Latin America. *Anthropological Theory, 17*(4), 474–496. doi:10.1177/1463499617735257

MIF. (2013). *The MIF, Cirque du Soleil and three Latin American social circus schools join forces to promote youth employability, press release.* Retrieved from http://www.fomin.org/en-us/Home/News/PressReleases/ArtMID/3819/ArticleID/995.aspx

Programa Circo Social Ecuador. (2012). *Mision y objectivos.* Quito. Retrieved from http://www.vicepresidencia.gob.ec/programas/sonrieecuador/circo-social-yartistico

Rice, P. L., & Ezzy, D. (1999). Qualitative research methods: A health focus. *Melbourne, Australia.*

Richman, C., Clark, M., & Brown, K. (1985). General and specific self-esteem in late adolescent students: Race× gender× SES effects. *Adolescence, 20*(79), 555–566.

Robitschek, C. (1998). Personal growth initiative: The construct and its measure. *Measurement and Evaluation in Counseling and Development, 30,* 183–198.

Rockwell, S. K., & Kohn, H. (1989). Post-then-pre evaluation: Measuring behavior change more accurately. *Journal of Extension, 27*(2). Retrieved from http://www.joe.org/joe/1989summer/a1985.html

Savolainen, A., & Suoniemi, S. (2015). *Hoitsusirkus Namibiassa-sosiaalisen sirkuksen voimauttava ja ryhmäyttävä vaikutus namibialaisten lasten keskuudessa.* Retrieved from https://www.theseus.fi/bitstream/handle/10024/98828/savolainen_aleksei.pdf?sequence=1&isAllowed=y

Secretaria Nacional de Planificación y Desarrollo. (2009). *Plan nacional para el buen vivir 2009–2013: Construyendo un estado plurinacional e intercultural.* Quito: Government of Ecuador.

Secretaria Nacional de Planificación y Desarrollo. (2013). *Plan nacional para el buen vivir 2013–2017.* Quito.

Spiegel, J. B. (2014). Social circus as an art for social change: Promoting social inclusion, social engagement and cultural democracy. In K. Kekäläinen (Ed.), *Studying social circus: Openings & perspectives* (pp. 70–75). Tampere: University of Tampere.

Spiegel, J. B. (2015). *The value of social circus: creative process, embodied critique, and the limits of 'capital'.* Canadian Association for Theatre Research, Montreal.

Spiegel, J. B. (2016a). Singular bodies, collective dreams: Socially engaged circus, arts and the "Quebec spring". In L. P. Leroux & C. Batson (Eds.), *Cirque global – Quebec's expanding circus boundaries* (pp. 266–283). Montreal: McGill-Queen's University Press.

Spiegel, J. B. (2016b). Social circus: The cultural politics of embodying "social transformation". *TDR: The Drama Review, 60*(4), 50–67. Retrieved from http://www.mitpressjournals.org/doi/pdfplus/10.1162/DRAM_a_00595

Spiegel, J. B. (in press-a). Creativity and the condition of precarity: Embodied social transformation in a changing socio-political landscape. In J. B. Spiegel & B. Ortiz Choukroun (Eds.), *The art of collectivity – Social circus and the cultural politics of a post-neoliberal vision*. Montreal: McGill Queen's University Press.

Spiegel, J. B. (in press-b). Social circus, *Buen Vivir*: A critical inquiry into one bold political vision. In J. B. Spiegel & B. Ortiz Choukroun (Eds.), *The art of collectivity – Social circus and the cultural politics of a post-neoliberal vision* (pp. 3–44). Montreal: McGill Queen's University Press.

Spiegel, J. B., Breilh, M., Campana, A., Marcuse, J., & Yassi, A. (2015). Social circus and health equity: Results of a feasibility study to explore the national social circus program in Ecuador. *Arts & Health: An International Journal for Research, Policy and Practice, 7*(1), 65–74. doi:10.1080/17533015.2014.932292

Spiegel, J. B., Ortiz Choukroun, B., Campaña, A., & Yassi, A. (in press). Cultural policy and the *Buen Vivir* debate: Politics of transition and the development of Circo Social Ecuador. In J. B. Spiegel & B. Ortiz Choukroun (Eds.), *The art of collectivity – Social circus and the cultural politics of a post-neoliberal vision*. Montreal: McGill Queen's University Press.

Spiegel, J. B., & Parent, S. (2017). Re-approaching community development through the arts: A 'critical mixed methods' study of social circus in Quebec. *Community Development Journal, 42*(3), 1–18. doi:10.1093/cdj/bsx015

Trotman, R. (2012). *Building character and community. Community circus: A literature review*. Retrieved from http://www.simplycircus.com/node/631

Twenge, J. M., & Campbell, W. K. (2002). Self-esteem and socioeconomic status: A meta-analytic review. *Personality and Social Psychology Review, 6*(1), 59–71. doi:10.1207/S15327957PSPR0601_3

Ugolotti, N., & Moyer, E. (2016). 'If I climb a wall of ten meters': Capoeira, parkour and the politics of public space among (post) migrant youth in Turin, Italy. *Patterns of Prejudice, 50*(2), 188–206.

UNICEF, Ecuador. (2002). *Observatory for the rights of children and adolescents*. Retrieved from http://www.unicef.org/ecuador/english/children_2991.htm

Walsh, C. (2009). *Interculturalidad, estado, sociedad: luchas (de) coloniales de nuestra época*. Quito: Universidad Andina Simón Bolívar.

Walsh, C. (2010). Development as Buen Vivir: Institutional arrangements and (de)colonial entanglement. *Development, 53*(1), 15–21. doi:10.1057/dev.2009.93

Weisbrot, M., Johnston, J., & Merling, L. (2017). *Decade of reform: Ecuador's macroeconomic policies, institutional changes, and results*. Retrieved from http://cepr.net/publications/reports/decade-of-reform-ecuador-s-macroeconomic-policies-institutional-changes-and-results

Yassi, A., & Campaña, A. (in press). The impact of Circo Social Ecuador and other community arts on health: A longitudinal comparative quantitative analysis. In J. B. Spiegel & B. Ortiz Choukroun (Eds.), *The art of collectivity – Social circus and the cultural politics of a post-neoliberal vision*. Montreal: McGill – Queen's University Press.

Yates, J., & Bakker, K. (2013). Debating the 'post-neoliberal turn' in Latin America. *Progress in Human Geography, 30*, 0309132513500372. doi:10.1177/0309132513500372

# 'Live Beautiful, Live Well' ('*Vivir Bonito, Vivir Bien*') in Nicaragua: Environmental health citizenship in a post-neoliberal context

Chris Hartmann ⓘD

**ABSTRACT**
The concepts *Vivir Bien* and *Buen Vivir*, often translated as 'living well' or 'collective well-being,' are central to contemporary social medicine reforms in Latin America. Owing to increasing social inequalities, notably in the public healthcare sector, Vivir Bien has regional significance as it redefines the neoliberal development goals from economic improvement to so-called post-neoliberal social goals of harmonious co-existence between society and the physical environment. To examine how this abstract concept is conceptualised, is incorporated into, and shapes state-sponsored public health strategies, I analyze the '*Vivir Limpio, Vivir Sano, Vivir Bonito, Vivir Bien … !*' ('Live Clean, Live Healthy, Live Beautiful, Live Well … !') national campaign in Nicaragua that began in 2013. The campaign promotes normative socio-political ideals around environmental health citizenship, including the adoption of indigenous grammars and solidarity. However, analyses of dozens of interviews and 143 household surveys in four historically impoverished, untidy, and unhygienic communities suggest that the campaign's discourses do not resonate with citizens or their socio-economic contexts. In highlighting discrepancies between state-sponsored normative sociopolitical ideals and citizens' lived realities and perspectives, this paper introduces the term 'post-neoliberal citizenship' to reflect contemporary – and changing – conceptualizations of health, wellbeing, and citizenship in post-neoliberal Latin America.

## Introduction

Governance is inextricably linked to population health and well-being, environmental matters, and development. In Nicaragua, as well as in other 'New Left' countries in Latin America (e.g. Venezuela, Bolivia, Ecuador, and El Salvador, among others), reducing social inequalities and reframing development discourses, particularly as they relate to health, well-being, and the environment, are at the core of progressive governance changes (see Nading, 2014). After nearly a two decades-long absence from office, during which time neoliberal discourses and policies firmly took root and drastically re-organized post-revolutionary Nicaragua, Daniel Ortega, who first governed the country from 1979–1990, was re-elected president in 2006 on a populist and self-described anti-neoliberal platform. In an attempt to move away from – but not entirely replace – neoliberalism, the Ortega administration has adopted several so-called 'post-neoliberal' ideals, including emphasis on equality and solidarity, an appreciation of indigeneity, and highlighting social over economic goals (Ettlinger & Hartmann, 2015).

This paper examines the emergence of the post-neoliberal concepts *Vivir Bien* and *Buen Vivir*, which are commonly translated from Spanish to English as 'living well' or 'collective well-being,' and the aesthetic concept *Vivir Bonito*, meaning 'living beautiful' or 'living nice,' in Nicaraguan state discourses. In particular, this study focuses on the '*Vivir Limpio, Vivir Sano, Vivir Bonito, Vivir Bien ... !*' ('Live Clean, Live Healthy, Live Beautiful, Live Well ... !') national campaign, which began in 2013. The national campaign, hereafter referred to as Live Beautiful, Live Well,[1] stresses transformation of the practices and 'culture of everyday life, putting emphasis on the necessary consistency between what we are, what we think and what we do' (Murillo, 2013). Besides focusing on Live Beautiful, Live Well's practical and material implications (e.g. cleaning up urban environments in order to increase tourism) (Fisher, 2016), this study critically examines the socio-political discourses around environmental and public health as well as social life at the core of the campaign. Further, to examine how the national campaign is understood by citizens at the subnational and local spaces it intends to 'beautify,' this article analyzes household surveys from four historically impoverished, untidy, and unhygienic communities. In doing so, the article seeks to add to the literature which examines contemporary Latin American social medicine reforms by addressing the emergence of a new form of environmental health citizenship, what is termed here as 'post-neoliberal citizenship.'

## Post-neoliberalism and environmental health governance in latin america

Latin America is widely recognised as 'the privileged birthplace of neoliberalism' and 'a laboratory for neoliberal experiments par excellence' (Sader, 2009, p. 172). Around the world, neoliberalism is a political economic model that regulates economies in favour of free and open markets, liberalises trade, privatises state-owned corporations and services, and curtails social spending (particularly in the healthcare sector) (Harvey, 2006). Neoliberal policies have exacerbated social inequalities, notably in the public healthcare sector (Homedes & Ugalde, 2005; ISAGS, 2012).

In recent years, several countries in the region (e.g. Venezuela, Bolivia, Ecuador, Brazil, Argentina, Nicaragua, and El Salvador, among others) have proposed, to varying degrees, governance strategies that counter neoliberal hegemony; in response, some academics have coined this new epoch the 'post-neoliberal' era.[2] To date, much focus has been paid to post-neoliberalism in terms of macro-economic policies, including South-South cooperation (Muhr, 2013), the nationalisation of the hydrocarbon and mining sectors (Kennemore & Weeks, 2011), and the redistribution of capital surplus to social policies (Macdonald & Ruckert, 2009), as well as strengthened state-civil society relations and attempts to democratize decision-making from the bottom-up (Grugel & Riggirozzi, 2012). Little attention has been paid to the implications of post-neoliberal governance for transforming environmental health governance, of which individual and population behaviours are integral. Therefore, the Live Beautiful, Live Well campaign provides an important opportunity to do so.

According to Gudynas (2011b) and Walsh (2010), the concept Vivir Bien ostensibly redefines the primary goal of state-sponsored development efforts from economic improvement to the social goal of 'living well.' Led by the political left and indigenous movements, post-neoliberal political economic discourses and strategies are framed by diverse orientations, including twenty-first century socialism and indigenous cosmovisions (Escobar, 2010). The concept Vivir Bien is central to the recently rewritten constitutions of Ecuador (2008) ('Constitución del Ecuador,' 2008) and Bolivia (2009) ('Constitución de Bolivia,' 2009). In these juridical documents, the Vivir Bien model is a relational vision in that individuals are inextricably linked to society, which is interconnected with broader socio-cultural and environmental processes per indigenous beliefs. For instance, the Preamble of the Ecuadorian Constitution States: 'We decided to construct a new form of citizen coexistence, in diversity and harmony with nature, to reach buen vivir' ('Constitución de Ecuador,' 2008, p. 15). Further, Vivir Bien is deeply tied to national development goals. In Ecuador and in Bolivia, meeting basic needs like access to a healthy environment, education, and housing, which have long been denied to the majority of citizens by colonial and more recently neoliberal development models, are fundamental to securing Vivir Bien and promoting political economic alternatives. Furthermore, Vivir Bien is central to the implementation of contemporary public health and social medicine reforms, including providing state-guaranteed public healthcare, promoting intercultural care, and democratising healthcare decision-making, to reduce long-standing health inequalities in Ecuador, Bolivia, and Venezuela (Hartmann, 2016). Despite the concept's importance to modern governance in the region, our understanding of how Vivir Bien is woven into and alters environmental health discourses and strategies remains limited.

In examining the deployment of the social goal of Vivir Bien alongside Vivir Bonito in Nicaragua, this paper heeds Radcliffe's call to critically analyze 'the discourses, institutions, rationales, practices, and forms of rule put into motion by anti-neoliberal political and electoral power' (Radcliffe, 2012, p. 240; see also Ghertner, 2010). Hence, the paper investigates the emergence of purported post-neoliberal state 'governmentalities,' a term Foucault defines as the study of the mentalities by which governance of populations, their environments, and their relations occur (Foucault, 2003, p. 245). For Foucault, his interest lie in understanding the technologies of power that seek to configure the habits, aspirations, and beliefs of individuals and communities, in relation to their environments, with the objective of improving population health (Foucault, 2003). Under neoliberalism we see the 'degovernmentalization' of the state but not a decline in government (Rose, 1996, pp. 40–41). Yet, across Latin America and particularly in Ecuador, Bolivia, Venezuela, and Nicaragua, the post-neoliberal present is characterised by claims of the re-emergence of a strong state in terms of engineering economic policy to social policy (Bebbington & Humphreys Bebbington, 2011; Grugel & Riggirozzi, 2009, 2012; Macdonald & Ruckert, 2009), strengthening state-society relations through the promotion of democracy and increased involvement of civil society in decision-making (Grugel & Riggirozzi, 2012), and adopting and promoting alternative conceptualizations regarding well-being and development goals (Escobar, 2010; Gudynas, 2011b; Walsh, 2010).

In the post-neoliberal present, it is necessary to examine the re-'"governmentalization" of the State' (Foucault, 2000, p. 220) to understand how the state's use of the concepts Vivir Bien and Vivir Bonito seek to 'conduct the conduct' of populations toward alternative social, political, and economic goals. From this perspective and in the context of Nicaragua, I ask: How do post-neoliberal governmentalities seek to alter local socio-political relations, particularly as they pertain to human-environment relations? What kind of citizen subjectivity is produced under contemporary governmentalities? How do persons living in targeted (i.e. impoverished, untidy, and unhygienic) communities perceive the Nicaraguan state's campaign slogans of living beautiful and living well?

## Methods

The evidence presented here draws from state-sponsored primary sources and peer-reviewed academic articles. Examples of official government documents include policy reports, speech transcripts, and development reports. Contemporary sources were located online from the website of the Government of Nicaragua (www.presidencia.gob.ni) as well as that of President Daniel Ortega and the Sandinista party (www.elpueblopresidente.com, www.el19digital.com). Secondary sources, including reports, analyses, and articles, were gathered from the two largest periodicals in Nicaragua – El Nuevo Diario and La Prensa.

In addition, this article draws from semi-structured interviews and household surveys completed during fieldwork stints of one month in 2013 and three months in 2015 in Managua, the capital city and political, cultural, and economic centre of Nicaragua. First, the analysis draws from more than 50 semi-structured interviews with community members and leaders, representatives of NGOs, and state officials. The purpose of the semi-structured interviews was to examine the role of community leaders in realising public health campaigns and changes to environmental health governance over time. Interviews were conducted in the native language of the interviewee (Spanish or English) and varied in length from 45–120 minutes.

Second, to understand citizens' perceptions of the Live Beautiful, Live Well campaign, the household survey was administered in four communities that, since the 1970s, have been heavily involved in the local recycling economy. In many respects, the four surveyed neighbourhoods exemplify the spaces targeted by the Live Beautiful, Live Well campaign because the communities are impoverished, untidy, and unhygienic spaces (Hartmann, 2018). According to guidelines developed by the Nicaraguan Government and World Bank (INIDE, 2015), at the time of the household surveys, an estimated 39% of residents in the surveyed communities lived in poverty, one-half of which lived in extreme poverty; in comparison, 29.6% of all Nicaraguans lived in poverty and 8.3% in extreme poverty, whereas in Managua 11.6% of the population lived in poverty and 1.8% in extreme poverty (Guerrero, 2015). These neighbourhoods thus represent an ideal context in which to investigate the implementation of the Live Beautiful, Live Well campaign.

In each neighbourhood, I approached homes selected by a computer-based random number generator. The survey addressed a range of topics including household composition, labour, and income; additionally, several open-ended questions gauged perceptions of what it means to live beautiful (vivir bonito) and live well (Vivir Bien). I administered the surveys in Spanish. One or two community residents accompanied me at all times to clarify key points and colloquialisms when pertinent and to assist in making contact with potential research participants. I handwrote survey responses, transcribed data verbatim, grouped responses by categories, and completed all Spanish-to-English translations.

I administered the household questionnaire survey to 146 households in March and April 2015; three participants did not respond to the open-ended questions. Surveys were completed in approximately one half-hour. The total participation rate was approximately 62% (n = 146); 13% of homes refused participation, and the head of household was absent in 25% of houses approached. Interviewees were more likely to be women (68.7%), and the average age of interviewees was 41.1 years. The majority of respondents reported being self-employed small business owners (21.0%), informal recyclers (20.8%), or public employees in the municipal recycling plant (16.9%); the remainder held other salaried jobs (11.2%), completed manual labour (8.1%), or were otherwise employed (8.8%) or self-employed (13.4%).

## Results

### State discourses & strategies

Environmental health discourses and strategies always are political insofar as they reflect current social and political economic framings, ideals, and goals (e.g. Evered & Evered, 2012; Nading, 2014; Petersen & Lupton, 1996). For example, during the revolutionary Sandinista period (1979–1990), health education materials explicitly supported the popular revolution and encouraged loyalty to the FSLN party. The educational materials aimed to increase health literacy and provide citizens with scientific knowledge to address health concerns (Donahue, 1986). Further, revolutionary health materials incorporated reflection and discussion, intending to 'empower people rather than control them from above' (Donahue, 1986, p. 64).

In the contemporary period, the concept Buen Vivir first appeared in written state discourses in the National Human Development Plan for 2012–2016. In the 203-page document, Buen Vivir is neither defined explicitly nor discussed at length; in fact, it is mentioned only five times and Vivir Bien appears zero times. Nor is the term mentioned in the Model of Family and Community Health, the conceptual and planning framework for the Sandinista Ministry of Health, written in 2007 (MINSA, 2007). As in Ecuador and Bolivia, Nicaragua's human development plan discusses 'living well' in the context of social *and* environmental processes: 'the ongoing search of constructing the Living Well (*Buen Vivir*) for each Nicaraguan and the Common Good (*Bien Común*) among and for all Nicaraguan women and men as a whole, in harmony with Mother Earth (*Madre Tierra*)' (PNDH, 2012, p. 14). Buen Vivir is briefly discussed in relation to both population health and environmental education. To the former, the 'main health policy' is 'to accomplish that people do not become sick, a healthy pueblo is happy within the framework of Buen Vivir' (PNDH, 2012, p. 84); to the latter, the state takes it upon itself to communicate to all Nicaraguans the importance of preserving and protecting Mother Earth. Finally, Article 98 of the Nicaraguan Constitution, amended in 2014, declares that Buen Vivir is the primary economic goal of the State:

> The principal function of the State in terms of the economy is to achieve human sustainable development in the country; to improve the conditions of the *pueblo* and to achieve a more just distribution of wealth in the search of *buen vivir*.

Furthermore, Article 5 was amended at the same time to 'recognize that original peoples and Afro-descendants possess their own identity under a single and indivisible State.' The inclusion of immaterial goals like living well in the PNDH 2012–2016 and the Nicaraguan Constitution – as well as the focus on indigenous peoples in the latter – occurred six years after Ecuador and Bolivia rewrote their constitutions. The timing is critical: it reflects a watershed moment in which indigeneity is celebrated and enshrined in several constitutions in Latin America. Indeed, it exemplifies the ways in which states deploy indigenous alternatives to Western development and materialism, what Zimmerer calls 'speaking like an indigenous state' (Zimmerer, 2015). In his analysis of Bolivia, Zimmerer argues that indigeneity is visible through its promotion of indigenous peoples' rights *and* the adoption of an environmental ethic; namely, through its use of terms such as Buen Vivir and 'Mother Earth.'

In January 2013, First Lady Rosario Murillo invited all Nicaraguans to participate in the Live Beautiful, Live Well campaign. The etho-politics orientation of the Basic Guide, the document written by the Nicaraguan government that outlines the campaign's aims around fourteen themes, is diverse. According to Murillo, the campaign draws inspiration from 'humanist, idealist, ethical, and evolutionary philosophies' (Murillo, 2013). Further, Fisher notes that the campaign's 'language of "love," "care," and "beauty," (are) important elements in the FSLN's re-visioned, 21st century political philosophy of *sandinismo*,' a term used to connote the political ideology of early twentieth century Nicaraguan revolutionary fighter Augusto Sandino (Fisher, 2016). In the present day, critics suggest sandinismo represents a cultural as opposed to a political economic revolution (Kampwirth, 2008; Torres Rivas, 2007). At its core, contemporary sandinismo remains an appeal to the masses (*el pueblo*), as evidenced by its continued embrace of anti-imperialist rhetoric that characterised it in the 1970s and 1980s.

The origins of the Live Beautiful, Live Well campaign are multifold. First, from a public health and urban planning perspective, the campaign responds to decades-long garbage mismanagement issues (e.g. lack of infrastructure, littering) in Nicaragua, particularly Managua and other urban areas (Nading & Fisher, 2017). Indeed, the country's two largest periodicals – *La Prensa* and *El Nuevo Diario* – frequently highlight the country's garbage woes and call attention to the connections among garbage mismanagement, public health concerns (e.g. mosquito-borne diseases and leptospirosis), and other crises such as flooding. Thus, the campaign's focus on cleanliness is widely appealing to Nicaraguans (Envío Team, 2013). Second, the campaign seeks to galvanise support for the neighbourhood-level Cabinets of the Family, Community, and Life (CFCLs), which were announced in conjunction with the campaign and evolved out of the Citizen Power Councils (2007–2013), themselves a reincarnation of the Sandinista Defense Committees from the revolutionary period (Gertsch Romero, 2010; Potosme & Picón, 2013). Under Live Nice, Live Well, the *barrio* (neighbourhood) is the preferred 'zone or space of governmental intervention' (Osborne, 1997, p. 176). A major focus of CFCLs is to raise citizen 'awareness' (*conciencia*), and the campaign has been largely grounded in neighbourhood anti-littering campaigns and clean-ups. Third, from an economic perspective, the campaign expects that cleaning up Nicaragua will stimulate foreign investment and international tourism (El 19 Digital, 2013). Finally, the campaign solidifies Nicaragua's sociocultural and political ties to other leftist Latin American countries – notably Venezuela, Bolivia, and Ecuador – as mentioned above and as will be discussed further below.

The campaign unites the Ministries of Health (MINSA), Environment and Natural Resources (MARENA), and Education (MINED), as well as the Nicaraguan Institute for Tourism (INTUR). Within weeks of its announcement, state institutions, along with volunteer members of CFCLs, distributed 500,000 copies of the Live Beautiful, Live Well Basic Guide (Figure 1) – in addition to 'Yo

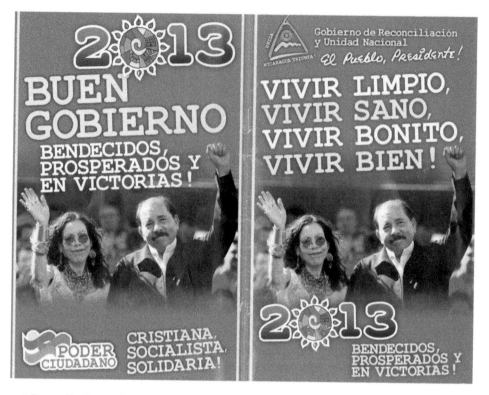

**Figure 1.** Front and back cover of the Live Beautiful, Live Well pamphlet distributed throughout Nicaragua by the national government in 2013.

*Vivo Bonito*' ('I Live Beautiful') bumper stickers, posters, and other Live Beautiful, Live Well-themed propaganda – across Nicaragua, including in state-run schools (Envío Team, 2013). The CFCLs, other groups sympathetic to the FSLN party (e.g. Sandinista Youth), and state institutions led litter cleanups, educational workshops, and other activities to promote the national campaign. Further, the campaign received extensive attention in state-run media outlets and social media.

Additionally, members of the FSLN party expect to rewrite Law 423, the General Health Law (Rugama, n.d.). It is plausible that the rewritten law will incorporate rhetoric from Live Nice, Live Well and the PNDH 2012–2016, thereby further linking Nicaraguan State discourses to indigeneity and the country's unique blend of etho-politics.

The campaign, described as encompassing a set of 'simple, easy, daily actions,' covers fourteen wide-reaching topics around environmental stewardship, personal and collective health, and civic duties and state-civil society relations. Instead of recognising the heterogeneity of Nicaraguan citizens' social, political, and ethnic identities, the Basic Guide homogenises them, preferring to use the singular in discussing 'culture,' 'heritage,' and 'community identity.' Despite the legal separation of state and Church per the Nicaraguan Constitution, it is not surprising that the Basic Guide references 'Christian and family values' given the Ortega administration's alliance with the Catholic Church and the political currency of embracing Christianity in a country where citizens overwhelming identify as Christian.[3] Live Beautiful, Live Well is not a juridical document and as such does not guarantee rights to human beings or nature as Buen Vivir does in the Ecuadorian constitution. Notably, neither Vivir Bien in Bolivia nor Buen Vivir in Ecuador tie ethical-moral values or rights to a specific religion.

In the following subsections, I examine specific themes of Live Beautiful, Live Well, including environmental health, pedagogy, the responsibilization of health and well-being, and indigeneity and environmental stewardship. Then, I examine lay perceptions of 'live beautiful' and 'live well.'

### Environmental health

In the contemporary period, Western public health discourses regularly reflect a broad understanding of the determinants of health, including social, psychological, and environmental elements (WHO, 2008). The same is true of the Live Beautiful, Live Well campaign. The Basic Guide's fourteen points reference health promotion and health education, nutrition, community participation, and hygiene, among others, as key factors contributing to individual and collective health and well-being. Commonly, modern public health campaigns conceptualise the physical environment as a biomedical risk or hazard to health and well-being (World Health Organization, 1989, p. 21). Live Beautiful, Live Well does this, too, though sparingly; for example, the risk posed by garbage to 'natural, environmental, cultural, personal, familial, and community rights' is the lone exception. Instead, the focus of the campaign – as evidenced by the Basic Guide and other state discourses – remains centred on altering the sociopolitical subjectivity of the Nicaragua population according to indigenous cosmovisions, as discussed below.

### Pedagogy

The contemporary health discourses of the Live Beautiful, Live Well campaign are distinct from those of the revolutionary period in that power is rigidly hierarchical. Power is unidirectional (top-down) and citizens do not collaborate with state entities in any meaningful manner; instead citizens – collectively or individually – alone are expected to meet the 'fulfillment of … all the plans, campaigns, and norms related to health, healthy living spaces, citizen education, environmental restoration, cleanups, and beautification' (Point 6). Consequently, such realities call into question the notion that post-neoliberalism signals the state's intention to democratize governance and 'make the state public' (Grugel & Riggirozzi, 2012, p. 15). Whereas revolutionary health material encouraged discussion around a specific health issue or environmental health problem (e.g. preventing diarrhea, illnesses linked to inadequate garbage management), the focus of the Basic Guide is broad, and its utility for addressing specific environmental health risks is extremely limited. Moreover, the campaign does not itself represent a transfer of medical knowledge as did revolutionary health materials. Finally, in a departure from traditional leftist-led social medicine efforts in Latin America (Waitzkin, Iriart, Estrada, & Lamadrid, 2001) and prior Sandinista discourses, Live Beautiful, Live Well eschews attention to economic class differences; instead, it homogenises citizens. In sum, seemingly the campaign reflects hierarchical and populist underpinnings over a radical and revolutionary approach to environmental health governance.

### Responsibilizing 'Health' and 'Well-being'

Collective action is germane – or ought to be (Beaglehole, Bonita, Horton, Adams, & McKee, 2004; World Health Organization, 1978) – to definitions of 'public health.' During the revolutionary years (1979–1990), citizens assisted in the development, planning, and carrying out of ambitious social welfare projects in consultation with the state (e.g. neighbourhood-level Popular Health Councils and Popular Health Work Days) (Donahue, 1986). Collective and solidarity action was a fundamental organising principle of the revolutionary Ministry of Health, which stated 'Health is a right of every individual and a responsibility of the State and the Popular organizations' (Donahue, 1986, p. 25), and was institutionalised in the Constitution in 1987. In the contemporary period, Live Beautiful, Live Well strategically uses collective rhetoric to spur individual action to secure health and well-being to 'promote the Beautiful and better Nicaragua that we all want' (Point 9). To incite and promote collective action, Murillo uses the 'we' verb tense. Additionally, the Basic Guide uses key concepts like 'unity' to speak of Nicaraguan citizens as a collective whole and citizens are expected to work with State institutions, neighbourhood groups, and religious leaders to prevent certain social problems.

In the Basic Guide of Live Beautiful, Live Well, collective responsibility slips into individual responsibility for securing health and well-being. Live Beautiful, Live Well outlines several sets of specific duties, including keeping a tidy home, maintaining clean and beautiful neighbourhoods and public spaces, and caring for Mother Earth. The individual responsibilization exhibited by the Live Beautiful, Live Well campaign exemplifies the notion that in the neoliberal present 'the individual has never been more important' as the individual citizen is germane to health governance and takes on an increasing number of responsibilities for their health and well-being (Brown & Baker, 2012, p. 1; Petersen & Lupton, 1996). Article 60 of Nicaragua's Constitution from 1987 guaranteed the right to a healthy environment and declared that the State would 'preserve, conserve, and rescue' the physical environment. In contrast, the new version of the constitution, which was rewritten in 2014, proclaims that 'Nicaraguans have a right to inhabit a healthy environment, (and) it is *their* obligation to preserve and conserve it' (emphasis added). Thus, in devolving juridical responsibility to citizens, the recent amendment dropped entirely language obligating the State to preserve and conserve the environment, which ironically was amended to the Constitution in 1987 under President Daniel Ortega.

In addition, in Live Beautiful, Live Well, references to indigeneity overlap with and are entangled in solidarity principles, other humanistic values, and neoliberal values, producing a uniquely Nicaraguan set of discourses. For instance, Point 11 seeks to produce 'good environmental citizens' who recognise their duties and responsibilities in relation to consumer activities: 'We promote the efficient use of water, energy and services that others still lack' and 'We promote a culture of simple living and without waste or ostentation, that hurts, excludes, or limits other citizens.' As such, Point 11 recognises the need for solidarity in the face of market inequalities.

### Indigeneity and environmental stewardship

Live Beautiful, Live Well departs from dominant public health discourses in its visible embrace of indigeneity and deep ecology. Here, 'indigeneity' is understood as the 'social, cultural, economic, political, institutional, and epistemic processes through which the meaning of being indigenous in a particular time and place is constructed' (Radcliffe, 2017). Indigenous knowledges often contrast with Western knowledges in that the latter are largely technocratic and science-oriented (Gregory, Johnston, Pratt, Watts, & Whatmore, 2009). Latin American indigenous conceptualizations of health, though numerous and diverse, often view individual life in harmony with community, the environment, and the universe (Montenegro & Stephens, 2006; WHO, 2007).

The Basic Guide of Live Beautiful, Live Well demonstrates the Nicaraguan State's attempt to 'speak like an indigenous State.' Zimmerer developed this concept to describe the Bolivian State's usage of indigenous grammars such as Living Well and Mother Earth, which he argues '[are] centred on widely common linguistic terms, rather than bureaucratic State-speak' (Zimmerer, 2015, p. 315). Regarding Nicaragua, indigeneity is invoked on the cover of the Basic Guide booklet through the use of the serpent feather deity, Quetzalcoatl (Figure 1). Since less than 9% of the national population identifies as indigenous (INIDE, 2005), the inclusion of the symbol, which also appears in a large memorial to the late Venezuelan President Hugo Chavez in the heart of Managua, is curious. Ettlinger and Hartmann (2015) suggest the deployment of the symbol is intended to connect Nicaragua to pink tide Latin American governments, including Bolivia and Ecuador.

Second, Live Beautiful, Live Well uses the terms Mother Earth (*Madre Tierra*), Mother Nature (*Madre Naturaleza*), and Nature (*Naturaleza*). The Nicaraguan campaign uses these indigenous terms for nature differently than the term 'environment' (*ambiente*), which it uses in discussing environmental hazards and risks. The campaign uses the terms Mother Earth, Mother Nature, and Nature in stating that nature must be cared for and in discussing the relationship between human beings and the physical environment. To the latter, Live Beautiful, Live Well conceives of the individual body, families, and communities as interconnected and coexisting with Mother Earth.

> Point 1: "We learn together … simple and practical norms of coexistence among us, between us and Mother Earth, and between family, community, public, and private spaces around cleanliness, hygiene, order, aesthetics, respect, loving care, and permanent solidarity."

In addition, the campaign inextricably links human well-being to harmonious relations with Nature and the well-being of Nature:

Point 10: "We learn to see in Nature and in natural environments, which we safeguard, as Gifts from God, temples of energy replacement, renewing our physical and spiritual strength and well-being in harmony and human comprehension."

Such perceptions highlight the campaign's simultaneous concern with environmental stewardship and its discursive connections to Buen Vivir in Bolivia and Ecuador.

The inclusion of indigenous discourses in Live Beautiful, Live Well seems to be influenced by the Universal Declaration of the Common Good of the Earth and Humanity and the constitutions of Ecuador and Bolivia. To the latter, concepts of citizen coexistence and harmony with nature, which are discussed in Live Beautiful, Live Well, are of particular importance in the Bolivian (Article 403) and Ecuadorian constitutions (Article 275) (Gudynas, 2011a; Walsh, 2010). The similarities in indigenous grammars demonstrate the transnational and networked flows of (indigenous) cultures and rhetoric among leftist governments in Latin America (Andolina, Laurie, & Radcliffe, 2009).

## Lay perceptions

To understand the ways in which government discourses align with and diverge from lay perceptions of 'live beautiful' (Vivir Bonito) and 'live well' (Vivir Bien), I asked heads of households in four communities in Managua to define each concept in their own words. As previous research elsewhere on views of health and well-being has found (Izquierdo, 2005; Richmond, Elliott, Matthews, & Elliott, 2005), it is not surprising that lay perceptions of 'living beautiful' and 'living well' varied widely.

Most definitions of 'live beautiful' fit into one of three categories: 1) cleanliness and the aesthetic environment, 2) social factors, and 3) economic factors (Table 1). First, many respondents equated 'live beautiful' with general cleanliness, tidiness, and orderliness (44.1%), as well as in the streets (27.3%) and in homes (25.2%) more specifically. For instance, a respondent, looking at her humble, government-provided home, stated:

If you clean the house, even if it isn't a mansion, is to live beautiful, to live clean and orderly. (Woman, 40 years old)

Similarly, several respondents related living beautiful to living in an environment free of garbage and litter (11.9%) or to environmental stewardship (e.g. planting trees) (6.3%). That many definitions of 'live beautiful' centred on cleanliness and the aesthetic environment is not surprising given the

**Table 1.** Lay perceptions of definitions of Live Beautiful (Vivir Bonito).

|  | # Mentions (a) | # Mentions/Total Respondents (a/ 143) | # Mentions/All Mentions (a/ 296) |
|---|---|---|---|
| Live Clean (*limpio*)/tidy/ordered | 63 | 44.1% | 19.3% |
| Clean street | 39 | 27.3% | 12.0% |
| Get along with neighbours | 37 | 25.9% | 11.3% |
| Clean house | 36 | 25.2% | 11.0% |
| Be in good health, live healthy (sano) | 29 | 20.3% | 8.9% |
| Formal/Beautiful house | 25 | 17.5% | 7.7% |
| Collect garbage | 17 | 11.9% | 5.2% |
| Meet basic needs | 17 | 11.9% | 5.2% |
| Live peacefully/tranquility | 16 | 11.2% | 4.9% |
| Social welfare programmes | 11 | 7.7% | 3.4% |
| Environmental stewardship | 9 | 6.3% | 2.8% |
| Collective participation | 8 | 5.6% | 2.5% |
| Doesn't know | 7 | 4.9% | 2.1% |
| Good job | 4 | 2.8% | 1.2% |
| Religion/spirituality | 4 | 2.8% | 1.2% |
| Education | 2 | 1.4% | 0.6% |
| Family relations | 1 | 0.7% | 0.3% |
| Improved life | 1 | 0.7% | 0.3% |
| Total | 326 | 100% | 100% |

regularity of neighbourhood clean-ups in each of the four neighbourhoods as well as the general abundance of state propaganda and media attention on the topic.

Second, many community members linked social features, such as getting along with neighbours (25.9%) – sometimes discussed as living in harmony with their community – as well as collective participation and solidarity (5.6%), to 'living beautiful.' Being in good health and having health (20.3%), which were nearly always discussed in relationship to cleanliness, were key to being able to 'live beautiful.' For example, a 42-year-old woman who was relocated by the government from a flood-prone squatter settlement to new government housing shared:

> Live tidy. If … you don't live like a pig and if we clean our house there won't be any illnesses. Flies come … and then you get vomiting.

Third, respondents often related 'living beautiful' to their economic condition; for example, several respondents associated living in a decent home (*casa digna*) (17.5%). Additionally, several respondents discussed the ability to meet basic needs (e.g. afford housing and food) (11.9%) and the availability of social welfare programmes (e.g. free education and healthcare) (7.7%) as key factors in 'living beautiful.' These perceptions are not surprising given persistent poverty and extreme poverty in the surveyed neighbourhoods.

Definitions of 'live well' (Table 2) differed from live beautiful in that descriptions largely revolved around economic and social factors. For example, respondents most frequently equated having a decent job, salaried position, or improved economic condition (29.4%) with living well. Moreover, several respondents defined living well as the ability to eat everyday (23.1%), meet their basic needs (e.g. afford housing and food) (18.2%), or live in a decent house (16.8%). For example, two men who previously worked informally in the garbage dump and secured salaried positions in the new municipal recycling plant shared similar sentiments:

> (To live well) is to not lack anything. At times, I don't live well because I lack food … I only eat beans." (Man, 54 years old)

> It is not only living beautiful (and) we would live not only rich, but be able to provide for us and other children." (Man, 63 years old)

**Table 2.** Lay perceptions of definitions of Live Well (Vivir Bien).

|  | # Mentions (a) | # Mentions/Total Respondents (a/143) | # Mentions/All Mentions (a/326) |
| --- | --- | --- | --- |
| Have job/fixed income/improved economic condition | 42 | 29.4% | 14.2% |
| Be in good health, live healthy (*sano*) | 33 | 23.1% | 11.1% |
| Have daily food | 33 | 23.1% | 11.1% |
| In harmony with neighbours | 28 | 19.6% | 9.5% |
| Meet basic needs | 26 | 18.2% | 8.8% |
| Have house | 24 | 16.8% | 8.1% |
| Live in peace | 17 | 11.9% | 5.7% |
| Don't know | 14 | 9.8% | 4.7% |
| Be clean | 13 | 9.1% | 4.4% |
| Education | 11 | 7.7% | 3.7% |
| Same as Live Beautiful | 11 | 7.7% | 3.7% |
| Harmony with family | 10 | 7.0% | 3.4% |
| Solidarity/community participation | 6 | 4.2% | 2.0% |
| Have basic services (e.g. access to electricity and water, paved streets) | 6 | 4.2% | 2.0% |
| Religion/spirituality | 6 | 4.2% | 2.0% |
| Be happy/feel well | 5 | 3.5% | 1.7% |
| Environmental stewardship | 4 | 2.8% | 1.4% |
| Secure neighbourhood | 3 | 2.1% | 1.0% |
| Own car or motorcycle | 2 | 1.4% | 0.7% |
| Be beautiful person | 1 | 0.7% | 0.3% |
| No garbage in sight | 1 | 0.7% | 0.3% |
| Total | 296 | 100% | 100% |

Respondents also equated 'living well' with being in good health and having health (23.1%). In this context, however, healthiness was not tied to cleanliness like it was for 'living beautiful'; rather, to 'live well' was described as a general state of well-being dependent on economic factors and social relations. Respondents believed getting along and living in harmony with neighbours (19.6%) and family (7.0%) as well as the ability to live in peace (e.g. tranquility, without fear of gangs or crime) (11.9%) to be key components of 'living well.'

It is notable that respondents were less likely to offer definitions for 'live well' (9.8%) than 'live beautiful' (4.9%); relatedly, several respondents described 'live well' as 'a huge word' and 'a very broad word' and, thus, difficult to define. Further, some participants equated 'live well' with 'live beautiful,' suggesting that there was not a difference between the two terms (7.7%). Finally, 'live well' was less likely than 'live beautiful,' albeit it slightly, to be linked to solidarity and community participation (4.2% vs. 5.6%) and environmental stewardship (2.8% to 6.3%).

Respondents had mixed feelings when asked whether they thought that they could 'live beautiful' and 'live well' in their neighbourhood. Most agreed that it was possible, but believed it depended on an individual person's demeanour and behaviours:

> Depends on the people themselves. (Woman, 18 years old)

> If one wants to, yes. If one doesn't want to, then no. (Man, 26 years old)

Moreover, many respondents stated that the solution to improving the quality of life among households and in the community was to make people aware of (*concientizar*) and change personal behaviours instead of addressing contextual, sometimes systemic factors.

In contrast, other respondents spoke about the importance of shared collective responsibility:

> Yes (I can live beautiful and live well) because of neighborhood solidarity. There are many *compañeros*. There is good communication among people. We support each other; not only Sandinistas. (Woman, 33 years old)

> Some—not all—participate in clean-ups of public areas and streets. We have to get people involved, meet with them regularly. (Woman, 31 years old)

In referencing neighbourhood solidarity, these responses echo Sandinista discourses of the revolutionary and contemporary periods.

Still other respondents tied health and well-being to structural processes not discussed in the Basic Guide of Live Beautiful, Live Well. Participants indicated that their ability to 'live beautiful' and to 'live well' was determined by political economic issues out of their control. Specifically, many participants referenced their lack of employment or underemployment and its impact on their ability to 'live well':

> Yes, but we have to have a good job. Yes, here we live beautiful, but we do not live well. (Woman, 34 years old, 3 members of her 9-person household work in informal recycling economy)

Another respondent, a 43-year-old man who previously worked informally in the garbage dump and secured a salaried position in the new municipal recycling plant, stated:

> There has to be a wage that conforms to the basic food basket, (if not) we can't live well.

Although Nicaragua is no longer formally subjected to IMF surveillance as part of its debt reduction plan, the Ortega administration continues to adhere to the development agency's suggestions, including the recommendation that the minimum wage not be increased. As a result, the monthly minimum wage of most sectors (US$200) is approximately one-half that of the estimated monthly cost of living (US$420) (i.e. basic food basket).

In summary, the data yield several noteworthy patterns. Survey responses are similar to the Nicaraguan state's key discourses about 'live beautiful,' as reflected by each mentioning cleanliness, tidiness, and living in social harmony with neighbours and families. Also, lay perspectives rarely associate environmental stewardship with conceptualizations of 'live beautiful' and 'live well.' Finally, several principal concerns that Nicaraguan citizens expressed – employment, income, meeting basic needs – are not discussed at all in the Basic Guide of Live Beautiful, Live Well, evidence of a potential disconnect between this national campaign and on-the-ground realities of everyday life in Nicaragua.

## Discussion and conclusion

The Live Beautiful, Live Well campaign aspires to a reformulated environmental health governance model to change the 'culture of everyday life'(Murillo, 2013) in Nicaragua. As a governmental technique (Ghertner, 2010), the campaign appeals to the masses with its focus on urban aesthetics (i.e. urban hygiene) while simultaneously instilling much broader socio-political and environmental expectations of a unique subjectivity, what I term 'post-neoliberal citizenship.' 'Post-neoliberal citizenship' demonstrates the complex and not-quite-neoliberal forms of idealised citizenship envisioned by the Nicaraguan state, or rather President Daniel Ortega and Vice President Rosario Murillo. Moreover, at a time when questions have arisen elsewhere in Latin America regarding the point of emergence of the concepts Vivir Bien and Buen Vivir (Hidalgo-Capitán, Arias, & Ávila, 2014), this study provides some evidence that Vivir Bien and Vivir Bonito, at least as framed by the Nicaraguan state, may be best understood as an 'invention' by those in power rather than the product of social movements from below.

In comparison to campaigns from the revolutionary period, Live Beautiful, Live Well highlights several changes to how environmental public health is conceptualised and practiced. First, key determinants of health are absent in Live Beautiful, Live Well, and its utility as an environmental health campaign, outside of encouraging citizens to tidy up their homes, is questionable. Specifically, critics point out that Live Beautiful, Live Well 'disguises,' or covers up, economic realities of Nicaragua's poor majorities (Potosme & Picón, 2013). Similarly, one survey participant, stated 'only in Rosario (Murillo)'s illusion and mind do people live beautiful because there are people that don't eat.' Second, the Live Beautiful, Live Well campaign is not, nor does it strive to be, liberating and empowering as was the objective of popular health education pedagogy of the revolutionary era. Neither does the campaign celebrate nor recognise the plurality of Nicaraguan citizenship, as guaranteed in the constitution. Instead, the campaign represents a set of top-down discourses aimed at normalising society (Foucault, 1980a) through a particular 'regime of truth' (Foucault, 1980b, p. 131). State discourses demand citizens adopt a particular set of normative etho-politics (Rose, 1999) focused on indigenous grammars and logics around nature-society relations applied to health and well-being. Taken as a whole, the Basic Guide of Live Beautiful, Live Well falls into a similar normalising trap as Buen Vivir / Sumak Kawsay in Ecuador: 'it unthinkingly reproduces a form of elite post-colonial modernity that continuously denigrates other ways of knowing and practicing development' (Radcliffe, 2012, p. 247).

This study examined whether state discourses around social, health, and environmental matters match perceptions of citizens living in communities targeted by the campaign. Notably, not one of the 146 surveyed participants spoke of the indigenous grammars discussed in the campaign. The results are not unexpected: incorporating indigeneity in everyday governmentalities may seem out of place in Nicaragua, since less than 9% of Nicaraguans identify as indigenous[4] (INIDE, 2005). References to indigeneity extend the perception that the Ortega administration is sensitive to inclusivity of diverse cultures and may assist in redirecting attention away from Nicaragua's continued involvement in environmentally destructive and neoliberal development projects (e.g. mining concessions, the proposed interoceanic canal), which negatively affect local populations, indigenous and non-indigenous alike (Hartmann, 2013). At the regional scale, sensitivity to indigeneity buys Nicaragua socio-political currency with other Latin American nations, notably Ecuador and Bolivia, where indigenous groups compose much larger percentages of national populations (Ettlinger & Hartmann, 2015; Gudynas, 2011a; Radcliffe, 2017; Walsh, 2010; Zimmerer, 2015).

Also, Live Beautiful, Live Well propagates notions of individual responsibility for health, a hallmark of neoliberal health governance in Latin America and globally. In Nicaragua, citizen participation is key for securing health and well-being in the contemporary period. Under the discourses of solidarity, individual citizens are made responsible for their health and well-being *as well as* that of their families, communities, and Mother Nature (Envío Team, 2013). Furthermore, citizens are expected to care for public and private spaces alike – while the role of the state is neither questioned nor discussed at any significant length – in the name of solidarity and shared responsibility. On one hand, participants' responses reflect revolutionary and contemporary Sandinista discourses that stated change begins at the household and street level (Donahue, 1986). On the other hand, reducing issues of health and well-being to personal (i.e. individualised) responsibility call to mind neoliberal rhetoric (Petersen & Lupton, 1996) that the Ortega administration often speaks against. Indeed, Dora Maria Tellez, former Minister of Health during the revolutionary period and historian, expressed concern that the campaign's slogan seems to be 'Don't ask me to solve your problems, change your attitude' (del Cid, 2013). Such mentalities, which permeated Nicaraguan society from 1990 to 2006, failed to take into consideration other contributing factors such as social, economic, and political determinants of health. Thus, the data demonstrate the difficulty in determining the origin(s) and entanglement of diverse governmentalities concerning environmental health citizenship. In sum, new duties and ways of thinking, which are expressed in the Basic Guide of Live Beautiful, Live Well, through state propaganda, and by members of neighbourhood-level CFCLs, communicate the expectations of 'post-neoliberal citizenship' to Nicaraguans.

In contemporary Nicaragua, post-neoliberal citizenship demands by the state demonstrate the tensions and contradictions between neoliberalism, socialism, and post-neoliberalism. On one hand, state discourses are centred around socialist notions of 'solidarity' and 'shared responsibility.' This matches the definition of liberal citizenship in the first half of the twentieth century: 'a social being whose powers and obligations were articulated in the language of social responsibilities and collective responsibilities' (Miller & Rose, 1993, p. 97). In the case of Nicaragua – as well as Ecuador and Bolivia – social/collective responsibility is paired with post-neoliberal indigenous grammars depicting harmonious nature-society relations whereby citizens are made responsible for the care of Mother Earth. Amidst liberal and post-neoliberal duties, the latter overlaps with neoliberal expectations of citizenship, too. Live Beautiful, Live Well discusses environmental duties such as water and energy conservation in relation to the market economy (and social solidarity), thereby exemplifying neoliberal rationalities (Petersen & Lupton, 1996). Thus, in being made responsible for individual health and well-being as well as that of their neighbours and community, 'citizenship is (understood) to be active and individualistic rather than passive and dependent' (Miller & Rose, 1993, p. 98). Survey data, too, indicate that consideration of social responsibilities, to which CFCL members in particular ascribe, is largely overshadowed by notions of individual responsibilization for personal health. While contemporary governance in Nicaragua seemingly grants citizens freedom and autonomy in a manner characteristic of neoliberal governmentalities (Miller & Rose, 1993; Petersen & Lupton, 1996), the state's normative ethos-politics simultaneously seeks to inculcate various post-neoliberal moral and political values, including solidarity, socialism, environmental stewardship, and indigeneity.

In conclusion, contemporary environmental health governance in Nicaragua, as examined through the lens of the Live Beautiful, Live Well national campaign, is entangled in specific normative socio-political agendas, representing an amalgam of diverse socio-political orientations. Under the Live Beautiful, Live Well campaign, health and well-being – both broadly defined – come under the purview of the modern state, which attempts to shape the habits, aspirations, and beliefs of citizens toward particular post-neoliberal goals. In doing so, the campaign – and the state more broadly – seeks to produce a normalised post-neoliberal citizenry that reflects the diverse antecedents of contemporary governance in Nicaragua and Latin America. Finally, the Live Beautiful, Live Well campaign demonstrates the diversity of conceptualizations of health, wellbeing, and citizenship in contemporary and post-neoliberal Latin America.

## Notes

1. The state and popular media outlets commonly refer to the campaign using the shorthand Vivir Bonito, Vivir Bien. 'Bonito' may be translated as 'pretty,' 'beautiful,' or 'nice.'
2. Still other academics consider recent changes as representing the rise of a socially conscious and aware variant of neoliberalism—labeled as 'inclusive neoliberalism,'(Craig & Porter, 2003) 'social neoliberalism,'(Andolina et al., 2009, p. 8) or 'adjustment with a human face'(Radcliffe, Laurie, & Andolina, 2004, p. 398).
3. In fact, Vice-President Murillo stated that she was 'very proud' that Nicaragua 'is the only country in the world that declares itself Christian' (Envío Team, 2013).
4. In contrast, more than 70% of Bolivians identify as indigenous; thus, invoking indigeneity-laden grammars is a way to consolidate the political and moral support of the masses (Zimmerer, 2015).

## Acknowledgements

Becky Mansfield, Kendra McSweeney, Nancy Ettlinger, and Jennifer Hartmann provided valuable feedback on this research. This research was made possible with the financial support from Ohio State University, Tinker Foundation, and Conference of Latin Americanist Geographers.

## Disclosure statement

No potential conflict of interest was reported by the authors.

## Funding

This research was made possible with the financial support from Ohio State University, Tinker Foundation, and Conference of Latin Americanist Geographers.

## ORCID

Chris Hartmann ⬥ http://orcid.org/0000-0002-8947-205X

## References

Andolina, R., Laurie, N., & Radcliffe, S. (2009). *Indigenous development in the Andes: Culture, power, and transnationalism*. Durham, NC: Duke University Press.
Beaglehole, R., Bonita, R., Horton, R., Adams, O., & McKee, M. (2004). Public health in the new era: Improving health through collective action. *The Lancet, 363*(9426), 2084–2086.
Bebbington, A., & Humphreys Bebbington, D. (2011). An Andean avatar: Post-neoliberal and neoliberal strategies for securing the unobtainable. *New Political Economy, 16*(1), 131–145.
Brown, B., & Baker, S. (2012). *Responsible citizens: Individuals, health, and policy under neoliberalism*. London: Anthem Press.
Constitución de Bolivia. (2009). *Ministerio de la Presidencia, Estado Plurinacional de Bolivia*. 178 pp.
Constitución del Ecuador. (2008). *Asamblea Constituyente*. 218 pp.
Craig, D., & Porter, D. (2003). Poverty reduction strategy papers: A new convergence. *World Development, 31*(1), 53–69.
del Cid, A. (2013, February 11). Batalla digital "vivir bonito." *La Prensa*. Retrieved from http://www.laprensa.com.ni/2013/02/11/nacionales/134201-batalla-digital-vivir-bonito.
Donahue, J. (1986). *The Nicaraguan revolution in health: From Somoza to the Sandinistas*. South Hadley, MA: Bergin & Garvey Publishers, Inc.
El 19 Digital. (2013, February 5). Companera Rosario invita a familias nicaraguenses a enfrentar juntos el desafio de vivir en una Nicaragua mejor (Companera Rosario invites Nicaraguan families to confront together the challenge to live in a better Nicaragua). Retrieved from http://www.elpueblopresidente.com/EL-19/15136.html.
Envío Team. (2013). Is it a bird? A plane? A cultural revolution … ? *Revista Envío*, (379).
Escobar, A. (2010). Latin America at a crossroads: Alternative modernizations, post-liberalism, or post-development? *Cultural Studies, 24*(1), 1–65.
Ettlinger, N., & Hartmann, C. D. (2015). Post/neo/liberalism in relational perspective. *Political Geography, 48*, 37–48.
Evered, K. T., & Evered, EÖ. (2012). State, peasant, mosquito: The biopolitics of public health education and malaria in early republican Turkey. *Political Geography, 31*(5), 311–323.

Fisher, J. (2016). Cleaning up the streets, Sandinista-style: The aesthetics of garbage and the urban political ecology of tourism development in Nicaragua. In M. Mostafanezhad, R. Norum, E. J. Shelton, & A. Thompson-Carr (Eds.), *Political ecology of tourism: Community, power and the environment* (pp. 231–250). London: Routledge.

Foucault, M. (1980a). Two lectures. In C. Gordon (Ed.), *Power/knowledge: Selected interviews and other writings, 1972-1977* (pp. 78–108). New York: Vintage Books.

Foucault, M. (1980b). Truth and power. In C. Gordon (Ed.), *Power/knowledge: Selected interviews and other writings, 1972-1977* (pp. 109–133). New York: Vintage Books.

Foucault, M. (2000). Governmentality. In J. Faubion (Ed.), *Michel foucault, power* (pp. 201–222). New York: The New Press.

Foucault, M. (2003). 17 march 1976. In *"Society Must be Defended": Lectures at the College de France 1975-1976* (pp. 239–264). New York: Picador.

Gertsch Romero, E. (2010, May 16). De los CDS a los CPC (From the CDS to the CPC). *La Prensa*. Retrieved from http://www.laprensa.com.ni/2010/05/16/politica/24768-de-los-cds-a-los-cpc.

Ghertner, A. (2010). Calculating without numbers: Aesthetic governmentality in Delhi's slums. *Economy and Society*, 39(2), 185–217.

Gregory, D., Johnston, R., Pratt, G., Watts, M., & Whatmore, S. (eds.). (2009). *The dictionary of human geography* (5th ed). Malden, MA: Blackwell.

Grugel, J., & Riggirozzi, P. (2009). Conclusion: Governance after neoliberalism. In *Governance after neoliberalism in Latin America* (pp. 217–230). New York: Palgrave Macmillan.

Grugel, J., & Riggirozzi, P. (2012). Post-neoliberalism in Latin America: Rebuilding and reclaiming the state after crisis. *Development and Change*, 43(1), 1–21.

Gudynas, E. (2011a). Buen vivir: Germinando alternativas al desarrollo. *América Latina En Movimiento*, 462, 1–20.

Gudynas, E. (2011b). Buen vivir: Today's tomorrow. *Development*, 54(4), 441–447.

Guerrero. (2015, October 7). Nicaragua es menos pobre, asegura BCN. *El Nuevo Diario*. Retrieved from http://www.elnuevodiario.com.ni/nacionales/372748-nicaragua-reduce-pobreza-aumenta-consumo/.

Hartmann, C. (2016). Postneoliberal public health care reforms: Neoliberalism, social medicine, and persistent health inequalities in Latin America. *American Journal of Public Health*, 106(12), 2145–2151.

Hartmann, C. (2018). Waste picker livelihoods and inclusive neoliberal municipal solid waste management policies: The case of the La Chureca garbage dump site in Managua, Nicaragua. *Waste Management*, 71, 565–577.

Hartmann, C. D. (2013). Garbage, health, and well-being in Managua. *NACLA Report on the Americas*, 46(4), 62–65.

Harvey, D. (2006). *A brief history of neoliberalism*. Oxford: Oxford Univ. Press.

Hidalgo-Capitán, A. L., Arias, A., & Ávila, J. (2014). El pensamiento indigenista ecuatoriano sobre el Sumak Kawsay [Ecuadorian indigenist thought about Sumak Kawsay]. In A. L. Hidalgo Capitán, A. Guillén García, & N. Deleg Guazha (Eds.), *Antología del Pensamiento Indigenista Ecuatoriano sobre Sumak Kawsay* (pp. 29–73). Huelva y Cuenca: FIUCUHU.

Homedes, N., & Ugalde, A. (2005). Why neoliberal health reforms have failed in Latin America. *Health Policy*, 71(1), 83–96.

INIDE. (2005). Censo de población (Population census). Inistituto Nacional de Información de Desarrollo. Retrieved from http://www.inide.gob.ni/censos2005/resumencensal/resumen2.pdf.

INIDE. (2015). Results of the national households survey on measurement of level of life, 2014. Instituto Nacional de Informacion de Desarrollo. Retrieved from http://www.inide.gob.ni/Emnv/Emnv14/Poverty%20Results%202014.pdf.

ISAGS. (2012). Sistemas de salud en suramerica: desafíos para la universalidad, la integralidad y la equidad. Instituto Suramericano de Gobierno en Salud.

Izquierdo, C. (2005). When "health" is not enough: Societal, individual and biomedical assessments of well-being among the Matsigenka of the Peruvian Amazon. *Social Science & Medicine*, 61(4), 767–783.

Kampwirth, K. (2008). Abortion, antifeminism, and the return of Daniel Ortega: In Nicaragua, Leftist Politics? *Latin American Perspectives*, 35(6), 122–136.

Kennemore, A., & Weeks, G. (2011). Twenty-First century socialism? The elusive search for a post-neoliberal development model in Bolivia and Ecuador. *Bulletin of Latin American Research*, 30(3), 267–281.

Macdonald, L., & Ruckert, A. (2009). *Post-neoliberalism in the Americas: An introduction*. New York: Palgrave.

Miller, P., & Rose, N. (1993). Governing economic life. In M. Gane, & T. Johnson (Eds.), *Foucault's New Domains* (pp. 75–105). London: Routledge.

MINSA. (2007). *Modelo de Salud Familiar y Comunitario* [Model of family and community health]. Nicaragua: Ministerio de Salud (Ministry of Health).

Montenegro, R. A., & Stephens, C. (2006). Indigenous health in Latin America and the Caribbean. *The Lancet*, 367 (9525), 1859–1869.

Muhr, T. (2013). *Counter-globalization and socialism in the 21st century: the Bolivarian Alliance for the Peoples of Our America*. London: Routledge.

Murillo, R. (2013, January 25). Estrategia Nacional para "Vivir Limpio, Vivir Sano, Vivir Bonito, Vivir Bien … !" [National strategy to "live clean, live health, live nice, live well … !"]. Retrieved from http://www.el19digital.com/articulos/ver/titulo:7428-estrategia-nacional-para-vivir-limpio-vivir-sano-vivir-bonito-vivir-bien.

Nading, A. (2014). *Mosquito trails: Ecology, health, and the politics of entanglement.* Oakland, CA: University of California Press.

Nading, A., & Fisher, J. (2017). Zopilotes, Alacranes, y Hormigas (Vultures, Scorpions, and Ants): animal metaphors as organizational politics in a Nicaraguan garbage crisis. *Antipode.* Advance online publication. doi:10.1111/anti.12376

Osborne, T. (1997). Of health and statecraft. In A. Petersen, & R. Bunton (Eds.), *Foucault, health, and medicine* (pp. 173–188). London: Routledge.

Petersen, A., & Lupton, D. (1996). *The new public health: Health and self in the age of risk.* London: SAGE Publications.

PNDH. (2012). *Plan nacional de desarrollo humano: 2012-2016* [National human development plan: 2012-2016]. Managua: Government of Nicaragua.

Potosme, R., & Picón, G. (2013, February 8). Ven fascismo en doctrina de Murillo. *La Prensa.* Retrieved from http://www.laprensa.com.ni/2013/02/08/politica/133883-ven-fascismo-en-doctrina-de-murillo.

Radcliffe, S. A. (2012). Development for a postneoliberal era? Sumak kawsay, living well and the limits to decolonisation in Ecuador. *Geoforum; Journal of Physical, Human, and Regional Geosciences, 43*(2), 240–249.

Radcliffe, S. A. (2017). Geography and indigeneity I: Indigeneity, coloniality and knowledge. *Progress in Human Geography, 41*(2), 220–229.

Radcliffe, S. A., Laurie, N., & Andolina, R. (2004). The transnationalization of gender and reimagining andean indigenous development. *Signs: Journal of Women in Culture and Society, 29*(2), 387–416.

Richmond, C., Elliott, S. J., Matthews, R., & Elliott, B. (2005). The political ecology of health: Perceptions of environment, economy, health and well-being among 'Namgis First Nation. *Health & Place, 11*(4), 349–365.

Rose, N. (1996). Governing "advanced" liberal democracies. In *Foucault and political reason: Liberalism, neo-liberalism and rationalities of government* (pp. 37–64). Chicago: University of Chicago Press.

Rose, N. (1999). Inventiveness in politics. *Economy and Society, 28*(3), 467–493.

Rugama, H. M. (n.d.). Priorizarán reforma a Ley General de Salud en 2016 [They will prioritize a reform to the General Health Law in 2016]. *El Nuevo Diario.* Retrieved from http://www.elnuevodiario.com.ni/politica/380400-priorizaran-reforma-ley-general-salud-2016/.

Sader, E. (2009). Post-neoliberalism in Latin America. *Development Dialogue, 51,* 171–179.

Torres Rivas, E. (2007). El retorno del sandinismo transfigurado [The return of transfigured sandinismo]. *Nueva Sociedad: Democracia Y Política En América Latina.* Retrieved from http://nuso.org/articulo/el-retorno-del-sandinismo-transfigurado/.

Waitzkin, H., Iriart, C., Estrada, A., & Lamadrid, S. (2001). Social medicine then and now: Lessons from Latin America. *American Journal of Public Health, 91*(10), 1592–1601.

Walsh, C. (2010). Development as Buen Vivir: Institutional arrangements and (de)colonial entanglements. *Development, 53*(1), 15–21. doi:10.1057/dev.2009.93.

WHO. (2007). *Health of indigenous peoples.* United Nations World Health Organization. Retrieved from http://www.who.int/mediacentre/factsheets/fs326/en/.

WHO. (2008). *Closing the gap in a generation: Health equity through action on the social determinants of health: Commission on social determinants of health final report.* Geneva: World Health Organization, Commission on Social Determinants of Health.

World Health Organization. (1978). *Declaration of Alma-Ata.* International Conference on Primary Health Care, Alma-Ata, USSR.

World Health Organization. (1989). *Environment and health: The European charter and commentary.* Frankfurt-am-Main: WHO Regional Publications.

Zimmerer, K. S. (2015). Environmental governance through "speaking like an indigenous state" and respatializing resources: Ethical livelihood concepts in Bolivia as versatility or verisimilitude? *Geoforum, 64,* 314–324.

# Rites of Resistance: Sex Workers' Fight to Maintain Rights and Pleasure in the Centre of the Response to HIV in Brazil

Laura Rebecca Murray, Deanna Kerrigan and Vera Silvia Paiva

**ABSTRACT**

Drawing on ethnographic research conducted from 2011 to 2015 and the authors' long-term engagement in diverse aspects of HIV and human rights advocacy in Brazil, this paper explores key elements of the Brazilian sex workers' movement response to HIV and the broader political factors that profoundly influenced its trajectory. We argue that the movement has constantly challenged representations of prostitution by affirming sex workers' roles as political actors, not just peer educators, in fighting the HIV epidemic and highlight their development of a sex positive and pleasure centred response that fought stigma on multiple fronts. Moments of tension such as the censorship of an HIV prevention campaign and implementation of 'test and treat' projects are analysed, as are the complex questions that Brazil's 2016 political and economic crisis evokes in terms of how to develop and sustain responses to HIV driven by communities but with material commitment from the State. We conclude with what we see to be the unique, central components of Brazilian sex workers' approach to HIV prevention and what lessons can be learned from it for broader collective health movements in Latin America and beyond.

## Introduction

In 2016, the founding principles that made Brazil's widely recognised response to HIV a success (Berkman, Garcia, Munoz-Laboy, Paiva, & Parker, 2005) came under direct threat. For the first time since the installation of Brazil's democratic constitution in 1988, the country had a Minister of Health, Ricardo Barros, who publicly positioned himself against the Universal Health Care System (SUS – acronym in Portuguese) and in favour of expanding private health care plans (Colucci, 2016). Michel Temer, Brazil's president after the impeachment of the country's first female president, Dilma Rousseff, acted quickly after taking power to pass a Constitutional Amendment that froze the already underfunded health and education budgets for 20 years. Denounced by UN officials as an 'affront to human rights' (Melo, 2016), many see the amendment as paving the way for the end of the SUS (Dias, 2016).

The dismantling of Brazil's public health system raises critical questions about sustaining a rights-based approach to health in times of political crisis. The SUS is an outcome of extensive civil society mobilizations after two decades of dictatorship (Paiva & Teixeira, 2014). It was formalised in Brazil's 1988 democratic constitution and has been a cornerstone of the AIDS response for a series of interrelated reasons, perhaps most importantly because mobilisation in response to the HIV epidemic in Brazil occurred in parallel to the influential public health reform movement to establish the SUS (Daniel & Parker, 1991; Parker, 2003). The National AIDS Programme (NAP) invited representatives from social movements active in fights against the dictatorship to be involved in designing the country's first HIV prevention actions for their peers soon after was founded, bringing together public health reform movements and social movements for sexual rights.

The sex worker movement was one of these movements. Founded amidst Brazil's redemocratization process in 1987, the movement has its roots in resistances to the military dictatorship and mobilizations against police violence. What contemporary literature refers to as 'structural determinants of HIV' (Gupta, Parkhurst, Ogden, Aggleton, & Mahal, 2008) have been the foundation of the movement's politics (and Brazil's response to HIV) since the beginning along with a strong defense of prostitution as work and a sexual right (Leite, Murray, & Lenz, 2015). As Lourdes Barreto, a sex worker from the state of Pará who co-founded the Brazilian Prostitute Network[1] stated in a 2012 interview, 'In prostitution, I learned to see how society has a lot of problems, and that I wasn't one of them'(Bogea, 2012). Lourdes' affirmation of not being one of the problems is emblematic of the movement's position that the heightened vulnerability of sex workers to HIV is more of an outcome of stigma, gender inequalities and the continued criminalisation of prostitution than their profession itself[2].

Sex worker movements around the world have taken a similar stance on rights-based approaches to HIV (Chateauvert, 2013; Mgbako, 2016). Researchers have focussed more specifically on structural and social determinants of sex workers' vulnerability to HIV publishing a series of studies conducted in the late 1990s and mid-2000s that emphasise the importance of policy and social contexts and community mobilisation responses (Basu et al., 2004; Kerrigan et al., 2006; Lippman et al., 2012). A growing body of literature has emphasised the role of criminalisation of sex work in increasing sex workers' vulnerability to HIV and violence (Decker et al., 2015; Shannon et al., 2015), with *The Lancet* 2014 special series on HIV and sex work explicitly calling for decriminalisation as the most effective way to fight the HIV epidemic among sex workers (Beyer et al., 2015).

These are important advances. There remains, however, little research examining the political dimensions of HIV intervention programmes in sex work contexts beyond legal and policy frameworks. Here, we suggest that the Brazilian sex worker movement's response to HIV is unique for the ways in which it has maintained sex and pleasure at the centre of its response. The decision by the national network to use the word *prostituta* (prostitute) in its name, while other international movements have shifted towards 'sex work,' is an example of how activists have chosen to reclaim, rather than alter, terminologies and aspects of the profession associated with transgression or immorality. More confrontational than conforming, this strategy is characteristic of many of the Brazilian Prostitute Networks' actions and illustrative of Jaques Ranciere's definition of politics as a mode of subjectification that provokes reconfigurations of broader systems of domination and inequality (Rancière, 1999).

In this article, we take a closer look at the political dimensions of the sex worker movement in Brazil's response to HIV. We focus primarily on their relationship with the Ministry of Health, contextualising it within the broader context through which both the movement, and its response to AIDS, grew. We suggest that the changes in taking place at the level of federal government in 2016 are a culmination of a series of setbacks in Brazil over the past decade, and reflective as well of broader neoliberal tendencies and the (re)medicalisation of the HIV response (Nguyen, Bajos, Dubois-Arber, O'Malley, & Pirkle, 2011). We highlight what we see to be the unique, central components of Brazilian sex workers' approach to HIV prevention that make it effective for activism and HIV prevention, and what lessons can be learned from it for broader collective health movements in Latin America and beyond.

## Methodology

The research presented in this article is based on the extended case method approach to data collection and analysis (Burawoy, 1998), drawing on the authors' unique and long-term engagement in HIV prevention and sex worker rights in Brazil. The first author has worked in Brazil since 2004 in a series of HIV prevention, advocacy, film and research projects with sex workers, collaborating frequently with the Brazilian Prostitute Network. In 2012, she began an ethnographic study as part of a dissertation on prostitute activism in Brazil that extended through 2014 and included archival research and ethnographic fieldwork with three sex worker organisations (Murray, 2015). The second author has worked on issues related to HIV and sex work since 1996, first in the Dominican Republic and then in Brazil, later coordinating international projects surrounding community empowerment as a cornerstone of HIV prevention among sex workers sponsored by WHO, UNFPA and The World Bank. The third author has focussed her research on sexuality and a human rights based approach to health. She has served on a series of Brazilian and WHO/UNAIDS commissions on HIV/AIDS since 1992, and in 2014 was elected to compose Brazil's National Human Rights Commission (CNDH – acronym in Portuguese), that oversees human rights violations in the country.

Drawing on these experiences allows us to comment on the intersections between the prostitute movements' activism, HIV policy shifts nationally and internationally, and the political and economic crises that have shaken Brazil. In this way, our analysis is inspired by Lorway and Khan's ethnography of a large HIV prevention intervention in India (2014). They argue that observing the project across diverse contexts and spaces permitted the 'opportunity to learn about the complex workings of [its] multiple components' (Lorway & Khan, 2014). We suggest that our viewpoints and engagement with sex work and HIV/AIDS policies in distinct local, national and international contexts allows us to identify both the unique contributions of the prostitute movement and the broader political factors that profoundly influenced their trajectory over the past decade.

The empirical data cited in this article derives from the archival research, participant observation and 65 in-depth interviews with sex workers, activists and government and non-governmental officials that the first author conducted as part of her ethnographic research on sex worker activism in Brazil (Murray, 2015). As part of this research process, interviews and field notes were coded, and data was organised into analytical memos to identify themes and systemic patterns (Emerson, Fretz, & Shaw, 1995). Analytic field notes were transformed into the conceptual frameworks, and the analysis presented in this paper derives from the theoretical frameworks developed to understand the movement's engagement and activism surrounding HIV/AIDS . This research was approved by the Columbia University Medical Centre Institutional Review Board, along with the Institute of Social Medicine at the State University of Rio de Janeiro (IMS/UERJ) and Brazil's National Ethics Review Board (CONEP).

## Beginnings

Brazil's first national HIV prevention programme with sex workers, prisoners and drug users was called PREVINA. Dr. Lair Guerra, the first director of the National AIDS Programme, invited prostitute activist and co-founder of the recently formed Brazilian Prostitute Network (RBP – acronym in Portuguese), Gabriela Leite, to Brasilia in the late 1980s to discuss the project. Despite a climate of broad civil society mobilisation and the emerging female sex worker movement, the original project design of PREVINA presented a morally charged vision of prostitution and activities that were more individual than community driven. The general objective was to,

> Implant a Program of Control and STD/AIDS Prevention in prostitution [contexts] seeking to raise the consciousness of those who work in it (men as well as women), or that have some sort of relationship with it and risk of contamination and transmission of disease through sexual acts (MOH, n.d.).

Roberto Domingues, a technical advisor to the Brazilian Prostitute Network who formed part of the PREVINA project team, shed light on the early discussions with the Ministry of Health regarding the prevention materials they had initially developed for the project:

> We had a life and death fight with the Ministry of Health because we arrived at the conclusion, the group on prostitution, led by Gabriela, that the materials couldn't have the biological focus that they were taking. We saw these questions of "[how] you get it [HIV], [how] you don't get it" that weren't resonant, and we stood firm … And we won, because it was the first large material produced that breaks with a biological approach. And we clearly see in these materials that they have a very large bias towards sex work as an identity.

Roberto is referring to the materials, *Fala, Mulher da Vida*, or literally, 'Speak, Woman of the Life' (to be 'in the life' is a slang, but not necessarily pejorative term for being in prostitution) (Figure 1). As Roberto notes, rather than focus on biological aspects of HIV, prevention is directly, and positively, located within a prostitution context across these materials. Statements such as 'Sex is good' and 'you are very important for people that seek you out' and whether you are 'in this life because of want or need, you can have many moments of pleasure' affirm a pleasurable, and professional, identity for sex workers.

Roberto also emphasised that the fight from the very beginning was about much more than health. At the time, sexuality and citizenship were fundamental components of any response to an epidemic. This was reflected across the broader AIDS movement as a whole (Parker, 2003). As Roberto said, 'the AIDS movement won me over as an activist when I perceived that it was part of a fight for democratization … it was a moment of reconstructing citizenship.' The openness to listening in the National AIDS Programme was also largely due to their connections to the broader social movements for public health reform in Brazil (Galvão, 2000; Parker, 1987, 1994). As Roberto said, 'It wasn't only through resistance that we lived. We had a lot of allies who made things happen. Inside the Ministry of Health, but specifically, inside the STD/AIDS [program].'

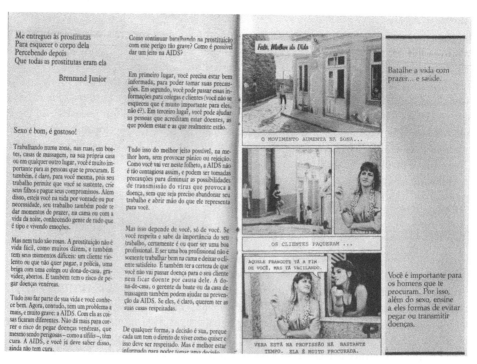

**Figure 1.** The first two pages of the brochure developed for the PREVINA project by the Prostitution and Civil Rights program at the Institute for Religious Studies (ISER) in Rio de Janeiro. The project was coordinated by Gabriela Leite and the material content written by Flavio Lenz Cesar. The material is called, 'Speak, Woman of the Life,' and begins with the phrase, 'Sex is good, it's delicious!'. © ISER, 1989. Image is a scanned copy of the original.

The PREVINA project team released the *Fala, Mulher da Vida* materials along with similar materials made specifically for male and transgender sex workers at a national meeting focussed on 'AIDS and Prostitution' in 1989. The meeting opened with doctors and specialists talking, but sex workers, led by Gabriela Leite, soon rebelled. As she was quoted by the Brazilian Prostitute Network's newspaper, *Beijo da rua* (A Kiss from the street) editor, Flavio Lenz, in an article about the event,

> I felt that people were distant from everything and that the doctors were, of course, involved in a debate with themselves. So the next morning, I came back in a low cut black dress, high heels, exaggerated make-up and I talked about my life (1990, p. 4).

Gabriela's intervention is illustrative of the movement's approach of refusing victimisation and bringing sexuality back to the centre of the conversation about prostitution and prevention. Rather than adjust her appearance to one that would be more 'appropriate' and consistent with the doctors' perspectives in order to be heard, Gabriela broke protocol and completely reversed the meeting's dynamic. After her intervention, sex workers at the event started speaking for themselves.

The sex-positive approach to prevention and the protagonist role of sex workers in developing and implementing HIV programmes were two of the defining features of the federally funded AIDS programmes during the 1990s. The Ministry of Health developed a manual to train peer educators maintaining the positive and inclusive tone towards prostitution that had characterised the *Fala, Mulher da Vida* materials. In the section on citizenship, they state:

> What ruins a prostitute, what takes away her health and dignity, is not having sex professionally, but the lack of working conditions, the right to personal security, the right to justice, respect for private and family life, liberty of expression and opinion, the right to marry and form a family continuing our profession, etc. (1996, p. 25)

The manual, once again, asserts that the issue at stake is not exchanging sex for money, but rather the social context in which sex workers live and work.

Government AIDS programmes and prostitute rights and AIDS advocacy organisations grew rapidly during the 1990s period with financial support from the World Bank and international foundations. The rapid expansion of NGOs was sanctioned by the government: from 1993 through 1997, the National AIDS Programme funded 564 projects with 181 AIDS NGOs nationally (Nunn, 2009, p. 176), 52 of which were for male, female or transgender sex workers, with the majority (44) for female sex workers (Rossi, 1998).

During the time period 1998–2003, a second World Bank loan funded even more projects with NGOs, with a total of 2,163 projects with 795 organisations (Nunn, 2009). *Esquina da Noite (Night Corner)*, a national-level project implemented as part of the second World Bank loan centred on expanding the number of sex worker-led organisations working in HIV prevention in rural areas and interior cities, where the epidemic was also spreading, and spanned 50 municipalities throughout the country. The project was strategic as it was implemented at a time that the Ministry of Health (MOH) started to increasingly decentralise its actions, meaning that organisations would be funded through municipal and state sources rather than the federal government. Given the climate of decentralisation, *Esquina da Noite* focussed its attention on forming partnerships between sex worker organisations and state and municipal AIDS programmes; a feat that *Beijo da rua* identified at the time as one of the largest challenges to implementing the project's activities.

The principles of solidarity, respect and citizenship that Brazil became so well known for in its HIV programmes made their way into a 2002 national prevention campaign centred around a character named *Maria Sem Vergonha* (Maria Without Shame). The campaign image has Maria over a row of flowers called *sem vergonhas* (referred to as shameless because they will grow anywhere), and was accompanied by a series of statements such as, 'No shame in being a prostitute' and 'No shame in valuing your work.' The campaign included radio spots and print materials distributed in prostitution contexts throughout Brazil.

The *Maria Without Shame* campaign had even more relevance given its timing. The government launched the campaign the same year that the Ministry of Labour recognised *profissionais do sexo* (literally, sex professionals) as an official profession within the Brazilian Classification System (CBO acronym in Portuguese) of formal occupations that qualify for federal government benefits such as retirement benefits and government assistance in case of illness. The Ministry of Labour was well aware of the Ministry of Health's successful HIV campaigns in partnership with sex worker organisations at the time, and invited the Brazilian Prostitute Network to participate in the development of the professional category in the CBO's database (ABIA & DAVIDA, 2013).

The movement's influence is clear in the definition of the profession's five main activities included on the Ministry of Labour's CBO database: finding dates, minimising vulnerabilities (which includes both condom use and combating stigma), attending to clients, accompanying clients, and promoting worker organising (CBO, 2017). References in the definition to 'minimizing vulnerabilities' are also demonstrative of the ways in which STD and HIV prevention influenced the very meaning of sex work in Brazil. This is another example of the impact of HIV on sex worker organising and of how the movement integrated AIDS as one of its pillars, alongside fighting discrimination and stigma and promoting sexual education and labour organising.

Not everyone in Brazilian society was pleased with these advances, however. Conservative religious organisations (both Evangelical and Catholic) that gained political influence throughout the decade organised large mobilizations against the inclusion of sex work in the classification of occupations. In 2007, the Ministry of Labour called another meeting to 'minimize the religious and societal pressures' surrounding the controversy, making small, but symbolic changes such as removing the word *puta* (whore) which had been included as a synonym, and attributes of the profession that were considered to be too sexual (such as, 'seducing clients with your eyes') (ABIA & DAVIDA, 2013). Lourdes Barreto and Gabriela Leite defended the importance of using the word *puta* from early on in the movement, seeing its usage as the most effective way to challenge the gender inequalities and hypocrisies at the core of the stigma around prostitution (Leite, 2013). Thus its removal from the CBO, after their hard fought victory years earlier to include it, was particularly symbolic of the changing times.

The 4th National Prostitute Network Meeting was held in Rio de Janeiro in December of 2008 in this tense climate. Rather than adjust their politics to the increasingly conservative and religious influences, the RBP confronted them. As can be seen in Figure 2, the official artwork displayed on a gigantic banner depicted Gabriela Leite as Jesus, surrounding by other leaders from the RBP. The banner states, 'Fourth Encounter of the Network of Prostitutes,' yet the designer, the late Sylvio Oliveira, organised the letters of *prostituta* in a way that highlights the word *puta*. The combination of the playful, yet transgressive, use of the religious symbolism and prominence of the word *puta* on the banner are an excellent example of how the movement responded to attempts to diminish aspects of their profession and activism that they understood to be central to advancing both health and citizenship.

An ally from the Ministry of Labour and Employment attended the meeting. In his official powerpoint presentation, however, he took the opportunity to affirm that, 'The CBO recognises the existence of an occupation, of a job, but does not regulate it. To recognise is different than to legitimize.' The Ministry's official stance distinguishing between recognition and legitimation is important and emblematic of how many state institutions had begun to adjust their discourses around prostitution. As the following section explores, the time period between 2005 and 2010 was bittersweet for many sex workers and AIDS activists, and one in which setbacks increasingly outweighed advancements.

## Reconfigurations

In 2002, Luiz Ignacio Lula da Silva 'Lula' was elected president in Brazil and ushered in an era of hope among the populations that had supported the labour union leader since his days organising for democracy. Lula took office in 2003 and with his election, many activists from Brazil's women's,

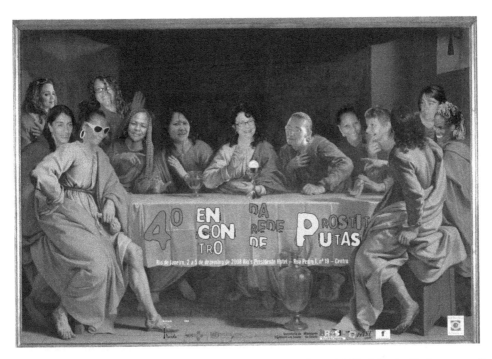

**Figure 2.** The artwork for the 2008 National Meeting of the Brazilian Prostitute Network in Rio de Janeiro. The banner says, 'Fourth Encounter of the Network of Prostitutes,' written in a way that also highlights the word 'Puta' (whore). It was created by the late Sylvio de Oliveira, artist and Davida member.

Lesbian, Gay, Bisexual and Transgender (LGBT), racial equality and AIDS movements took government office in Ministries and the newly established secretariats such as the Special Secretariat for Women's Policies (SPM) and Special Secretariat for Racial Equality. Lula's government initially was active in addressing issues of income, racial, gender and sexuality inequalities and did so through tactics that included programmes and plans designed at the federal level, involving large consultations in regional and national conferences with community-based organisations, civil society and social movements.

His first term coincided with several events that had a profound symbolic effect on sex worker activism and HIV prevention. First, in 2005, as part of President Bush's Emergency Plan for AIDS Relief (PEPFAR), the United States government introduced a contractual clause stipulating that all entities receiving US government funds have a statutory clause explicitly opposing prostitution. In partnership with the RBP, the Brazilian government refused to implement this mandate, eventually rejecting nearly US$40 million in HIV prevention funds that had been allocated to the country. Brazil's decision was heralded by the international community (Okie, 2006) and applauded by sex worker activists globally. Second, UNAIDS held a Global Consultation on Sex Work in Rio de Janeiro in 2006 as part of its process to draw up global guidelines for member states to address HIV/AIDS and sex work (Csete, 2013). Subsequent meetings were held regionally, in Lima in 2007, and nationally in 2008 (MOH, 2008).

The National Consultation on STD/AIDS, Human Rights and Prostitution resulted in the definition of sixty recommendations, largely focussed on broadening the HIV response to structural factors and demanding inter-sectorial committees to move forward a rights-based agenda of HIV prevention with sex workers. The Ministry of Health and National Secretariat of Women's Policies incorporated more than half of these recommendations into a revised version of a plan they developed in partnership with a variety of civil society groups to confront the increasing prevalence of HIV/AIDS among women in Brazil. The original plan (called 'Integral Plan to Confront the

Feminisation of the AIDS Epidemic and other STDs') had been launched in 2008 and only mentioned prostitutes once. The Ministry of Health revised it, however, in 2009, including a series of *agendas afirmativas*, or affirmative agendas, for specific populations, including sex workers (where 34 recommendations from the national consultation were incorporated). The prostitute movement considered the affirmative agenda a victory when it was launched, however, it did not *sair do papel* (expression meaning 'leave the paper,' or turn into action) (ABIA & DAVIDA, 2013).

To some extent, the civil society – government partnerships during Lula's government resulted in the conversion of sexual rights and AIDS activism into federal level secretariats, working groups, and plans that then relied on federal oversight mechanisms to enforce them at the state and municipal levels (Rich, 2013). This proved to be quite challenging, despite the work of what Jessica Rich refers to as *activist bureaucrats,* or 'reform-minded bureaucrats' that mobilised civil society groups to (attempt to) implement progressive federal policies and plans on a local level as the AIDS response was increasingly decentralised (Rich, 2013). Decentralisation also meant that NGOs had to abide by the extensive and complicated rules and regulations associated with receiving state and municipal level funding. Such requirements substantially increased the administrative burdens on NGOs and gave state administrators ample bureaucratic reasons to justify not funding them. According to Estela Scandola, an activist from the Feminist Health Network, state and municipal governments sought excuses not to fund the organisations perceived as trouble-makers. As she stated:

> [A]n NGO that wants to be civil society and autonomous, it is going to be a watchdog, and monitor the councils it participates in. So for example, state governments hate us. For example there was a project request and we did one for sex workers and our project wasn't approved because it was missing page 2, which is where we described our objectives, etc. In other times, they would have called us, [and said] "look you're missing page 2." An organization linked to the church won the money. This was in 2007, 2008.

As Estela points out, the issue was not just increased administrative burdens, but also related to increased influence of religious lobby groups. The Evangelical population expanded locally and regionally during Lula's two terms, comprising 22.2% of the country's population by 2010 (Instituto Brasileiro de Geografia e Estatística [IBGE], 2010), and forming a powerful Congressional lobby with 77 representatives. The expansion of religious fundamentalist movements within federal and state level governments led to recurrent waves of backlash in all matters related to gender and sexuality (Corrêa, 2016). Health and educational policies of the previous decades were challenged and extracted from local policy plans and speaking about sexuality and prevention in schools was eventually prohibited (Paiva & Silva, 2015).

Brazil's economy and position in the global political landscape was also changing rapidly. In 2007, when Brazil was selected to be the host for the 2014 World Cup, and two years later for the 2016 Olympics, the country was still being held up as an emerging global economic power. The economy weathered the 2008 international crisis, yet as Brazil came to be seen as middle income, large funders pulled out of the country. Funders (erroneously) assumed that sexual rights and HIV/AIDS were under control and firmly installed as government priorities; their decision had significant effects on the movements dedicated to these causes. The first decade of 2000 thus ended with a large number of progressive plans and initiatives for HIV in place, yet many organisations were either on the brink of losing funding or lacked the local support from their municipal or state level governments to implement them.

The HIV response with sex workers arguably reached its peak in 2002 when both the social movement and the federal AIDS programme were strong. While the development of the diverse plans and programmes during Lula's administration had a strong symbolic effect and reflected participatory processes, challenges posed by decentralisation and the increasing power of Evangelical fundamentalists made implementing them nearly impossible as fewer and fewer Ministries and secretariats were willing defend sex worker rights. Parallel to these processes, biomedical approaches to prevention, propelled by global pharmaceutical markets, gained steam on the global health landscape (Biehl, 2014; Nguyen et al., 2011) and were viewed as economically advantageous under the neoliberal logics governing public health systems (Parker & Aggleton, 2014). This provided the government with programmatic justification, and funding, for a shift in approaches. As the following section explores, sex worker activists sensed the government's support waning and became frustrated, leading to ruptures with the Ministry of Health, and later, within the movement (Leite et al., 2015).

## Ruptures

In 2011, the Brazilian Prostitute Network made a decision to no longer apply for federal funding for AIDS projects. The decision was made at the Network's regional conference in Belém, in a statement that began with the phrase, 'We are professionals of sex, not the government.' The statement makes various references to the difficulties organisations encountered with state funding and reporting mechanisms and, while it recognises the importance of the partnership with the National AIDS Programme, expresses their dissatisfaction with the directions the Programme was going. In particular, a sense that the 'risk group' mentality they had fought so vehemently against in the late 80s had returned through projects that 'reinforce prostitutes as spreaders of disease and distributors of condoms' (Leite et al., 2015, p. 18).

In 2013, the extent to which the MOH's approach to HIV prevention had changed became even clearer when the MOH censored a campaign developed in a workshop with leaders from prostitute organisations throughout Brazil. The campaign, developed for International Sex Worker Rights Day on June 2nd, lasted less than 24 hours online. The most controversial of the posters, which featured a sex worker with the sentence 'I'm happy being a prostitute,' provoked immediate and angry reactions from conservatives in Brazil's Congress. The Director of the STD and HIV/AIDS Department was fired and the entire campaign was taken offline just two days after its release. An altered campaign was put up in its place and only the posters with phrases about condom use were retained. Figure 3 shows one of the original campaign posters alongside an altered version.

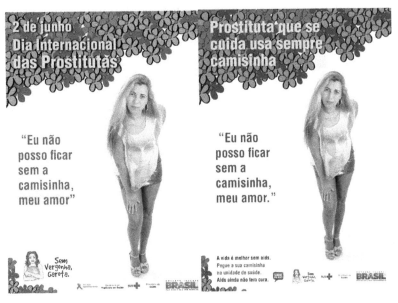

**Figure 3.** Ministry of Health original (left) and altered campaign (right), both downloaded from the www.aids.gov.br website. The top left of the original image states, 'June 2nd, International Prostitute's Day.' In the altered image, this is replaced with 'A prostitute who takes care of herself always uses a condom' and a text on the bottom left stating, 'Life is better without aids. Get your condom at the health center. AIDS still doesn't have a cure.' Pictured is Cida Vieira, president of the Minas Gerais Prostitutes' Association (APROSMIG). ©Governo do Brasil. No changes were made to the images.

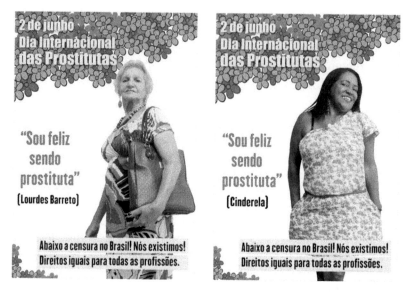

**Figure 4.** GEMPAC protest campaign. Both posters state (from top to bottom) June 2nd, International Prostitute's Day. 'I'm happy being a prostitute.' And in yellow: 'Down with censorship in Brazil! We exist! Equal rights for all professions.' Pictured are Lourdes Barreto and Cinderela. Downloaded from social media campaign. ©GEMPAC. No alterations were made to the images.

Although the Minister of Health at the time, Alexandre Padilha, expressed concern about the content (Rovai, 2013), the official reason for taking down the campaign centred upon a technicality: the campaign had not passed through the appropriate bureaucratic channels for approval. The mass mobilisation protesting the decision to dismantle the campaign disagreed. It was the third time in a year and a half that materials referring to HIV prevention and sexuality had been censored (these included a kit against homophobia designed for schools in 2011 and a Carnival campaign targeting gay youth in 2012). Sex worker organisations responded with strong statements and public actions (Figure 4). The RBP's statement makes a direct connection to violations of the SUS principles, drawing attention to what they saw to be political negotiations and agreements:

> What arrangements are behind these movements? Is there a project for happiness? Why can only they [politicians] be happy? What is the price to be paid by prostitutes? Our bodies, desires and lives are what are paying the prices of political agreements and party negotiations. This is the cost of the censorship and cutting off dialogue (Brazilian Prostitute Network, 2013).

The mobilizations against the campaign were an important time of broad based mobilisation for the movement, yet sadly, it was relatively short lived. Gabriela Leite's death four months later had a profound effect on the movement and was followed by discord over the first project to be implemented with RBP organisations with funding from the Ministry of Health since the 2011 decision in Belém to stop accepting MOH funding.

The motive of the reactivation of the partnership was a project called *Live Better Knowing* [your HIV status], a 'test and treat' project directed at sex workers, MSM, and people who use drugs. The project caused divisions within the Network because several organisations saw it as contrary to the clause of the RBP's *Letter of Principles,* which repudiates the 'offering of exams and other medical procedures in locations where prostitution is practiced, except in cases that involve the general population.' Indeed, HIV testing projects have had a long and contentious history with the Brazilian Prostitute Network. The clause against testing was closely connected to their resistance to HIV testing in work locations as they saw such initiatives as further stigmatising prostitution areas. The *Live Better Knowing* project was distinct from previous projects, however, as rather than researchers or health care staff, testing and counselling was to be conducted by sex workers themselves.

Such 'test and treat' actions are part of what Patton (2011) refers to as the Treatment as Prevention (TasP) regime, in which the right to dignity and quality of life has been truncated 'into a conveyed right to treatment read through the lens of uncontested and falsely promised scientific solutions,' that, according to Patton, actually violates, rather than protects, rights (263). Patton's observation regarding the use of rights language in TasP can be seen in the artwork on the rapid HIV testing van that was parked outside the World AIDS Day event in Rio de Janeiro in 2013 (Figure 5). The text reads, 'Get tested here for AIDS, Syphilis and Hepatitis B and C. It's quick and your right.' Underneath are cartoonish drawings of two male symbols together, a syringe, a condom, Maria Without Shame (the symbol of sex worker campaigns) and a boot with butterfly wings, the symbol of the government's campaign for *travestis*. The images of these past rights-based campaigns are resignified as endorsements of the rapid test campaign. Placed against condoms and syringes, populations are turned into prevention methodologies. Rights are reduced to the right to choose a prevention method.

As the Ministry of Health's actions moved further away from a human rights agenda (Basthi, Parker, & Terto Júnior, 2016), organisations increasingly turned towards cultural actions to sustain their activism and advocate for sex worker rights from a place of irony and pleasure, rather than as victims or vectors of disease. For example, Davida, a Rio de Janeiro based sex worker rights organisation, founded the clothing line *Daspu* (as in *das putas* – of the whores) in 2005 and their playful and provocative fashion shows continue to draw national and international media attention (Lenz, 2008). In 2012, the Belém based sex worker rights organisation GEMPAC started *Puta Dei* (as in 'day'), a day of cultural and advocacy activities to mark International Sex Workers Rights Day (June 2nd) that by 2014 had spread throughout Brazil. Such cultural actions are emblematic of sex worker activists' ability to transform and adapt to diverse political contexts. Yet as we've attempted to show, their insistence on the central roles of sexuality, stigma and pleasure in preventing HIV has paradoxically been their greatest strength in weathering political upheavals and economic crisis (though they have not gone unscathed), and also their largest challenge to sustaining their organisational structures. The challenges presented by decentralisation, the growing power of the Evangelical lobby and

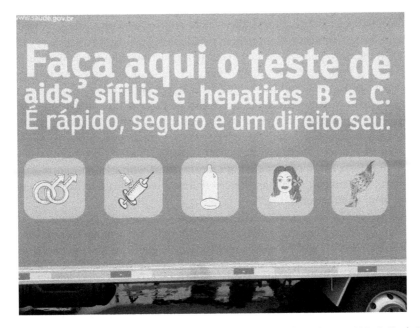

**Figure 5.** Ministry of Health rapid HIV testing truck, parked at the December 1st World AIDS Day activities in Rio de Janeiro, 2013. Photo by Laura Murray.

(re)medicalisation of the epidemic made maintaining the affirmative stance towards prostitution in government funded actions difficult.

## Pleasure and *Putas* at the Centre of a Response to HIV

In conclusion, we would like to highlight what we see to be unique aspects of the Brazilian prostitute movement's approach to HIV prevention. First, by confronting stigma as the primary driver of the AIDS epidemic among sex workers early on, they made respecting sex work a bottom line for collaboration. It is critical to note that this meant affirming the right be a *puta*, both in the sense of a positive affirmation of a whore identity, and also the right to break with normative gender and sexuality stereotypes of what it means to be a woman. Second, affirmative cultural actions such as *Puta Dei* and *Daspu* brought the multiplicities of sex workers' subjectivities to light and involved partners from a diverse range of fields. While increased dependence on conservative municipal and state governments for funding made maintaining organisational structures difficult (and in some cases, impossible), such strategies were critical to keeping sex worker rights visible and building key alliances outside state structures. Finally, through their advocacy and cultural actions, sex workers constantly shifted attention to the structural factors such as gender, sexuality and economic inequalities that influence sex workers' vulnerability to HIV. From the focus on pleasure in *Fala, Mulher da Vida* to their recommendations for cross-sector alliances in the global and national consultations, the movement consistently called for sex workers rights as full citizens to be respected and promoted by the State.

Fighting stigma as a key driver of HIV has been central in social movements' responses to the epidemic for decades (Gamson, 1989). Rather than sanitise sex, the movement's approach to reducing sex work stigma was to associate it with both pleasure and professionalism. The affirmations that 'sex is good' and 'you will have many moments of pleasure' in the PREVINA materials is an example of how they addressed the stigma surrounding prostitution and women's right to pleasure (and to charge for it). Examples of cultural activism (Crimp & Bersani, 1988; Ginsburg, 1997), *Daspu* and *Puta Dei* draw upon fashion, humour, and the body to engage culture as a site of contention and resignify prostitution. One of Daspu's top selling t-shirts summarises their provocative approach to challenging prostitution stigma: 'We're bad, but we could be worse.' Similar to the word whore in English, in Brazil, *puta* is also a fluid and transgressive category used to describe any woman who doesn't conform to normative paradigms of gender and sexuality (Olivar, 2013). The reclaiming of the word *puta* and sexual behaviour associated with the subjective category connects the prostitute movement to broader feminist movements and vindications regarding women's sexuality and sexual rights. As Roberto Domingues notes, sex workers have long demanded to be seen as women with health needs that go beyond 'the waist down,' yet their health and rights have continued to be addressed by the State exclusively in the context of HIV/AIDS, and often, as a separate group from cisgender women (Domingues, 2017, p. 17). Rather than confine the issue of prostitution to red light districts or HIV/AIDS, prostitute activist strategies such as *Daspu* and *Puta Dei* formed allies and partnerships with a variety of social actors from the fashion world, universities, media and artists that became even more important as State support for sex worker rights dwindled.

Michael Warner (1999) has argued for the importance of counter-hegemonic discourses in the gay and lesbian rights movements, emphasising that until behaviours considered deviant are recognised and respected outside the spaces they have been confined to, larger scale social change, including the reduction of stigma and sexual freedoms, will be compromised. The word 'whore,' has also been important to sex worker activism in English speaking countries (Chateauvert, 2013; Gira Grant, 2014; Leigh, 2004; Pheterson, 1989). Over time, however, many activist groups in contexts like the United States where prostitution is completely criminalised chose to adopt the term 'sex work' in their political advocacy as a way to reinforce the idea of sex work as labour and be more inclusive of all people who engage in sexual commerce (Chateauvert, 2013, p. 193). The

Brazilian Prostitute Network, on the other hand, has thus far chosen an approach similar to that of Warner. As we've attempted to argue here, however, they go beyond word choice to a *way* of organising and implementing HIV prevention actions that constantly challenge representations of prostitution by affirming their roles as political actors, not just peer educators, in fighting the epidemic. While the project based funding mechanisms created other problems for their actions in terms of sustainability (Galvão, 2000), we know both from experience and research that this sort of protagonist role is the backbone to any successful and human rights based response to HIV (Kerrigan et al., 2015; WHO, 2012).

Indeed, human rights approaches to health depend on a political environment in which all rights – not just those that have financial and political advantages – can be fully realised. At a time when such approaches have been incorporated into the international system, with groups such as the World Health Organisation endorsing structural approaches and decriminalisation of sex work as a way to fight HIV (WHO, 2012), we've shown how Brazil is going in the opposite direction. The (re)medicalisation of HIV prevention alongside the increased presence and power of the conservative lobby and neoliberalization of Brazil's public health care system (Seffner & Parker, 2016) has meant that previous human rights discourses in prevention have been reduced to the right to be tested. This shift to individual, as opposed to more collective rights (such as legal changes and professional recognition) may contribute to increasing, rather than decreasing sex workers' vulnerability to HIV.

In this context, we believe that it is increasingly important that there be a shift from looking *up* to the State, to looking *across* to other social movements. It was this type of wide mobilisation across the health, political activist and women's movements that formed the foundation of Brazil's response to HIV. The Brazilian Prostitute Network's rights and pleasure based approach is precisely one that invests in fighting multiple fronts with creativity and conviction. Not only does such an approach build allies, it also forces a more structural as opposed to individual response by seeking points of convergence between movements. At a time when austerity measures threaten Brazil's public health system, such alliances are critical not just for sex workers, but for the health of the population as a whole.

## Notes

1. Anthropological research has been important to uncovering the nuances of the terms used to refer to sex work in Brazil (Kulick, 1998; Mitchell, 2016; Piscitelli, 2007; Silva & Blanchette, 2005) and noted how *prostituta* (prostitute) and *puta* (whore) are the terms preferred by the organised movement, although other terms such as *trabalhadora sexual* (sex worker) and *professional do sexo* (sex professional) are also used (Olivar, 2013; Williams, 2013). This remains an active discussion within the movement today. Do to the diversity of preferences and terms among activists and those not in the organised movement, we will use 'prostitute/s' and 'sex worker/s' interchangeably. We've chosen to leave the word *puta* in Portuguese due to its specificity as a subjective category in Brazil (Olivar, 2013).
2. Sex work is a recognized profession in Brazil in accordance with the Ministry of Labour's Classification of Brazilian Occupations, yet all third party involvement, including brothel ownership, is illegal.

## Disclosure statement

No potential conflict of interest was reported by the authors.

## Funding

This research was supported in part by the Gender Sexuality and Health Training Grant [grant number T32HD049339] awarded to the Department of Sociomedical Sciences at Columbia University by the Eunice Kennedy Shriver National Institute of Child Health and Human Development.

# References

ABIA, & DAVIDA. (2013). *Analysis of prostitution contexts in terms of human rights, work, culture, and health in Brazilian cities*. Rio de Janeiro: Brazilian Interdisciplinary AIDS Association - ABIA.

Basthi, A., Parker, R., & Terto Júnior, V. (Eds.). (2016). *Myth vs. reality: Evaluating the Brazilian response to HIV in 2016*. Rio de Janeiro: Brazilian Interdisciplinary AIDS Association (ABIA) - Global AIDS Policy Watch.

Basu, I., Jana, S., Rotheram-Borus, M., Swendeman, D., Lee, S. J., Newman, P., & Weiss, R. (2004). HIV prevention among sex workers in India. *Journal of Acquired Immune Deficiency Syndromes, 36*(3), 845–852.

Berkman, A., Garcia, J., Munoz-Laboy, M., Paiva, V., & Parker, R. (2005). A critical analysis of the Brazilian response to HIV/AIDS: Lessons learned for controlling and mitigating the epidemic in developing countries. *American Journal of Public Health, 95*(7), 1162–1172.

Beyer, C., Crago, A.-L., Bekker, L.-G., Butler, J., Shannon, K., Kerrigan, D., ... Strathdee, S. A (2015). An action agenda for HIV and sex workers. *The Lancet, 385*(9964), 287–301.

Biehl, J. (2014). Patient value. In E. Fischer (Ed.), *Markets, values and moral economies* (pp. 67–90). Santa Fe: SAR Press.

Bogea, H. (2012, May 25). *Na prostituição, aprendi a ver que a sociedade tem muitos problemas, e eu não era a errada da história*. Retrieved from http://www.hiroshibogea.coms.br/lourdes-barreto-na-prostituicao-aprendi-a-ver-que-a-sociedade-tem-muitos-problemas/

Brazilian Prostitute Network. (2013). Statement from the Brazilian Prostitute Network of Prostitutes about Censorship and the Federal Government's Intervention and Alteration of the AIDS Prevention Campaign. Retrieved from: http://www.akissforgabriela.com/?cbg_tz=180&cat=3&paged=6

Burawoy, M. (1998). The extended case method. *Sociologial Theory, 16*(1), 4–33.

CBO. (2017). 5198:05 - Profissionais do Sexo. Retrieved from: http://www.mtecbo.gov.br/cbosite/pages/pesquisas/ResultadoFamiliaDescricao.jsf

Chateauvert, M. (2013). *Sex workers unite: A history of the movement from stonewall to slutwalk*. Boston: Beacon Press.

Colucci, C. (2016, May 17). *Tamanho do SUS precisa ser revisto, diz novo Ministro da Saúde, Folha de São Paulo*. Retrieved from http://www1.folha.uol.com.br/cotidiano/2016/05/1771901-tamanho-do-sus-precisa-ser-revisto-diz-novo-ministro-da-saude.shtml

Corrêa, S. O. (2016). The Brazilian response to HIV and AIDS in troubled and uncertain times. In A. Basthi, R. Parker, & V. T. Júnior (Eds.), *Myth v reality: Evaluating the Brazilian response to HIV in 2016* (pp. 7–15). Rio de Janeiro: Brazilian Interdisciplinary AIDS Association - ABIA - Global AIDS Policy Watch.

Crimp, D., & Bersani, L. (1988). *AIDS: Cultural analysis, cultural activism* (1st ed.). Cambridge, MA: MIT Press.

Csete, J. (2013). Victimhood and vulnerability: Sex work and the rhetoric and reality of the global response to HIV/AIDS. In L. Murthy (Ed.), *The business of sex* (pp. 45–80). New Dehli: Zubaan.

Daniel, H., & Parker, R. (1991). *AIDS: A terceira epidemia (ensaios e tentativas)*. São Paulo: Iglu.

Decker, M., Crago, A.-L., Chu, S., Sherman, S., Seshu, M., Buthelezi, K., ... Beyer, C. (2015). Human rights violations against sex workers: Burden and effect on HIV. *The Lancet, 385*(9963), 186–199.

Dias, B. (2016). Golpe fatal: PEC 55 é aprovada em meio a manifestações e brutal repressão policial. Retrieved from: https://www.abrasco.org.br/site/noticias/movimentos-sociais/golpe-fatal-pec-55-e-aprovada-em-meio-a-manifestacoes-e-brutal-repressao-policial/24431/

Domingues, R. (2017). A Batalha Entre Sujeito e Objeto no Sertão da Saúde. *Beijo da Rua, 28*(2), 15–17.

Emerson, R. M., Fretz, R. I., & Shaw, L. L. (1995). *Writing ethnographic fieldnotes*. Chicago: University of Chicago Press.

Galvão, J. (2000). *AIDS no Brasil: A agenda de construção de uma epidemia*. Rio de Janeiro: ABIA.

Gamson, J. (1989). Silence, death, and the invisible enemy: AIDS activism and social movement newness. *Social Problems, 36*(4), 351–367.

Ginsburg, F. (1997). From little things, big things grow: Ingidenous media and cultural activism. In R. Fox & O. Starn (Eds.), *Between resistance and revolution: Cultural politics and social protest* (pp. 188–144). New Brunswick: Rutgers University Press.

Gira Grant, M. (2014). *Playing the whore*. London and New York: Verso.

Gupta, G. R., Parkhurst, J. O., Ogden, J., Aggleton, P., & Mahal, A. (2008). Structural approaches to HIV prevention. *The Lancet, 372*, 764–775.

IBGE (Instituto Brasileiro de Geografia e Estatística) (2010). Censo Demográfico. Retrieved from: http://www.ibge.gov.br/home/estatistica/populacao/censo2010/default.shtm

Kerrigan, D., Kennedy, C., Morgan-Thomas, R., Reza-Paul, S., Mwangi, P., Win, K. T., ... Butler, J. (2015). A community empowerment approach to the HIV response among sex workers: Effectiveness, challenges, and considerations for implementation and scale-up. *The Lancet, 385*(9963), 172–185.

Kerrigan, D., Moreno, L., Rosario, S., Gomez, B., Jerez, H., Barrington, C., ... Sweat, M. (2006). Environmental-structural interventions to reduce HIV/STI risk among female sex workers in the Dominican Republic. *American Journal of Public Health, 96*(1), 120–125.

Kulick, D. (1998). *Travesti*. Chicago: University of Chicago Press.

Leigh, C. (2004). *Unrepentant whore*. San Francisco: Last Gasp.

Leite, G., Murray, L. R., & Lenz, F. (2015). The peer and non-peer: The potential of risk management for HIV prevention in contexts of prostitution. *Revista Brasileira de Epidemiologia, 18*(Suppl 1), 7–25.

Leite, G. (2013). Why Gabriela prefers the word whore? (YouTube video). Retrieved from: https://www.youtube.com/watch?v=CvKkGPiXv0o

Lenz, F. (2008). *Daspu: Moda Sem Vergonha*. Rio de Janeiro: Objetivo.

Lippman, S., Chinaglia, M., Donini, A., Kerrigan, D., Reingold, A., & Diaz, J. (2012). Findings from encontros: A multilevel STI/HIV intervention to increase condom use, reduce STI, and change the social environment among sex workers in Brazil. *Sexually Transmitted Diseases, 39*(3), 209–216.

Lorway, R., & Khan, S. (2014). Reassembling epidemiology: Mapping, monitoring and making-up people in the context of HIV prevention in India. *Social Science & Medicine, 112*, 51–62.

Melo, D. (2016). Toda uma geração está condenada diz relator da ONU sobre a PEC 55. *Carta Capital*. Retrieved from: http://www.cartacapital.com.br/politica/toda-uma-geracao-esta-condenada-diz-relator-da-onu-sobre-a-pec-55

Mgbako, C. A. (2016). *To life freely in the world: Sex worker activsim in Africa*. New York: New York University Press.

Mitchell, G. (2016). *Tourist attractions*. Chicago: University of Chicago.

MOH. (2008). *Consulta nacional sobre DST/AIDS, Direitos Humanos e Prostituição*. Brasilia: Ministry of Health.

MOH. (n.d.). *Projeto PREVINA*. Brasilia: Ministry of Health.

Murray, L. (2015). *Not fooling around: The politics of sex worker activism in Brazil* (PhD). Columbia University, New York.

Nguyen, V.-K., Bajos, N., Dubois-Arber, F., O'Malley, J., & Pirkle, C. M. (2011). Remedicalizing an epidemic: From HIV treatment as prevention to HIV treatment is prevention. *AIDS, 25*, 291–293.

Nunn, A. (2009). *The politics and history of AIDS treatment in Brazil*. New York: Springer.

Okie, S. (2006). Fighting HIV-lessons from Brazil. *New England Journal of Medicine, 354*, 1977–1981.

Olivar, J. M. (2013). *Devir puta: Políticas de prostituição de rua na experiência de quatro mulheres militantes*. Rio de Janeiro: Ed UERJ.

Paiva, C. H. A., & Teixeira, L. A. (2014). Reforma sanitária e a criação do Sistema Único de Saúde: notas sobre contextos e autores. *História, Ciências, Saúde-Manguinhos, 21*, 15–36.

Paiva, V., & Silva, V. (2015). Facing negative reactions to sexuality education through a multicultural human rights framework. *Reproductive Health Matters, 23*, 96–106.

Parker, R. (1987). Acquired immunodeficiency syndrome in Urban Brazil. *Medical Anthropology Quarterly, 1*, 155–175.

Parker, R. G. (1994). *A AIDS no Brasil, 1982–1992*. Rio de Janeiro, RJ: ABIA: IMS-UERJ : Relume Dumará.

Parker, R. G. (2003). Building the foundations for the response to HIV/AIDS in Brazil: The development of HIV/AIDS policy, 1982–1996. *Divulgação em Saúde para Debate, 27*, 143–183.

Parker, R., & Aggleton, P. (2014). Test and treat from a human rights perspective. *Global AIDS Policy Watch*. http://gapwatch.org/news/articles/test-and-treat-from-a-human-rights-perspective/118

Patton, C. (2011). Rights language and HIV treatment: Universal care or population control? *Rhtetoric Society Quarterly, 41*(3), 260–266.

Pheterson, G. (1989). *A vindication of the rights of whores*. Seattle: Seal Press.

Piscitelli, A. (2007). Shifting boundaries: Sex and money in the North-East of Brazil. *Sexualities 10*(4), 489–500.

Rancière, J. (1999). *Disagreement: Politics and philosophy*. Minneapolis: University of Minnesota.

Rich, J. (2013). Grassroots bureaucracy: Intergovernmental relations and popular mobilization in Brazil's AIDS policy sector. *Latin American Politics and Society, 55*, 1–25.

Rossi, L. (1998). *Prevencao das DST/Aids e a Prostitucao Feminina no Brasil*. Brasilia: Ministerio de Saude: Coordenacao Nacional de DST e Aids.

Rovai, R. (2013, June 6). *Padilha explica por que não permitiu campanha "sou feliz sendo prostituta"* [Padilha explains why he didn't permit the campaign, "I'm happy being a prostitute]. Retrieved from http://revistaforum.com.br/blogdorovai/2013/06/11/padilha-explica-porque-nao-permitiu-o-sou-feliz-sendo-prostituta/

Seffner, F., & Parker, R. (2016). The neoliberalization of HIV prevention in Brazil. In A. Basthi, R. Parker, & V. Terto Júnior (Eds.), *Myth vs. reality: Evaluating the Brazilian response to HIV in 2016* (pp. 22–30). Rio de Janeiro: Brazilian Interdisciplinary AIDS Association (ABIA) - Global AIDS Policy Watch.

Shannon, K., Strathdee, S., Goldenberg, S., Duff, P., Mwangi, P., Rusakova, M., ... Boily, M. (2015). Global epidemiology of HIV among female sex workers: Influence of structural determinants. *The Lancet, 385*(9962), 55–71. doi:10.1016/S0140-6736(14)60931-4

Silva, A. P., & Blanchette, T. (2005). Nossa Senhora da Help: Sexo, Turismo, e Deslocamento Transnacional em Copacabana. *Cadernos Pagu, 1*(25), 249–280.

Warner, M. (1999). *The trouble with normal*. Cambridge: Harvard University Press.

WHO. (2012). *Prevention and treatment of HIV and other sexually transmitted diseases for sex workers in low and middle income countries*. Geneva: World Health Organization. http://apps.who.int/iris/bitstream/10665/77745/1/9789241504744_eng.pdf?ua=1

Williams, E. L. (2013). *Sex tourism in Bahia: Ambiguous entanglements*. Urbana, Chicago and Springfield: University of Illinois Press.

# Confluent paths: Research and community participation to protect the right to health among transgender women in Peru

Ximena Salazar ⓘ, Arón Núñez-Curto, Jana Villayzán Aguilar, Miluska Lusquiños, Angélica Motta Ochoa ⓘ and Carlos F. Cáceres

**ABSTRACT**

The recognition of transgender women (TGW) as the most vulnerable population to HIV/AIDS in Peru and their inclusion as a specific key affected population in health research was the outcome of an extended process that culminated when TGW community organisations succeeded in articulating themselves as a population separate from men who have sex with men (MSM) and, in alliance with some academic research groups, documented their HIV prevalence and vulnerability factors. Prior to that process, TGW remained subsumed under the epidemiological category of men who have sex with men (MSM), invisible in the context of public health policies. Based on a growing body of academic research evidence, coupled with the increasing number and capacities of TGW representatives in technical and policy-related gatherings, a consensus emerged for the establishment of TGW health statistics separate from MSM by 2010. During the past decade, social and health research has contributed conclusive evidence on the living conditions of TGW and the structural barriers they face, beyond the focus of HIV/AIDS research. Despite such progress, pervasive barriers in public policies continue to hinder the use of existing research evidence and community experience in the development of sensitive HIV prevention and care strategies as part of a comprehensive health model for TGW in Peru.

## Introduction

Two decades ago a *transgender women's* (TGW) social movement did not yet exist in Peru. So called *travestis* (an emic term used mostly in the 90's) were considered by the public health sector and academia to be a small fraction of the male homosexual collective and one heavily marginalised (Salazar, Silva Santisteban, Villayzán, & Caceres, 2010; Silva-Santisteban et al., 2012). From 2006 onwards, Peruvian academic research has generated evidence that has allowed the recognition of TGW as one of the most HIV affected populations (Sánchez, Peinado, & Lama, 2011; Silva-Santisteban et al., 2012). These data have also highlighted barriers to TGW's gender affirmation, to access to health services, and to HIV treatment (Poteat et al., 2015), as well as other contextual factors this population experiences on a daily basis that heighten their HIV risk. Simultaneously, this scientific literature has produced broader insights with regard to the social reality of TGW, and TGW leaders and organisations have drawn on this evidence in becoming distinct actors in the field of HIV politics (Reisner et al., 2016), delineating confluent paths between trans activism and scientific research.

In this way, the devastating impact of the AIDS epidemic did not render TGW immediately visible. Instead, we argue, it contributed to an ongoing process of transformation in the sexuality and gender landscape in Peru. This process began with the gay liberation movement in the 1980's and ended up providing the basis for claims, among a number of early TGW activists. With time, such activists articulated needs of the trans population that were fundamentally different from those of gay men and that required the constitution of a new movement, the transgender women's movement.

Globally, partnerships between LGBT organisations and academic partners are at present utilised as a vehicle to conduct community health interventions (Chillag et al., 2002; Griffith et al., 2010; Wilson, Lavis, & Guta, 2012). These partnerships have also been counted among the 'critical enablers' of combination HIV prevention programmes (Skovdal, Magutshwa-Zitha, Campbell, Nyamukapa, & Gregson, 2013). However, interactions among these partners are under-studied. Here we reflect on the relationship between the field of transgender health research and the strengthening of TGW organisations. This collaborative work cannot and need not be generalised to the entire local trans community and all academic institutions, but provides a basis for reflection on the processes of coalition formation between researchers and TGW organisations, which may bear political effects, despite their unresolved tensions. One example of these tensions is the ambiguous construction of the category transgender within academia evident in the persistence of gender dysphoria as a psychiatric disorder, while TGW are accepted as a legitimate community within the field of public health. Another issue is the instrumental use of TGW in HIV research, although, clearly, TGW activists who mediate the relationship between academics, funders and TGW organisations also have complex interests that play a role in these processes. Additionally, despite the wealth of health research that has been carried out so far, some concerns (violence, discrimination, civil and identity rights) expressed by TGW in diverse gatherings remain invisible and marginal in much research focused on HIV.

The goal of this paper is to explore the confluence of academic research and allies with processes of strengthening and consolidation of the TGW movement. We analyse the role of research and researchers in both building knowledge about and the enhancement of the TGW movement beyond HIV. Finally, while a full discussion of the role of funders and state parties in defining the TGW activist agenda is beyond the scope of this paper, we will briefly address their impact, as well.

## Methods

We conducted an assessment that considered: (1) The evidence-base on TGW articulated in both peer-reviewed scientific papers and books and grey literature published in Peru between 2006 and 2011 (a period in which the most significant production of Peru-specific research on TGW took place). Importantly, many of these publications were authored by the first author of this paper along with other researchers of the Cayetano Heredia University. (2) This paper also benefits from the contribution of two TGW leaders, Jana Villayzan and Miluska Luzquiños, activists with long trajectories in social activism and co-authors of this article. Both are part of Red Trans Peru, an organisation that has been active from the start of a more articulated social trans movement. The first author of this paper has conducted research and has shared in meetings, discussions and activism with these leaders to address the problems of TGW in Peru.

Publications were tabulated to indicate authors, methodology and key findings. Grey reports were identified to help define milestones in the development of TGW activism. Data deemed useful in defining this history were identified and tabulated. Data sources and methods were triangulated to build understanding of the TGW movement in Peru, describe the contribution of research in such process, and identify the confluences and tensions between the roles and motives of both scientific and community actors. Quotes included in this paper come from the grey literature or from personal communications between the authors, involving Ms. Villayzan and Ms. Luzquiños (indicated as personal communications).

## Findings

### Research on TGW in Peru (2006–2011): A new population emerges in the field of health research

Health-related research on TGW in Peru began soon after 2000, with the first publications focused on TGW taking place around 2006. Table 1 lists key publications that engaged Peruvian TGW between 2006 and 2011. Most publications listed are focused on HIV, with some additional issues gaining attention as of 2008.

Approximately a decade before the emergence of the TGW population, this group remained subsumed within the overarching category of Men who have Sex with Men (MSM) in HIV/AIDS studies and global reports (Kaplan, Sevelius, & Ribeiro, 2016). As a concept that sought to describe homogenous sexual practices or sexual behaviours, the notion of 'biological sex' (as stable and homogenous) (Kaplan et al., 2016), together with the concept of sexual orientation, were seen as

**Table 1.** Methodological approach and key findings of scientific publications focused on TGW in Peru (2006–2011).

| Authors/Year | Research method | Key findings/Conclusions |
|---|---|---|
| Salazar et al. (2006) | Qualitative | The study emphasises the importance of the socio-cultural environment for the prevention of HIV / AIDS by its influence on the social norms of gender in the construction of identity, in relationship forms, in sexual negotiation and in the meaning of risk. |
| Caceres et al. (2008) | Secondary information analysis | The study identifies that risk behaviours in the transvestite population are associated with adverse socio-economic and psychological conditions, contributing to the existence of a population highly vulnerable to HIV infection. |
| Salazar and Villayzán (2007) | Qualitative | One of the most important findings of this study was that prostitution in a transvestite population has as its indispensable condition the assumption of a female identity. |
| Montalvo, Andía, and Rodríguez, (2009) | Qualitative | The study proposes that violence against TGW comes with great force from public order institutions, such as the municipal and the national police. |
| Salazar and Villayzán (2009) | Qualitative | The study highlights TGW's efforts to achieve their desired identity in their bodies, and with family. The study also refers to the exercise of their human rights and few job opportunities, while a large number are engaged in prostitution. |
| Salazar (2009) | Qualitative | The study delineates the types of violence TGW suffer in several regions of the country |
| Salazar (2010) | Qualitative | The author argues that there are no laws, policies, norms and / or regulations regarding the social inclusion of TGW and that there are no capacity building mechanisms in trans organisations, which makes it difficult to participate in civil society forums. |
| Salazar et al. (2010) | Qualitative/ Quantitative | The study discusses the importance of institutions to recognising TGW identity. It highlights gender discrimination and violence as well as the difficulties experienced by women in their relationships with partners that influence condom use and HIV prevention. This is in addition to the problems TGW have in accessing health services. |
| Segura et al. (2010) | Quantitative | The study estimates 22,456 transgender women in the city of Lima |
| Bayer, Paca, and Garvich (2011) | Qualitative/ Quantitative | The study concludes that TGW sex workers experience greater vulnerability than TGW who are not engaged in sex work. Being sex work a factor of vulnerability. A significant minority has never been tested for HIV and therefore require specialised services to their needs. |
| Sánchez et al. (2011) | Quantitative/ Epidemiological | This study provides epidemiology of TGW in Lima, finding 20.8% HIV prevalence, 36.2% prevalence of syphilis. It argues that the HIV epidemic among MSM and transgender women is becoming increasingly young, with a higher incidence among the population under 25 years of age. This epidemiological data from a sentinel study is the data used by the Ministry of Health. |
| Silva-Santisteban et al. (2012) | Quantitative/ Epidemiological | This study developed with the Responding Driven Sampling methodology in the UPCH provides epidemiology of TGW in Lima, finding 29.6% HIV prevalence, 22% syphilis prevalence. It confirms that TGW represent the group most affected by the HIV / AIDS epidemic in Peru. |
| Velarde (2011) | Qualitative | The study concludes that the health system does not give attention to the need for body modification, nor for sexual health of TGW living with HIV |

providing all relevant information for epidemiologic purposes. Even though several studies began to identify new populations at risk of contracting HIV (Caceres et al., 2008), for the calculation of prevalence, as well as for behavioural and qualitative studies, TGW were considered part of the MSM category. As of 2005, for the most part, international references to TGW still included them as part of the 'gay and other MSM' collective, as did the Peruvian Ministry of Health. Likewise, most local academic papers kept these groups together, although some started to distinguish a group of so-called 'MSM with female gender identity', or simply *travestis* (Salazar et al., 2006). During this period, the term 'vulnerable populations' was still being used, highlighting the structural determinants of HIV risk, beyond risks resulting from individual behaviours. In a study on alcohol and drug use published in 2007 (Caceres, Salazar, Rosasco, & Salazar, 2007), MSM and *travestis* appeared as separate groups. In this study, risk behaviours in the *travestis* population were closely associated with adverse psychological and social/structural conditions, resulting in their high vulnerability to HIV infection. At that point, interest emerged on the topic of sex work among TGW, known as one of the few economic activities available to *travestis*' livelihood (Salazar, 2009; Salazar & Villayzán, 2007; Salazar & Villayzán, 2009).

In 2010, a mixed methods study on TGW took place, focused on social and epidemiological dimensions of their vulnerability to HIV/AIDS (Salazar et al., 2010; Silva-Santisteban et al., 2012). The qualitative component of this study revealed, once again, the importance of the recognition of TGW and the need for their inclusion and legitimation. This study discussed how, in conditions of poverty and exclusion, TGW face health (including HIV-related) outcomes that cannot be isolated from other important experiences such as institutional violence, exclusion from the job market, poor housing conditions, and others. The quantitative study showed that TGW represented the group most affected by the HIV/AIDS epidemic in Peru, with an HIV prevalence of almost 30% (Silva-Santisteban et al., 2012).

Another publication focused on the STI and HIV Epidemiological Surveillance Study conducted in 2011 (Sánchez et al., 2011), raised concerns about the fact that the HIV epidemic among MSM and TGW was affecting increasingly younger people, with a higher incidence among populations under 25 years old. A study on HIV prevention and access to sexual and reproductive health services among people living with HIV carried out in eight Peruvian cities (Salazar et al., 2013) revealed that the TGW population had the lowest level of completed schooling in all geographical areas. With regard to experiences in health services, the majority of TGW was usually not offered information regarding the lack of interaction between hormonal treatment and the use of antiretroviral therapy (ART), so that fears about ART interfering with their feminisation process prevailed (Salazar et al., 2013).

Importantly, much of the qualitative research conducted (and even some mixed-methods efforts [Silva-Santisteban et al., 2012]) represented unintended examples of participatory research (PR), a paradigm in which activists work together with researchers and use the outcomes of research to improve living conditions of the TGW community (Currah & Spade, 2007). Such successful experiences have not only represented a learning experience for researchers and TGW activists alike; they have also demonstrated the critical role that research can play in advancing policy and advocacy work in the most vulnerable communities (Currah & Spade, 2007).

### *The development of the TGW's movement in Peru (2005–2011)*

TGW organisations emerged less than 20 years ago in the context of the Peruvian LGBT movement. The first gay and lesbian organisations were founded in the early 80s (Bracamonte, 2011). During that decade, when the use of 'gender identity' as driving political mobilisation of gender non-conforming people had not started at a global scale, only a few TGW participated in actions promoted by gay groups in Peru (Jaime, 2013).

It is since the advent of the new millennium that TGW groups emerged, in the context of their participation in discussions for HIV/AIDS prevention organised by the Peruvian gay movement,

UNAIDS and the projects of The Global Fund to Fight AIDS, Tuberculosis and Malaria, and also in discussions of gender and sexuality within academic spaces. One of the first TGW organisations was Angel Azul, which appeared in 2002, growing from demands among some TGW for their own space in order to reflect on social aspects of their vulnerability beyond HIV risk. In those years, the term 'transgender women' was not well known among members of academia and the Ministry of Health, and TGW's specific needs (i.e. concerning social inequalities, such as lower access to health, non-availability of hormone therapy, human and sexual rights among others) was still an unexplored field.

In the specific case of Angel Azul, their contact during 2002 with Lohana Berkins, a brilliant trans activist from Argentina, helped them reflect on the structural drivers of their vulnerability to HIV, given that their non-conforming gender identification increased their social exclusion and stigmatisation, as compared to gay men, and they developed a new collective discourse on that basis. Another early group, 'Claveles Rojos', emerged out of the friendship among TGW coping with isolation and adversity in a hair salon in a poor district in Lima (La Mestiza Colectiva, 2008). These foundational groups focused their efforts on dealing with violence against TGW (Montalvo et al., 2009).

It was not until the year 2006 that the academic and political discussion about gender and sexuality influenced some TGW leaders, motivating their decision to strengthen their organisations. In 2006, Red Trans Peru started its activities as a national network of transgender women. This organisation led several activities aimed at creating a community, which now remain milestones of the TGW organisations' trajectory. As of 2007 meetings and activities that brought together TGW from all over the country and Latin America were organised in order to consolidate a coalition in Peru similar to those that had previously been formed in Argentina or Brazil. These milestones are summarised in Table 2.

Towards the second decade of the millennium, the TGW movement also started to receive support from international donors, who became conscious of their increasing visibility and demands, signaling the assumption of a political identity as the group most affected by HIV infection (Salazar et al., 2010). In those meetings, the concepts of 'transgender' (transgénero) and 'trans' (trans), originating in American academia and activism, began to be used to name body and gender experiences under a single term, and to articulate collective demands vis-à-vis international donors and the State.

### The visibility of TGW as a vulnerable group and their participation in HIV interventions

During the last five years of the first decade of the new millennium, evidence produced by epidemiological and transgender health research, describing and explaining the high prevalence of HIV among TGW, played a significant role in articulating the demands of activism in this new context of convergence between organisations and the national HIV programme. This research provided, on the one hand, information to activists to support their demands for social recognition as distinct from 'MSM.' On the other hand, this scientific evidence was used to support their lobbying for self-representation before the Peruvian government.

HIV policies entered a stage characterised by technological sophistication and the establishment of specific goals in HIV prevention and treatment. Simultaneously, CONAMUSA – the name adopted in Peru by the Country Coordinating Mechanism (CCM) established to manage the activities related to the Global Fund to Fight AIDS, Tuberculosis and Malaria (GF) in Peru – promoted a

**Table 2.** Milestones of early transwomen activism in Peru (2005–2007).

| Year | Milestones of early transwomen activism in Peru (2000–2007) |
|---|---|
| 2005 | First Transvestite, Transgender and Transsexual Encounter in Peru |
| 2006 | National Workshop on Stigma and Discrimination in the Transvestite, Transgender and Transgender Population |
| 2006 | Birth of the RedTrans Peru |
| 2007 | Regional Consultation on Sex Work and HIV/AIDS in Latin America and the Caribbean (in Lima) |
| 2007 | National Consultation on Sex Work, Human Rights and HIV and AIDS |

distinct participation of TGW alongside other vulnerable communities introducing some capacity building activities among them (Jaime, 2013). These activities contributed to the visibility of the TGW population in Peru.

In this way, the HIV agenda not only became a field in which TGW's demands were articulated for social recognition; it also operated as a setting where technical and political capacity building for some TGW took place, resulting in strengthened political leadership. The technical capacity building took place in the areas of transgender health, project management, human rights training, and international networking. As a TGW leader noted in an interview for a 2010 report about the participation of transgender women in the Peruvian Global Fund Country Coordinating Mechanism (CCM):

> Regional networks of sex workers (RedTraSex) and trans (RedLacTrans) have played a crucial role in raising awareness among their members about the importance of getting involved in projects funded by the Global Fund. Moreover, they [the networks] have supported the local and regional advocacy work of their members to achieve representation at the CCM. (Salazar, 2010, p. 48)

However, TGW activists have also pointed out the tensions in the type of community participation facilitated by the GF. For example, they indicated that the GF's utilitarian (i.e. HIV-restrictive, funding-driven) view of participation left no room for other rights claims beyond HIV (Salazar, 2010); they also indicated that the assistance-focused project implemented by local NGOs created dependence among TGW rather than helping them develop capacities for self-maintenance.

> The Global Fund has created an assistance-focused project: We are supposed to expect to get support to rent a house, to be paid a space, to wait for the work of peer promoters (…). It has not contributed to strengthening the leadership of Trans people who stand in the regions and who have managed to get groups of twenty girls to follow them, perhaps supporting them to self-manage an organization. (Comment made by co-author Jana Villayzán during a training workshop funded by GIZ (German Cooperation) for Peruvian trans women, July 2016)

## *The trans movement and Its ongoing struggle for comprehensive health*

In Peru, the confluence between academic research and activism reveals that an overwhelming emphasis on HIV-focused public policy has not allowed for the recognition of other TGW's human rights needs and demands (Jaime, 2013). Currently the fundamental link between the health system and TGW in Peru remains HIV-focused, while in some other regional experiences, HIV services have been integrated with other TGW needs (Salazar et al., 2016).

On one hand the demand for comprehensive health has been expressed by TGW activists as a critical posture vis-à-vis the approaches of the Ministry of Health and clinical research: only HIV prevention and treatment are visible. As a TGW in a focus group noted in the same 2010 report about the participation of transgender women in the Peruvian CCM:

> We can also have other diseases, like stomach aches; we can get sick, we can have a migraine, in the hospital we look like 'guinea pigs' because they will only see you as if you have HIV … (Salazar et al., 2010, p. 19)

On the other hand, a claim that comes from transgender activists is the need to address structural problems identified by research in public policies which are intertwined with HIV (Bayer et al., 2011):

> I think that … I mean, I've always said, HIV is not only a health issue, it's a social issue, right? The [main] issue is different: they [the state and society] do not provide them [TGW] access to education, they do not let them work, they do not let them do thousands of things, they are being discriminated against, they are being hit from all sides, and they are being put far away. Their needs are still primary: food, housing, and love maybe. Don't you think so? (Comment made by co-author Miluska Lusquiños during an informal conversation about the demands of the trans population at a meeting in Bolivia, 2017)

Considering these claims, TGW's expectations toward health policies seek the integration and expansion of health services that can address TGW health needs and can tackle stigma, discrimination and social exclusion.

## Discussion

After the long process described above, recently the exclusion of TGW from civil life has been problematised and addressed through some initial policy measures like the release of technical health standards for transgender women. During the early, most critical years of the HIV epidemic, they became visible, yet only as 'a group of high-risk MSM' who 'dressed as women' and were 'mostly involved in prostitution' (Segura et al., 2010). Twenty years later, the confluence between academic research and activism together with an international trend to make visible the situation of trans women in the world provided them with the opportunity to articulate a discourse that allowed TGW to emerge as a political group (and as a social actor) quite distinct from MSM, with their own culture and needs. In this paper, we have presented evidence of this process in Peru, of the role played by research conducted from a sexual rights/human rights perspective, and of the impact of collaboration between researchers and TGW organisations.

Health research focused on TGW in Peru has contributed to the constitution and consolidation of TGW organisations. Initially, such research fundamentally addressed biomedical/epidemiological concerns (i.e. HIV/sexually transmitted infections and associated 'risk factors') and operated mainly within a biomedical framework where the pathologizing view of non-conforming gender identity was accepted (Hausmann, 1995). Such a pathologizing view, we argue, led to TGW only being seen by policy makers, specialists in public health, international cooperation representatives and some academics through the lens of HIV. Over time, an increasing number of social science endeavours started to emerge. Initially, these were centred on HIV public policy (Ministerio de Salud del Perú, ONUSIDA, & Universidad Peruana Cayetano Heredia, 2014; Sánchez et al., 2011). However, a detour has been observed when social scientists started to work with TGW activists on at least two other themes: (a) human rights and structural vulnerability of TGW (Caceres et al., 2007; Salazar, 2009; Salazar et al., 2010, 2013; Salazar & Villayzán, 2009); and (b) sexuality, gender, and identity. Now, although the biomedical discourse and the discourse of human and sexual rights coexist, we have a more conscious and demanding TGW movement.

In our experience, working on human rights and structural vulnerability was not only useful from an advocacy perspective; it also helped depathologize TGW-focused research by both looking beyond disease and explaining the complex social determination of HIV risk. In turn, evidence produced by epidemiological and social research has been useful for TGW activists in their advocacy work, for example by using evidence to support their claim for recognition as a genuinely distinct constituency concerning the elaboration and oversight of GF projects (Salazar, 2010). Research evidence and academic discussion have also contributed to internal discussions about gender identity and organisational efforts as a TGW collective (Jaime, 2013; La Mestiza Colectiva, 2008). Finally, the demand among TGW for comprehensive transgender health research sheds light on the various social and subjective issues that still need to be addressed by research (Velarde, 2011).

## Conclusion

The onset of the new millennium represented a period of change in the social response to HIV in Peru. In the context of: (a) changing international perspectives on sexuality, gender and diversity, and (b) an evolving response to HIV in Peru, with both TGW-focused research and activism-related components, the community of transgender women – previously assumed by researchers, public health decision makers and international HIV agencies to be a part of the MSM constituency – made the case for their independent participation in HIV policy and human rights discussions.

Research evidence initially reinforced the concept of TGW as the group most affected by HIV, without questioning pre-existing pathological views of TGW in the biomedical field, and possibly naturalising their HIV burden. Subsequently, and in light of the HIV burden they face, a wave of social science research, often undertaken in collaboration with TGW, produced new evidence that, by focusing on their vulnerability, human rights and additional health needs, directly questioned the pathologizing paradigm and contributed to considerable growth of the TGW movement.

As we have shown, there are remaining issues that TGW activists are demanding should be seriously considered by government authorities, as well as by researchers. For example, body transformation procedures, transgender adolescence, transgender people's access to education, housing and employment, extreme poverty, internalised stigma among the community, social support, cohesiveness and community bonds – all are factors that influence TGW health outcomes, including HIV infection.

We firmly believe that by paying careful attention to TGW's social demands, and by assessing them with the participation of the community (as well as by reflecting on new ways to make that participation possible and ethical), research can contribute to resolving the substantial inequalities that continually repress TGW's quality of life.

## Disclosure statement

No potential conflict of interest was reported by the authors.

## ORCID

*Ximena Salazar* http://orcid.org/0000-0003-4998-8251
*Angélica Motta Ochoa* http://orcid.org/0000-0001-8506-4182

## References

Bayer, A. M., Paca, A., & Garvich, M. (2011). *Necesidades relacionadas a la prevención, atención y soporte en VIH y SIDA en jóvenes vulnerables en el Perú*. Lima: UNESCO.
Bracamonte, A. (Ed.). (2011). *De amores y luchas: diversidad sexual, derechos humanos y ciudadanía*. Lima: Programa de Estudios de Género de la Universidad Nacional Mayor de San Marcos.
Caceres, C. F., Konda, K. A., Salazar, X., Leon, S. R., Klausner, J. D., Lescano, A. G., Maiorana, A., Kegeles, S., Jones, F. R., Coates, T. J., & NIMH Collaborative HIV/STI Prevention Trial Group. (2008). New populations at high risk of HIV/STIs in low-income, urban coastal Peru. *AIDS and Behavior, 12*(4), 544–551. doi:10.1007/s10461-007-9348-y
Caceres, C. F., Salazar, X., Rosasco, A. M., & Salazar, V. (2007). *A lo que Venga! Alcohol, Drogas y Vulnerabilidad en el Perú actual*. Lima: USSDH-UPCH, ONUDD, ONUSIDA.
Chillag, K., Bartholow, K., Cordeiro, J., Swanson, S., Patterson, J., Stebbins, S., … Sy, F. (2002). Factors affecting the delivery of HIV/AIDS prevention programs by community-based organizations. *AIDS Education and Prevention, 14*(3 Suppl. A), 27–37.
Currah, P., & Spade, D. (2007). Introduction to special issue. The state we're in: Location of coercion and resistance in trans policy, part I. *Sexuality Research and Social Policy, 4*(4), 1–6.
Griffith, D. M., Ober, A. J., DeLoney, E. H., Robinson, K., Lewis, Y., Campbell, B., … Reischl, T. (2010). Community-based organizational capacity building as a strategy to reduce racial health disparities. *The Journal of Primary Prevention, 31*(1-2), 31–39. doi:10.1007/s10935-010-0202-z
Hausmann, B. L. (1995). *Changing sex, transsexualism, technology, and the idea of gender*. Durham, NC: Duke University Press.
Jaime, M. (2013). Diversidad sexual, discriminación y pobreza frente al acceso a la salud pública: demandas de la comunidad TLGBI en Bolivia, Colombia, Ecuador y Perú, Ciudad Autónoma de Buenos Aires: CLACSO.
Kaplan, R. L., Sevelius, J., & Ribeiro, K. (2016). In the name of brevity: The problem with binary HIV risk categories. *Global Public Health, 11*(7-8), 824–834. doi:10.1080/17441692.2015.1136346
La Mestiza Colectiva. (2008). "¡No me va a vencer el sistema, primero muerta!" *entrevista con Belissa Andia. Lima. La Mestiza, revista feminista, 1*, 16–19.
Ministerio de Salud del Perú, ONUSIDA, & Universidad Peruana Cayetano Heredia. (2014). Consulta Nacional: Construyendo Capacidades para la Prevención Combinada del VIH en el Perú. Informe de Relatoría. Retrieved from http://www.iessdeh.org/usuario/ftp/Consulta_nacional_Prevencion_Combinada_Peru_nov2014.pdf
Montalvo, J., Andía, B., & Rodríguez, R. (2009). *Realidades Invisibles. Violencia contra travestis, transexuales y transgéneros que ejercen comercio sexual en la ciudad de Lima*. Lima: Runa instituto de desarrollo y estudios sobre género.

Poteat, T., Wirtz, A. L., Radix, A., Borquez, A., Silva-Santisteban, A., Deutsch, M. B., … Operario, D. (2015). HIV risk and preventive interventions in transgender women sex workers. *The Lancet*, *385*(9964), 274–286. doi:10.1016/S0140-6736(14)60833-3

Reisner, S. L., Poteat, T., Keatley, J., Cabral, M., Mothopeng, T., Dunham, E., … Baral, S. D. (2016). Global health burden and needs of transgender populations: A review. *The Lancet*, *388*(10042), 412–436. doi:10.1016/S0140-6736(16)00684-X

Salazar, X. (2009). *Diagnóstico de la violencia contra los y las trabajadores/as sexuales, mujeres, transgénero y varones y su vulnerabilidad frente a las ITS y el VIH*. Lima: CARE PERU, FONDO MUNDIAL.

Salazar, X. (2010). *Estudio sobre la efectiva participación de mujeres y personas transgénero en los procesos del Fondo Mundial Perú*. Lima: AID for AIDS.

Salazar, X., Caceres, C. F., Maiorana, A., Rosasco, A. M., Kegeles, S., Coates, T., & NIMH Collaborative HIV/STI Prevention Trial Group. (2006). Influencia del contexto sociocultural en la percepción del riesgo y la negociación de protección en hombres homosexuales pobres de la costa peruana. *Cadernos de Saúde Pública*, *22*(10), 2097–2104.

Salazar, X., Maguiña, J., Villayzán, J., Anamaria, P., Sandoval, C., Ceccarelli, M., … Lugo, E. (2013). *"Y me dí cuenta que el SIDA no es sinónimo de Muerte". Diagnóstico del acceso a servicios y programas de Prevención de Salud Sexual y Reproductiva de las Personas Viviendo con VIH*. Lima: IESSDEH/UPCH, PERUANOS POSITIVOS, RED TRANS, ONUSIDA - UNFPA.

Salazar, X., Núnez-Curto, A., Villayzán, J., Castillo, R., Benites, C., Caballero, P., & Cáceres, C. (2016). How Peru introduced a plan for comprehensive HIV prevention and care for transwomen. *Journal of the International AIDS Society*, *19*(Suppl. 2), 20790. doi:10.7448/IAS.19.3.20790

Salazar, X., Silva Santisteban, A., Villayzán, J., & Caceres, C. F. (2010). *Las Personas Trans y la Epidemia del VIH/sida en el Perú: Aspectos Sociales y Epidemiológicos*. Lima: IESSDEH, UPCH, ONUSIDA, AMFAR.

Salazar, X., & Villayzán, J. (2007). Resultados de los Grupos Focales con Trabajadoras Sexuales Travestis sobre el Trabajo Sexual y los Clientes. Lima (not published).

Salazar, X., & Villayzán, J. (2009). *Lineamientos para el Trabajo Multisectorial en Población Trans, Derechos Humanos, Trabajo Sexual y VIH/sida*. Lima: IESSDEH, UNFPA, RedLacTrans.

Sánchez, J. L., Peinado, J. E., & Lama, J. R. (2011). *Estudio de Vigilancia Epidemiológica de ITS y VIH en Hombres que Tienen Sexo con Hombres Comparando las Metodologías de Reclutamiento: Muestreo por Conveniencia, Muestreo por Tiempo y Espacio y el Muestreo Dirigido por Participantes*. Lima: CARE PERÚ, CONAMUSA, FONDO MUNDIAL.

Segura, E., Cáceres, C., Mahy, M., Ghyos, P., Leyrla, R., & Salganik, M. (2010). Estimating the size of populations of men who have sex with men, transgender people and people living with HIV/Aids in Lima, Peru: A study using the Network Scale-Up Method. USSDH - UPCH. (Not published).

Silva-Santisteban, A., Fisher, R., Salazar, X., Villayzán, J., León, S., McFarland, W., & Caceres, C. F. (2012). Transgender women of Lima, Peru: Results from a sero-epidemiologic study using respondent driven sampling. *AIDS and Behavior*, *16*(4), 872–881. doi:10.1007/s10461-011-0053-5

Skovdal, M., Magutshwa-Zitha, S., Campbell, C., Nyamukapa, C., & Gregson, S. (2013). Community groups as 'critical enablers' of the HIV response in Zimbabwe. *BMC Health Services Research*, *13*, 195. doi:10.1186/1472-6963-13-195

Velarde, C. (2011). *La Igualdad en Lista de Espera: Necesidades, Barreras y Demandas en Salud Sexual, Reproductiva y Mental en Población Trans, Lesbiana y Gay*. Lima: PROMSEX.

Wilson, M. G., Lavis, J. N., & Guta, A. (2012). Community-based organizations in the health sector: A scoping review. *Health Research Policy and Systems*, *10*, 36. doi:10.1186/1478-4505-10-36

# Santo Domingo's LGBT social movement: At the crossroads of HIV and LGBT activism

H Daniel Castellanos

**ABSTRACT**
The emergent Dominican LGBT movement in Santo Domingo, Dominican Republic, has been embedded in local and global structures and discourses related to HIV/AIDS, women's health, and identity. This article explores how ongoing sociocultural changes, increased international HIV funding, and elite support facilitated a surge of collective actions and the institutional reconfiguration of the movement. However, the entry of new cohorts of leaders and the alignment of leaders with global discourses of gender and human rights exposed some rifts within the movement, including over the framing of identity, confrontational tactics, and the role of health issues. While creating political opportunities, international HIV/AIDS funding also consolidated the social movement around HIV at the expense of other issues. The rapid consolidation of the LGBT movement towards HIV issues in the Dominican Republic raises questions about the role of international health funding and health-related NGOs on a movement's discourses, strategies, and consolidation, and about the recruitment of social movement leaders as public health professionals. I suggest that the trajectories of new movements, when social and political opportunities arise, are ultimately defined by their ability to bridge over generational and ideological rifts, engage in a broader spectrum of strategies, and embrace intersectional collective actions.

The first public gay event in the Dominican Republic occurred in 23 March 1999, in Santo Domingo, when fifteen gay men and transgender individuals marched along the main shopping street in *Zona Colonial* carrying rainbow flags to protest police harassment (Padilla & Castellanos, 2005). Two years later in July 2001, about 100 people paraded along the same avenue. These early actions, however, found themselves eclipsed a few years later. Windows of political opportunities sparked by sociocultural changes, an influx of international HIV funding, and support from governmental elites changed the institutional configuration of the LGBT movement by re-energizing established LGBT groups and fostering new ones. A surge of LGBT collective actions between 2005 and 2006 increased the movement's visibility and encouraged its consolidation. As successful as these events were, they also exposed rifts within a movement deeply embedded in local and global discourses of feminism, HIV, and sexual orientation. Competing perspectives emerged on the role of new and younger leaders, mobilisation discourses and tactics, and the role of health issues.

The defiant and progressive nature of LGBT and HIV activism of the 80s and early 90s resulted in great political, medical, and sociocultural achievements for LGBT individuals, particularly in the United States and Europe. However, the current HIV political landscape has seen the transformation of HIV activists into institutional experts and increasingly shifted the focus from solidarity and justice to treatment adherence and access to pre-exposure prophylaxis or PrEP (Aggleton & Parker, 2015; Kenworthy & Parker, 2014). The former close connections of LGBT individuals to a 'gay community' and to their service organisations cannot be taken for granted any longer (Lewis et al., 2015; Rowe & Dowsett, 2008). As biomedical responses to HIV prevention (e.g. test and treat, PrEP) continue expanding across the globe, the progressive relationship between LGBT social movements and HIV organisations must be closely inspected, particularly in those countries with emerging LGBT movements and pervasive anti-LGBT policies.

Based on my involvement as a non-local activist during this period, I will examine the factors leading to the consolidation of the LGBT Dominican movement on HIV. I will also seek to examine how the stability and direction of this relatively new social movement became highly dependent on global HIV funding, local and global discourses of activism, and the historical material and ideological rifts within the Dominican society. Finally, I will explore how HIV non-governmental HIV organisations (NGOs) shaped the types of leadership, ideological frameworks, resources available, and framing and mobilisation strategies for the LGBT movement. While health-related resources and NGOs provide opportunities for the strengthening of a social movement, they also shape the discourses and mobilisation strategies of the movement into a less confrontational one, centred more on health than political or civil rights.

While attending to the particular Dominican experience, the analysis of these events draws from analytical tools and concepts from social movement theory to understand the socioeconomic and political landscape in which these collective actions were embedded (See Diani & Bison, 2004; Morris & Mueller, 1992; Tarrow, 2011; Whittier, 1997). Specifically, I used social network theory (Wasserman & Faust, 1994) to elucidate the connections among different social movement actors within the Dominican LGBT movement as well as between institutions serving, training, and engaging these leaders. The concept of discourse framing (Snow & Benford, 1988) was also key for understanding how most collective actions were framed within broader, national social and political discourses such as women's reproductive rights, universal access to HIV medication, or LGBT civil rights. Finally, the concepts of political generations and social movement cohorts (Whittier, 1997) helped me establish qualitative distinctions in the worldviews of the various leaders. As a new wave of collective action restarted, many LGBT individuals (regardless of age) joined or returned to the movement (political generation). Equally important, new cohorts of young people entered the movement at a time in which social media and international networks were transforming the daily lives of Dominican LGBT youth.

## The socioeconomic and political landscape of Santo Domingo circa 2005

Like other Latin American countries, the Dominican economy suffered sharp economic upheavals throughout the 80s (Lozano, Duarte, & Reyes, 1997). Over the next two decades, the Dominican economy would come to rely on export-lead manufacturing and tourism. By 2004, 20% of the Dominican Republic GDP came from the hosting of 3.4 million tourists a year (World Tourism Organization, 2005). The increased visibility of gay tourists and sex workers created anxiety over HIV contagion and the importation of homosexual mores (De Moya & García, 1999; Padilla & Castellanos, 2008). This created a backlash among the most conservative sectors of the Dominican society, including the Catholic Church (Padilla & Castellanos, 2008).

The LGBT movement started in the early 70s in Argentina and Mexico, and in the mid 70s in Colombia. In the case of Argentina, Brazil, Mexico, and Colombia, the LGBT movements shared a historical moment with left-leaning social movements, including armed ones, emerging from struggles for more democratic processes (Amaya, 2012; Diez, 2011; Facchini & França, 2013). While similar calls for democratisation were happening in the Dominican Republic, the LGBT movement only started at the very end of the 80s. It is possible that the right-leaning democracies of the 70s and 80s and the collective discourses of hyper masculinity, homophobia, and conservatism advocated by Trujillo and his successor Balaguer, mainstream society, and the Catholic Church delayed the emergence of Dominican LGBT activism.

While the general population still had negative views on homosexuality (Corcino, 2006), societal changes were increasing the ability of LGBT leaders to obtain elite support in the legal, cultural, and media circles. Newspapers began running stories in a more neutral tone towards LGBT issues as they became more receptive to the lobbying of LGBT activists for a more positive portrayal. LGBT artists and writers also began to mobilise against the state's and the church's control of discourses on homosexuality. The First Anthology of Gay Literature in the Dominican Republic was presented in 2004 at a popular bookstore with the participation of 43 writers (Caballero, 2004), and the formal censorship of LGBT literature at the 2004 International Book Fair generated considerable press and an opportunity for contesting negative discourses.

The HIV/AIDS epidemic forced a public discussion on homosexuality that challenged public officials and leaders to take public health, political and legal actions. By 2000, there were 50,000 documented cases of HIV infection in the Dominican Republic, with 7.6% of them assigned to homosexual/ bisexual contact (UAIDS, 2007). However, the rate could be higher due to lack of HIV testing or disclosure among men who have sex with men for fear of stigmatisation and homophobia (Caceres, 2002). The Dominican Presidential Council on AIDS, created in 2001, coordinated the national efforts to address HIV/AIDS. Nonetheless, several NGOs had responded earlier than that to the challenge of providing HIV services, including *Amigos Siempre Amigos* (ASA), the only gay-identified organisation in the Dominican Republic. HIV prevention in Santo Domingo was primarily conducted at gay bars and clubs, and depended heavily on peer educators from the targeted communities. The training of peers through curricula focused on self-esteem and positive gay identity had increased the number of youths involved in the LGBT movement (field notes, discussions with NGO representatives).

In June 2004, the Dominican Republic received a 5-year grant from the *Global Fund to Fight HIV/ AIDS, Tuberculosis, and Malaria*, including US$48.5 million for HIV/AIDS. Developed by the Presidential Commission on AIDS (COPRESIDA) in collaboration with other NGOs, the proposal included funding for men who have sex with men and required a strategy to create a political environment that favoured human rights for the prevention and treatment of STDs (Global Fund, 2004, 2015). Lagging behind in the implementation of this project, in early 2005 Global Fund officials increased the pressure on COPRESIDA to speed up the implementation of the five-year project (personal communication). As a result, COPRESIDA dramatically increased AIDS-related spending around June 2005, close to a year after the approval of the proposal (Global Fund, 2015).

## Methodology

This article is based on my participation as an activist in the Dominican LGBT movement in Santo Domingo between June 2005 and July 2007. I did not continuously reside in the Dominican Republic but I spent approximately 8 months in total and maintained contact with LGBT leaders during this time and after. As this article is not based a research project nor was it a part of an institutional effort, there was not a research proposal submitted to an Institutional Review Board. However, I strongly argue that research methodologies can guide activists in the development and documenting of collective action, strategies, and discourses, particularly in emerging social movements. Furthermore, social movement activities are often 'knowledge-practices,' processes of knowledge creation, reformulation, and diffusion (See Casas-Cortés, Osterweil, & Powell, 2008).

As an insider and an outsider and as a non-local activist, I relied on intersubjective tenets for conducting engaged ethnography (Demmer & Hummel, 2017). I tried as much as possible to protect the confidentiality and safety of these social actors, including utilising private settings for interviews, de-identifying personal information, and maintaining field notes private. Methodologically, it also meant placing greater attention to member checking and triangulation, being attentive to shifting roles, and ensuring a conscious critique of my perspective as one among many others. Therefore,

I tried to ensure that my interpretations were sound and grounded in local interpretations by presenting my initial thoughts privately to LGBT activists and academicians, including some whose work is cited here.

I utilised ethnographic strategies to guide the activities I was involved in and to document the processes and events taken place, including participant observations at gay-identified social venues and formal and informal interviews with LGBT leaders, gay youth, and researchers. Observations and informal interview notes were recorded in three small notebooks (approximately 160 pages). Formal 30-minute interviews with 10 young key informants on socio-cultural changes, globalisation processes, and the formation of a LGBT social movement were recorded and transcribed. I selected these informants based on their central leadership roles within the movement and their ability to provide both a descriptive and analytical perspective of the events. They were not compensated for their participation. Finally, I conducted a secondary analysis of media portrayals of LGBT issues in Dominican newspapers, published elsewhere (Padilla & Castellanos, 2008).

My involvement in the Dominical LGBT movement took a variety of forms. During the summer of 2005, I served as a foreign-student intern at an HIV NGO in Santo Domingo. I adapted and provided an HIV prevention intervention I had developed for Latino gay men in the USA. Having previously participated in LGBT activism in New York City for over a decade, I soon became engaged in similar activities in Santo Domingo. In particular, I participated in the planning and implementation of the public events celebrating the 2005 and 2006 LGBT pride. I also attended the public events organised for the 2007 LGBT pride.

As a participant, I became friends with many of the people involved in the movement, which allowed to meet many leaders within the LGBT community, including key young LGBT leaders. This role provided me with a broad range of information sources and engagement opportunities, including meetings with key informants, participation in private discussions, and access to internal documents. In collaboration with three experienced activists, I organised and facilitated a three-day Leadership retreat with 14 young gay and lesbian leaders right after the 2005 pride events. I presented initial drafts of the ideas contained in this article in Santo Domingo, including at a panel organised for the 2005 Gay Pride (presentation entitled 'Gay Communities and Globalization') and at a panel I co-organised at FLACSO in 2007 (presentation entitled 'At the crossroads of feminist, HIV, and LGBT activism'). A few years later, June 2009, I was invited to facilitate and document the IV Annual Forum on LGBT Human Rights, a two-day meeting of Dominican LGBT groups held in Santo Domingo.

## A new generation of LGBT leaders

The opening of the Dominican economy and the liberalisation process of the mid 90s had begun changing the Dominican society's relation to homosexuality. As stated by a 33 -year -old gay leader,

> To the extent that the Dominican Republic has opened up to the world, in the same way, it has had the chance to see other cultures, to analyse the gay issue, among other things, from perspectives different from the ones we had before these globalization processes.

These cultural and sexual exchanges fostered a different worldview on the LGBT young leaders who saw the European and American societies as models to emulate. As stated by a 27 -year -old gay man,

> All those [international] tourists come here. There is a cultural exchange. There is an exchange of information; there is an exchange about the lifestyle abroad and the lifestyle here. Then we would like to not so much copy but live a lifestyle similar to that of certain countries, like in Europe, one of the places where gay life is more open.

The impact of these changes was noticeable in the adoption of more public displays of gender non-conformism, an issue noticed as well by the Catholic church (Padilla & Castellanos, 2008) and LGBT leaders.

> In fact, I'm surprised the number of young people today that never went through something so common for my generation as "the crisis." Kids today assume their homosexuality [private and publicly] in such a natural way that it does not carry any type of identity crisis (ASA volunteer, 33 years).

As LGBT youth, including young leaders, adopted a more public persona, their lived experiences would become one of the fault lines in the community as visibility became a contentious point when discussing the need for public actions.

Cohorts are 'clusters of participants who enter a social movement within a year or two of each other and are shaped by distinct transformative experiences that differ because of subtle shifts in the political context' (Whittier, 1997, p. 762). This was also the case for LGBT youth. By 2005, a great number of youths were visible in the Dominican LGBT movement. *Colectiva Mujer y Salud and ASA,* two health-focused organisations, had been producing cohorts of receptive young activists over many years.

In 'La Urbanización de la Pobreza,' Lozano et al. (1997) argue that in most Latin American societies, including the Dominican Republic, youth have higher levels of injustice consciousness, political militancy, and participation in community activism. Although linked to feminism and HIV prevention, the new cohorts were, nonetheless, part of networks working on a variety of issues and more sympathetic to confrontational strategies such as public kiss-ins, demonstrations, boycotts and 'illegal' gatherings (field work). They were also more willing to bring their LGBT identity to other social movements such as the youth and labour movement (field work). In fact, they had extensive electronic-based supportive networks which were located in what Bennett (2003) calls 'polycentric (multi-hubbed) issue networks.'

Borrowing from the feminist emphasis on intersectionality, these networks saw the LGBT issue as one more interrelated issue connected to human rights violations (personal conversations). The issue of race, for instance, was closely related to LGBT leaders' engagement in community activism (See Curiel, 2004) and ran deep through the LGBT young leadership. Some of them had connected their LGBT activism with ongoing struggles over discrimination based on race or Haitian descent.

> Right now, the attacks on Black Dominicans, particularly Haitian Dominican, are in full force. I can't devote myself to 'gay equal HIV' while the oppression of Black Dominicans continues and it's not spoken in the gay community (lesbian and racial minority activist, 24 years).

In fact, they often had to battle the perception that the presence of dark-skin and gender non-conforming youth in public venues was associated with *peligro social* (actions or groups seemed as questioning or subverting traditional socio-cultural norms) (Tineo Durán, 2014).

Equally important to their movement, LGBT leaders saw changes happening at the societal level that created opportunities for action.

> I don't think that there has been a key change in the police as an institution. I think the individuals who are in the police have changed as a result of the same changes in society. The police as an institution is still repressive, abusive, and what not. But many police officers, as individuals within the society, have changed with it (ASA male volunteer, 33 years).

> The internet has helped change gay people's minds because the internet is an influential place. Information flows and you know what is happening here and internationally with respect to the gay life. And you find out how things are there and want the same things happening here. And there are many people trying to make that possible (ASA young activists, 18 years).

These societal changes, nonetheless, had also begun changing the political institutions. In 2000, as part of a larger advocacy and legislative process, the President signed the 'Ley General de Juventud 49.2000' (General Law on Youth), which included the creation of a Ministry of Youth and the only legal reference to LGBT protection at the time (*Article 27.- Gender equality*). The process led to the enactment of the law and the youth development projects of the newly created National Ministry of Youth which fostered a new generation of young leaders in the Dominican society, some of whom were gay and lesbian.

## The diversification of organisational structure and event-based coalitions: 2005

With the Global Fund project behind schedule and an upcoming performance evaluation, an urgent meeting, which I attended, was arranged for 30 May 2005, with representatives from HIV NGOs in the Dominican Republic. Attendees agreed on expediting the spending in HIV activities to ensure that the funding from the Global Fund was preserved. They also agreed to create strategies for integrating civil society in the development and implementation of the Global Fund proposal to ensure its success (field notes).

The sudden influx of funding from 2005 to 2006 created opportunities for a surge in collective actions within the LGBT movement by existing groups. It also supported the strengthening of two new LGBT groups associated with HIV prevention, *REVASA (Red de Voluntarios de ASA)* and *Trans Siempre Amigas (TRANSSA)*. Table 1 presents the main institutional actors involved in or associated with this surge. It also shows the interconnections between different groups, particularly in relation to HIV and leadership and volunteer development.

In the summer of 2005, ASA and REVASA called for a coalition of gay and lesbian activists to plan a gay pride celebration, the third in the history of the Dominican Republic; COPRESIDA decided to provide funding for the events. At first, the group advocated for social events at an open-air bar frequented mostly by young gay men. After joining the coalition, CAP members demanded the inclusion of political and lesbian issues in the celebration as well as the inclusion of non-bar-oriented events (meeting notes). Through lengthily and arduous negotiations, in which I participated, the coalition decided on three events that would incorporate diverse interests and encourage participation of all LGBT constituencies: an academic event, a public celebration, and a cultural event.

The academic event, organised by ASA, featured a review of LGBT history, a discussion on LGBT youth and globalisation (which I presented), and a presentation on pre-Hispanic Caribbean

**Table 1.** Institutional landscape in the period 2005–2006.

| Organization | Focus | Role in social movements | Year started | Year ended |
|---|---|---|---|---|
| Colectiva Mujer y Salud (Women's Health Collective) – NGO | Women's health; sexual & reproductive rights; and leadership development | Connected to feminist groups; trained lesbian leaders | 1984 | – |
| Centro de Orientación e Investigación Integral (COIN) – NGO | Health services to sex workers and MSM, including HIV | Developed LGBT health leaders | 1988 | |
| Amigos Siempre Amigos (ASA) – Only gay-identified NGO | HIV/AIDS education Social and cultural events | Trained hundreds of young gay men as peer educators; maintained extensive social network; organised collective actions; provided institutional support to smaller LGBT groups | 1989 | |
| CAP LGBTIR (Comité de Acción Política de Lesbianas, Gays, Bisexuales, Transexuales, Transgéneros, Intersexuales, Raros y Raras) – Non-partisan political group | advocating for public policies and legislation to guarantee rights for sexual minorities | Between 15 and 18 active gay and lesbian leaders; connected to the Dominican academia and research centres | 2004 | 2006 |
| REVASA (Red de Voluntarios de ASA) – Volunteer group | Volunteer HIV network of ASA Provided also a non-HIV social space | Over 50 active volunteers, mostly young gay men Key planner and implementer of most of the LGBT events | 2005 | |
| Trans Siempre Amigas (TRANSSA) – Transgender volunteer network of ASA | Provided a non-HIV social space | Between 10 and 15 active transgendered individuals | 2006 | |
| Los Muchachos and Muchachas de la Mesa de Atrás (The boys and girls of the back table, MMMA for simplicity) – Non-affiliated group | Struggled to define itself along the continuum of protest, advocacy, and service | Closed group of 12 young lesbian and gay activists; Members had participated in the Leadership Retreat aforementioned | 2005 | 2007 |

homosexuality. Held at ASA, the panel attracted about 35 individuals, mostly young men. Organised by CAP and held at ASA, an art exhibit with folk singers attracted close to 50 people and included the presence of Eric T. Schneiderman, then New York State Senator. Finally, REVASA and ASA organised a public celebration at 'El Boulevard,' a pedestrian boulevard near a shopping area. Despite fear of police harassment, the public event attracted a crowd of close to 400 people. While initially closing the area, the police allowed it, albeit without music, after the organisers mentioned that COPRESIDA sponsored the event as part of an HIV prevention effort.

In addition, a group of young gay leaders and I developed two social marketing materials to link the celebration with national and global legal discourses on human rights. A small sticker simply stated 'Gay Rights = Human Rights. Gay Community of Santo Domingo, 28 June 2005.' The selection of the word gay over the term LGBT tried to address the lack of awareness in the general public about the term LGBT, but understandably slighted many of the lesbian leaders. By selecting 'human rights' over 'civil rights,' the group tried to link the sticker with ongoing national and international discussions on human rights. Over 30 young gay men volunteered to place 5,000 stickers overnight in public spaces, including the Colonial District and twelve universities. Two of these volunteers were detained by the police while doing so.

Another 5,000 small cards with the slogan 'It's the Law. Know it' on the front and the text of Article 27 of the 'Ley General de Juventud' on the back were distributed throughout the summer at gay and non-gay venues. This card linked a legal argument to their collective actions and became a tool against police harassment when celebrating the gay pride events of 2005. Soon after, a newspaper highlighted the existence of the law in the Dominican Republic and its use during these events (Redacción Clave Digital, 2005).

## Consolidation of the field on HIV: 2006

The increased funding and support from AIDS government officials provided political opportunities that motivated the formation of a coalition. The newly-formed coalition decided to formalise the annual gay pride celebrations and, after the summer, it began discussing the upcoming 2006 events. The most influential LGBT leaders advocated for shifting strategies towards collaboration with COPRESIDA and realigning themselves more closely with HIV discourses to capitalise on the increased access to political elites and HIV (personal communication). At the same time, some female leaders expressed concerns about the presence of HIV funding and governmental involvement and worried about co-optation, lack of intersectionality, and conservative strategies (personal communication).

Over time, the public and private meetings showed both a consolidation of the field on HIV and fractures in the coalition's framing and strategies. HIV-affinity groups, officials at COPRESIDA, and some academic leaders played a central role in shaping the movement's ideological frameworks. At an organising meeting, a key leader involved in HIV work stressed his preference for a 'more engaging path to social change through their partnership with COPRESIDA' (meeting notes). On the other hand, leaders involved in other social issues argued for a broader agenda and confrontational strategies. A leader of CAP argued that 'you can create social change without challenging the power of the church and the existing laws penalizing gay people' (meeting notes).

After CAP disbanded at the end of 2005, the overtly political component of the coalition disappeared from the formal conversations. Furthermore, there were few lesbian leaders involved in the actual planning of the events, alienating and frustrating some of the remaining female activists (personal communication). Some young activists have for some time felt alienated by the lack of an intersectional approach and more confrontational strategies.

As we focus our actions around gay men's main issue, HIV, the fundamental issues impacting women, particularly lesbians, are relegated to second place. The current emphasis on gay rights as sexual expression is leaving unquestioned the patriarchal pillars of the Dominican society. The feminist struggles, since the 70s, on reproductive health, abortion, and gendered violence are not part of the current LGBT agenda (lesbian activist, 29 years).

Ultimately, the coalition decided to celebrate gay pride with a public forum to assess the status of LGBT individuals in the Dominican context and a party at a local club. Sponsored by COPRESIDA and coordinated by ASA and REVASA, the forum was held at a hotel in Santo Domingo on 23 June 2006. The forum had panelists from a variety of groups, and about 150 people attended the forum (Ortiz-Gomez, 2006). While the forum focused on human rights and diversity and political engagement, the event was still centred on HIV.

A week after the forum and again with the sponsorship of COPRESIDA, the *Alianza Nacional de Hombres Gay, Transgéneros, Transsexuales y Hombres que tienen Sexo con Hombres* (*Alianza GTH*) was formed at an event attended by the Director of COPRESIDA and with positive media coverage. *Alianza GTH* was charged with coordinating the national response to HIV/AIDS among sexual minorities; promoting human rights as a way of reducing risk; and providing institutional support to the groups of the coalition, including ASA, MMMA, REVASA, and Transsa (Sosa, 2006). As pointed out by several young lesbian leaders (personal correspondence), the absence of lesbians as a sexual minority in the *Alianza GTH*, the framing of human rights in function of HIV risk, and the incorporation of smaller groups within this Global Fund project formalised the consolidation of the field on HIV.

## Generational and gender rifts: Strategies of confrontation and intersectionality

As a member of the United Nations' Human Rights Commission, the Dominican Republic voted in 2005 to include sexual orientation as a human right, and some activists saw political opportunities in expanding the movement through the alignment of LGBT activism along global discourses on human rights (See Carvajal Diaz, 2005; Espinoza, 2005; Polanco, 2006). However, as discussed earlier, young leaders and lesbians working on other issues were dissatisfied with the strategies of collaboration with the state and with HIV as the focus of governmental responses to LGBT needs. Within this context, the generational and gender rifts among LGBT leaders became more evident.

### Generational rifts: The younger LGBT cohorts challenge the old order

After Gay Pride 2005, several young leaders and I discussed the need for leadership development among young LGBT cohorts to address sources of discrimination in the Dominican LGBT movement (e.g. heterosexism, sexism, racism, classism, and ageism). With a team of three experienced LGBT leaders from ASA, REVASA, and *Colectiva Mujer y Salud*, I facilitated a 3-day leadership retreat on 19–21 August 2005. We explicitly recruited 6 young gay men and 5 young lesbians who were already publicly involved as activists in various social movements, including those related to youth, women's health, HIV, and Afro-descendent rights. Although funding was a major issue, the group did not want to accept government money for fear of being co-opted. Instead, funding was obtained through our personal social networks in the United States.

After returning from the retreat, the group maintained close contact and openly challenged existing organisations to broaden the issues being addressed. However, dissatisfied with their inability to shape the direction of CAP and REVASA, eight of them created *Los Muchachos and Muchachas de la Mesa de Atrás* (MMMA, The boys and girls of the back table), a tongue-in-cheek comment on their resentment to the lack of opportunities to participate in decision-making processes or positions of power in the movement.

Yes, I have hope that young people will change things. I'm young. I believe that I am one of those that can help change things or that are changing them. This generation is more liberal than the previous one. They had a bad experience, and they always think that what happened before to them will happen again. We, young people, have not lived those experiences. Perhaps something will happen, but we still have to be active (ASA male volunteer, 18 years).

New cohorts also resented older leaders for the lack of strategies to contest openly broader social structures. But they also understood the challenges of the past generation and the role of youth in the new socio-political landscape.

> The gay community is young because this generation is the one that has opened up ("destapado"). A new phase has begun. We understand that gay people ten years ago came from a society in which the Dominican Republic suffered the aftermath of a dictatorship and then a semi-dictatorship. We had a difficult political situation due to the lack of freedom of speech ('expression"). Even journalists couldn't express their opinions without appearing dead on the streets the next morning. Imagine saying that you were gay. And then, we had a homophobic president, Joaquin Balaguer, for a long time. That explains a lot (ASA male volunteer, 22 years).

A week before gay pride 2006, the police had closed several gay bars and detained between 16 and 20 patrons (Redacción Clave Digital, 2006), creating fear and discontent among many LGBT individuals. As mentioned above, the central gay pride 2006 event was the aforementioned forum on LGBT Diversity, funded by COPRESIDA and with an emphasis on HIV education. Furthermore, organisers had previously eliminated street forms of celebration from the list of events out of concern to governmental reaction (private communications and meetings' notes). At a private meeting with 13 young gay and lesbians, they expressed their dissent with the excessively conservative and narrow agenda for the events. They advocated for a stronger reaction to the recent police actions and for holding street events based on identity rather than HIV.

To take advantage of the heightened interest on LGBT activism, this small group of young dissenters, many of whom had attended our 2005 retreat, and I decided to hold a rally at *Parque Duarte* the same night of the forum, June 23rd. This small square in the colonial area, popular with LGBT individuals and young nonconformists, is often their place for public protests. *Parque Duarte* was also selected because it is a site of contention between Cardinal Nicolás de Jesús López, a main spokesman for homophobic discourses in the Dominican Republic, and LGBT individuals and youth (See Padilla & Castellanos, 2008).

The rally was kept secret until 36 h before it took place due to concerns over a lack of a permit, the risk of police harassment, and co-optation from other leaders or COPRESIDA (meeting notes). Nonetheless, youth organisers discussed and utilised mobilisation strategies from other youth movements abroad. A press release was sent anonymously to supportive media, particularly to youth-oriented electronic media outlets (See Servicios de Clave Digital, 2006). They reached out to central individuals in international organisations of Santo Domingo to serve as deterrents of police harassment at the event (human shields). They lit up their extended and dense electronic social networks through hundreds of text messages, postings in list-servers, and messages in chat-rooms sent during collective sessions at internet cafés. While several leaders publicly distanced the forum from the rally and argued against attending it to avoid police entrapment, the rally attracted over 300 people in less than 36 h.

According to Armstrong, contexts of collective creativity are 'characterized by the intersection of multiple cultural strains, dense interaction, and uncertainty of a kind that produces optimism about the possible success of alternatives' (Armstrong, 2002, p. 362). I argue that these young leaders were positioned within a context of collective creativity, at the intersection of multiple cultural models of organising and engaged in different fields of collective actions (e.g. women's issues, Haitian struggles, youth issues). They were able to come together as an impromptu organising cadre, bypassing some of the existing rifts between gay and lesbian leaders and co-opting their pre-existing communication networks to create alternative collective actions.

While the field was consolidating on HIV, the youth who had participated in the leadership retreat created MMMA and, later, joined others to implement the collective action at *Parque Duarte*. Through these actions, young leaders openly challenged Dominican society and the central leaders of the LGBT. More importantly, the adoption of information communication technologies for rapid mobilisation and multi-sector collaborations showcased the young leaders' innovative strategies to circumvent centralised authority and obtain diverse sources of support.

### Gender rifts: Feminism, HIV

Lesbian and gay leaders had for some time maintained a close relation to international social movements and organisations, particularly those related to feminism, HIV, sexual orientation, and women's health (See Alvarez, 2000; Rohrleitner & Ryan, 2013). Dominican diasporas in New York and Boston had for some time shaped the political discourse in the Dominican Republic by creating a dialogue between Dominican feminists living or commuting within the diasporas (Polanco, 2006). A considerable number of feminist leaders had adopted intersectionality as a framework of reference for analysing the situation of LGBT activism. In particular, the new cohorts of lesbian leaders in the Dominican Republic had questioned the oversight of racism and classism in the discourses of women's oppression and distrusted LGBT leaders and their focus on HIV and reliance on international funding.

On the other hand, the connections to international HIV networks were relatively newer to the Dominican activists and were often connected to technical assistance projects, research studies, and conferences (informal interviews). NGO leaders connected to the movement usually linked LGBT activism to community awareness, self-acceptance, human rights, and anti-discrimination efforts, often the recommended framework of international HIV funding. Since the early 90s, most gay male leaders in the Dominican Republic had been trained at ASA, the only gay-identified organisation, and fully embraced the central role of HIV in the framing of community organising and mobilisation. Through their work, they had successfully engaged large constituencies across gender, class, and race (informal interviews with young gay activists).

While transgender women had been present throughout the years in the movement's actions, they were often absent from discussions about the role of transgender women or the direction of the movement (field observations, informal interviews, and media analysis). However, transgender women had become more and more integrated within the movement as inter-personal violence, sex work, and needle use for hormones were integrated within the broader view of HIV prevention for sexual minorities. The lack of information on transgender issues, primarily due to my limited engagement in transgender-related work and lack of primary data, constitutes a serious shortcoming of this article.

The different health issues and ideological discourses created rifts along gender lines. Many of these rifts were connected to deep historical gendered structures that favoured males, including the shift of the LGBT movement towards HIV. In a personal interview a young lesbian activist (23 years), stated,

> If we [lesbian Dominicans] have to create alternative spaces for confronting the state, so be it. I don't see a role for me in a movement enamoured with COPRESIDA-sponsored events. The meetings [to organize these events] just mirror the Dominican society, silencing women's voices and ignoring our long history of resistance. I also think that those spaces are already there in the alliances that we, lesbian feminists, have established for many years with other groups here in the Dominican Republic and in Latin America.

Most of the active lesbian leaders had participated in efforts of the *Colectiva Mujer y Salud* to develop a social movement centred on women's reproductive rights. Located at the crossroads of the LGBT movements and the Caribbean feminist diaspora, these leaders usually linked issues of heterosexism and gender oppression within the discourse of LGBT identity. However, while the youth were challenging the old guard, some older and younger feminists were also challenging Dominican feminism in regards to strategies to address structural inequalities based on class. As stated by Polanco, CAP founder, (2004, p. 7),

> Lesbian sexual activism has been led by radical feminist women. The majority of non-feminist and moderate feminist-lesbians accept the rules of the dominant heterosexual group. Most of them are closeted. They fear the

family rejection and maintain clandestine sexual relations with other women. Many of them are fervid critics of the LGBTQ movement. They reject the fact that activism breaks the class-boundary that guarantees a privileged position to the small elite in an exclusive unequal society.

CAP's rhetoric often resembled community organising models more common in the USA, namely political action committees, and collective actions rooted in political science. CAP's more confrontational approach, underlying class analysis, emphasis on legal action, and lesser focus on health, generated conflict with key lesbian and gay leaders (Polanco, 2006). CAP members, in particular, held a critical view of the role of these different gay groups and NGOs. As stated by a CAP lesbian activist (45 years),

> We need to create and push a broad social and economic policy agenda that codifies our rights in the Dominican legal system. Other than that, we will be merely tolerated but without rights. But no one, especially the leaders of NGOs, would want to risk the breadcrumbs given through the Global Fund.

Strong disagreements over pursuing a more confrontational and political agenda had led to the folding of CAP in early 2006. Yet, the work of CAP over its two years introduced a different organisational form within the Dominican LGBT movement with a focus on class-based critiques separate from health.

## Conclusions

The socio-political changes and availability of HIV funding had an impact on the institutional configuration of the LGBT movement in Santo Domingo between 2005 and 2007, including the emergence of new groups and opportunities and funding for collective actions. In this period, there was an opportunity for the LGBT movement to coalesce into a more stable and diverse coalition in the Dominican Republic. Instead, the field consolidated rapidly on HIV issues and less confrontational strategies. I suggest that this was possible because of the monopoly of the field by a few service-oriented organisations; the absence of funding to create a diversified leadership and organisational structure outside HIV; the lack of lesbian and youth leadership inside groups able to contest the overt focus on HIV; and the dependence of smaller groups to the HIV organisational structure of the movement. Like in other Latin American countries, Dominican progressive movements have struggled to address the impact of the HV epidemic and advance the civil rights for LGBT individuals, women, and racial minorities. The achievements of these progressive movements received a blow when the constitutional changes in 2010 banned abortion and same-sex marriage and stripped hundreds of thousands of Haitian Dominicans of their citizenship.

At the aforementioned IV Annual Forum on LGBT Human Rights in 2009, which I facilitated at the request of the organisers, leaders stressed the need for diversifying the movement's agenda and strategies. In addition to affirming the term 'LGBT community' in a broad, diverse, and pluralistic manner, participants affirmed the need for addressing the lack of formal political power and for developing a common, multi-issue and intersectional political discourse (private final report delivered to organisers). While there has been some progress in forcing the political system to discuss formally LGBT rights, there is not currently any substantive legal protection for LGBT Dominicans. Nonetheless, leaders have been effective at increasing public mobilisation and visibility, enlisting local and international figures as advocates in local actions, and stating their case before international organisations.

This analysis of the LGBT Dominican movement does not constitute a complete narrative of the events in this period. It cannot either fully explicate the local and global processes running through them. On the contrary, this article is a call for multiple voices to document the history of the movement and for more theoretical analyses of its challenges and successes.

The HIV/AIDS epidemic definitely brought political opportunities for the development of organisations and identity discourses across Latin American (Parker, Barbosa, & Aggleton, 2000), including the strengthening and institutionalisation of the movements and professionalisation of their leaders. However, there has been a variety of ways in which the HIV and LGBT social movements interacted across countries. In Colombia, for instance, the passing of a new constitution in 1991 provided a constitutional framework and legal tools for contesting the state regarding both universal access to HIV treatment and legal protection for minorities (Maldonado, 2006). In Argentina, HIV/AIDS provided some opportunities for LGBT activists. But it was the intersectional work developed through the sustained fight against the dictatorship that brought elite support from a broad range of constituencies (Brown, 2002). In Mexico, the right-leaning social and political backlash connected to the HIV/AIDS epidemic had a detrimental impact on the visibility and agenda of its LGBT social movement (Diez, 2011). But, the political transitions in the early 90s re-energized the social movement under the more encompassing framing of identity and diversity rather than HIV (Diez, 2011). Same sex unions were legally recognised in Colombia in 2007 and in Mexico in 2010. Same sex marriage became legal in Argentina in 2010.

In their analysis of the Brazilian LGBT movement, Facchini & França in (2013) argue that there is not enough information on the recruitment of HIV activists, as public experts and managers, increasingly specialised and professionalised, and on how this recruitment impacts public policies and the advance of LGBT social movements. The rapid consolidation of the Dominican movement on HIV raises also questions about the potential of health-focused NGOs and public health officials to accelerate or hinder the efforts of non-health social movements when social and political opportunities arise, e.g. increased funding, shifts in power structures, or international pressure. Given aforementioned changes in the HIV epidemic, these questions are particularly relevant as the responses to the HIV epidemic rest more and more on biomedical interventions and prevention work is conducted within medical settings and by career health professionals.

More broadly, there is a need for a more thorough examination of whether and how social movements and health efforts can promote and sustain critical activism at times of political constraint, as well as political opportunity. As pointed out by Minkoff (1999), professionalisation and institutionalisation of social movement organisations does not necessarily entail conservatism. Given the ongoing discourses linking human rights and health deployed across the globe, there is a need for critical analysis of the spatial and temporal conditions in which health-related NGOs can support progressive social movements, particularly in countries with developing or newly emerging civil societies.

## Disclosure statement

No potential conflict of interest was reported by the author.

## ORCID

H Daniel Castellanos  http://orcid.org/0000-0003-0057-6168

## References

Aggleton, P., & Parker, R. (2015). Moving beyond biomedicalization in the HIV response: Implications for community involvement and community leadership among men who have sex with men and transgender people. *American Journal of Public Health, 105*(8), 1552–1558.

Alvarez, S. E. (2000). Translating the global effects of transnational organizing on local feminist discourses and practices in Latin America. *Meridians, 1*(1), 29–67.

Amaya, J. F. S. (2012). El olvido recobrado: Sexualidad y políticas radicales en el Movimiento de Liberación Homosexual en Colombia. *Revista CS, 10*, 19–54.

Armstrong, E. (2002). Crisis, collective creativity, and the generation of new organizational forms: The transformation of lesbian/gay organizations in San Francisco. In M. Lounsbury, & M. Ventresca (Eds.), *Social structure and organizations revisited* (Vol. 19, pp. 361–395). Oxford: Elsevier.

Bennett, W. L. (2003). Communicating Global activism: Strengths and vulnerabilities of networked politics. *Information, Communication & Society, 6*(2), 143–168.

Brown, S. (2002). Con discriminación y represión no hay democracia' The lesbian and Gay movement in Argentina. *Latin American Perspectives, 29*(2), 119–138.

Caballero, M. (2004). El que ataca a un gay es porque teme serlo: Miguel De Camps presenta hoy, junto a Mélida García, la primera Antología de la Literatura Gay en la República Dominicana. *El Caribe.* Retrieved from http://www.elcaribe.com.do/articulo_multimedios.aspx?id=821&guid=3A774969B8B84AB69B0AAD911A87790D&Seccion=71

Caceres, C. F. (2002). HIV among gay and other men who have sex with men in Latin America and the Caribbean: A hidden epidemic? *Aids (London, England), 16*, S23–S33.

Carvajal Diaz, M. (2005). Diversidad sexual, a propósito de las modificaciones legislativas. *Vértice: Revista de Ciencias Sociales, 3*(1), 16–19.

Casas-Cortés, M. I., Osterweil, M., & Powell, D. E. (2008). Blurring boundaries: Recognizing knowledge-practices in the study of social movements. *Anthropological Quarterly, 81*(1), 17–58.

Corcino, P. (2006). ENCUESTA CLAVE-CIES: El 60% de los dominicanos repudia la homosexualidad. *Clave Digital.* Retrieved from http://www.clavedigital.com/Portada/ClaveH.asp?offset=-1.

Curiel, O. (2004). Identidades esencialistas o construcción de identidades políticas: El dilema de las feministas negras. *Otras Miradas, Universidad de Los Andes (Venezuela), 2*(2), 96–113.

Demmer, U., & Hummel, A. (2017). Degrowth, anthropology, and activist research: The ontological politics of science. *Journal of Political Ecology, 24*, 610–622.

De Moya, E. A., & García, R. (1999). Three decades of male Sex work in Santo Domingo. In P. Aggleton (Ed.), *Men who sell sex. International perspectives on male prostitution* (pp. 117–129). London: Taylor & Francis.

Diani, M., & Bison, I. (2004). Organizations, coalitions, and movements. *Theory and Society, 33*, 281–309.

Diez, J. (2011). La trayectoria política del movimiento Lésbico-Gay en México. *Estudios Sociológicos, 29*, 687–712.

Espinoza, Y. (2005). Feminismo y lesbianismo en América Latina: Una vinculación necesaria. *Vértice: Revista de Ciencias Sociales, 3*(1), 42–50.

Facchini, R., & França, I. L. (2013). On hues, tints and shades: Subjects, connections and challenges in the Brazilian LGBT movement. In H. Sívori, S. r. Carrara, J. Russo, M. L. Heilborn, A. P. Uziel, & B. Zilli (Eds.), *Sexuality, Culture, and Politics: A South American Reader* (pp. 89–108), Rio de Janeiro: CEPESC.

Global Fund. (2004). Program Grant Agreement between The Global Fund to Fight AIDS, Tuberculosis, and Malaria (Global Fund) and Consejo Presidencial del SIDA (COPRESIDA) of the Government of the Dominican Republic ('Principal Recipient'). Retrieved from https://www.theglobalfund.org/en/portfolio/country/grant/?k=4ddffad2-febe-49c7-a34e-fb5795ac40b8&grant=DMR-202-G01-H-00

Global Fund. (2015). *Grant Performance Report: DMR-202-G01-H-0.* Retrieved from https://www.theglobalfund.org/en/portfolio/country/grant/?k=4ddffad2-febe-49c7-a34e-fb5795ac40b8&grant=DMR-202-G01-H-00

Kenworthy, N. J., & Parker, R. (2014). HIV scale-up and the politics of global health. *Global Public Health, 9*(1–2), 1–6.

Lewis, N. M., Bauer, G. R., Coleman, T. A., Blot, S., Pugh, D., Fraser, M., & Powell, L. (2015). Community cleavages: Gay and bisexual men's perceptions of gay and mainstream community acceptance in the post-AIDS, post-rights era. *Journal of Homosexuality, 62*(9), 1201–1227.

Lozano, W., Duarte, I., & Reyes, O. F. (1997). *La urbanización de la pobreza: urbanización, trabajo y desigualdad social en.* Santo Domingo: FLACSO, Programa República Dominicana.

Maldonado, D. B. (2006). *La constitución multicultural: Siglo del Hombre Editores.* Bogota: Universidad de Los Andes.

Minkoff, D. C. (1999). Bending with the Wind: Strategic change and Adaptation by women's and racial minority organizations. *The American Journal of Sociology, 104*(6), 1666–1703. Retrieved from http://links.jstor.org/sici?sici=0002-9602%28199905%29104%3A6%3C1666%3ABWTWSC%3E2.0.CO%3B2-O

Morris, A. D., & Mueller, C. M. (1992). *Frontiers in social movement theory.* New Haven: Yale University Press.

Ortiz-Gomez, A. (2006). Homosexuales reclaman sus derechos. *Hoy Digital*, June 23, 2006. Retrieved from http://hoy.com.do/homosexuales-reclaman-sus-derechos/

Padilla, M., & Castellanos, D. (2005). Orgullo gay Dominicano: Políticas culturales de identidad en Santo Domingo. *Vértice: Revista de Ciencias Sociales, 3*(1), 51–59.

Padilla, M., & Castellanos, D. (2008). Discourses of homosexual invasion in the Dominican global imaginary. *Sexuality Research & Social Policy, 5*(4), 31–44.

Parker, R., Barbosa, R. M., & Aggleton, P. (2000). *Framing the sexual subject: The politics of gender, Sexuality and power.* Berkeley: University of California Press.

Polanco, J. J. (2004). The lesbian, gay, bisexual, trans, and queer (LGBTQ) movement in the Dominican Republic: A sociopolitical and cultural approach. *Retrieved May 7*, 2007. Retrieved from http://www.globalgayz.com/domrep-JP-news.html

Polanco, J. J. (2006). *Pájaras y maricones 'llegó la hora': un relato de mi experiencia en el movimiento LGBTIR dominicano.* Paper presented at the Latin American Studies Association Forum.

Redacción Clave Digital. (2005, July 3). ORGULLO GAY: Homosexuales y lesbianas dominicanas celebraron su fiesta con éxito. *Clave Digital*, Retrieved from http://www.clavedigital.com/Noticias/Articulo.asp?Id_Articulo=5914

Redacción Clave Digital. (2006, June 19). BATIDA CONTRA LOS SITIOS GAYS: Cierran discoteca Arena, bar Punto y colmadón Omar en la Zona Colonial. *Clave Digital*, Retrieved from http://www.clavedigital.com/Portada/Articulo.asp?Id_Articulo=7656

Rohrleitner, M., & Ryan, S. E. (2013). *Dialogues across diasporas: Women writers, scholars, and activists of Africana and Latina descent in conversation*. Lanham: Rowman & Littlefield.

Rowe, M. S., & Dowsett, G. W. (2008). Sex, love, friendship, belonging and place: Is there a role for 'Gay community'in HIV prevention today? *Culture, Health & Sexuality, 10*(4), 329–344.

Servicios de Clave Digital. (2006, June 22). Convocan a los gays a una protesta por el derecho a la diversidad sexual. *Clave Digital*, Retrieved from http://www.clavedigital.com/Noticias/Articulo.asp?Id_Articulo=10832

Snow, D. A., & Benford, R. D. (1988). Ideology, frame resonance, and participant mobilization. *International Social Movement Research, 1*(1), 197–217.

Sosa, J. R. (2006, July 1). Proclaman Alianza Nacional de Hombres Gay, Transgeneros, Transexuales y Hombres que tiene Sexo con Hombres (Alianza GTH). *El Nacional*.

Tarrow, S. G. (2011). *Power in movement: Social movements and contentious politics*. Cambridge: Cambridge University Press.

Tineo Durán, J. (2014). *Imaginarios de género en juventudes dominicanas: aportes para el debate desde la colonialidad del poder*. Santo Domingo: Instituto Tecnológico de Santo Domingo.

UAIDS. (2007). *Caribbean: 2006 AIDS epidemic update*. Retrieved from http://data.unaids.org/pub/EpiReport/2006/07-Caribbean_2006_EpiUpdate_eng.pdf

Wasserman, S., & Faust, K. (1994). *Social network analysis: Methods and applications* (Vol. 8). Cambridge: Cambridge university press.

Whittier, N. (1997). Political generations, micro-cohorts, and the transformation of social movements. *American Sociological Review, 62*(5), 760–778. Retrieved from http://links.jstor.org/sici?sici=0003-1224%28199710%2962%3A5%3C760%3APGMATT%3E2.0.CO%3B2-P

World Tourism Organization. (2005). *Tourism Market Trends, 2005 Edition*. Retrieved from http://www.e-unwto.org/doi/pdf/10.18111/9789284411139

# Social Class for Collective Health Research: A Conceptual and Empirical Challenge

Adriana Gisela Martinez-Parra, César Ernesto Abadía-Barrero ⓒ, Chiharu Murata, Ignacio Méndez Ramírez and Ignacio Méndez Gómez-Humaran

**ABSTRACT**
Social Determination of Health (SDH)/Collective Health is a Latin American framework that sees the Marxist core concept of social class as fundamental for understanding health inequalities. In contrast to social stratification approaches, Marxist proposals seek to understand health as part of the historical transformations of capitalism's mode of production. In this article we aim to analyze the relationship between social class and health inequalities using data from the IV Oral Health National Study in Colombia. We conducted hierarchical cluster analyses to classify the population in five class positions and three living conditions clusters, which reflect how the spheres of production and social reproduction relate to social classes in Colombia. To measure oral health we use DMFT, as well as care and treatment needs indexes. Through variance analysis models we found that people from more exploited class positions and worse living conditions have more active disease and higher treatment needs. Despite technical and conceptual challenges, we conclude that a social class analytical framework can be operationalised via the interrelated spheres of production and social reproduction, which sheds light on the relationship between health inequalities and the class structure of the capitalist system.

This article is dedicated to the memory of Dr. Ignacio Méndez Ramírez, for his kindness and generosity sharing his wealth of knowledge.

## Introduction

Even though Rudolph Virchow is considered the father of Social Medicine, Frederick Engel's The Condition of the Working Class in England, published in 1845, stands as the pioneer study that merged critical political economy with morbidity and mortality analyses. Engels demonstrated with great level of quantitative and qualitative detail how the capitalist class structure at the hype of the industrial revolution in England not only influenced the poor health outcomes of workers (from the industrial, mining and agricultural sectors), but also affected the whole living conditions of the working class. At the factories, mines, or fields, men women and children faced over exploitative working conditions. In their neighbourhoods, they confronted misery, filth, famine, and disease. The prolific friendship between Engels and Marx gave rise to the most powerful theory to explain the contradictory nature of the capitalist system given that the two socially constituted classes, the capitalist and the proletariat, have opposing interests. It is precisely the Marxian grounding of social medicine which has allowed this interdisciplinary tradition to continue illuminating the relationship between capitalist accumulation patterns, class formation and struggle, and the health of the population.

While some social theorists have proposed ways to update the Marxian social class analysis considering the transformation of labour relationships, mode of production and class structure within the last fifty years (Portes & Hoffman, 2003; Wright, 2000), social medicine scholars have continued to unveil how the transformation of capitalist accumulation patterns influences health (Birn, Nervi, , & Siqueira, 2016; Breilh, 2007, 2010; Iriart & Emerson-Elias, 2017; Navarro, 1976, 2007; Waitzkin, 2016; Waitzkin, 2018). In particular, mental health, self-reported general health, health behaviours, and mortality are all health domains that exhibit differential outcomes with those whose employment relationships indicate higher rates of labour exploitation (the proletariat) exhibiting worse health in comparison to those who own the means of production (the capitalist) (Muntaner et al., 2010, 2012; Rocha et al., 2013). Importantly, however, several studies support Wright's theoretical category of 'contradictory positions' of the 'intermediary class' that Marx characterised as the petit bourgeoisie (Wright, 2000). Middle managers and supervisors, the petit bourgeoisie, have less-favorable mental health outcomes than workers without authority or higher managers (Muntaner et al., 2010, p. 2138), which is very likely the result of their responsibilities to increase profits to the companies' owners (the capitalists) by inflicting enhanced exploitation techniques on the workers (the proletariat). Given that a proper class analysis requires analytical abstractions from social relationships of production to the workings of the capitalist system, the studies that aim to unveil how social class influences health need to use 'proxy' indicators such as 'employment relations', 'class position', or 'social insertion'.

While it is challenging to think of direct relationships between oral health and social class, we do know that the development of the capitalist system has shaped historical processes that influence oral health epidemiological profiles. Sugar, the most important cariogenic food, was perhaps the first transnational agribusiness built around slave work within the plantation economy of the Caribbean colonies (Mintz, 1985). Importantly, sugar consumption patterns around the world changed between 1650 and 1900. Sidney Mintz's (1985) groundbreaking ethnographic and historical study showed how sugar as a commodity went from being a privileged and pricy food consumed only by the monarchy and the imperial elites, or because of its 'medicinal properties', to becoming a cheap and popular ingredient constitutive of people's diets around the world. Studies that inquire about changes in sugar consumption and presence of dental caries do demonstrate that the rates of this oral pathology grow hand in hand with higher patterns of sugar consumption and inadequate exposure to fluoride (Duque Naranjo & Mora Díaz, 2012). Currently, the WHO indicates that 'the burden of oral disease is particularly high for the disadvantaged and poor population groups in both developing and developed countries' (Petersen, Bourgeois, Ogawa, Estupinan-Day, & Ndiaye, 2005, p. 661). Epidemiological studies in different countries demonstrate an association between socioeconomic variables and the greater presence and severity of oral diseases among poor and marginalised social sectors (Bernabe & Hobdell, 2010; Medina-Solís et al., 2006; Vettore, Marques, & Peres, 2013; Zurriaga, Martínez-Beneito, Abellán, & Carda, 2004).

While we know that these stratification indicators, such as level of poverty, do not correspond to a social class analysis, we find them informative as they show that oral health inequalities do exist between social groups hierarchically differentiated by income and property assets. Hence, our task for this study is to bring a social class analysis to oral health and inquire if the social structure of the capitalist system does or does not reflect unequal patterns in oral health.

In order to advance in our task and before moving on to the methods and results sections, the remaining of the introduction presents: first, a brief synthesis of the historical transformation of the class structure in Latin America and Colombia. Then, we offer a summary of how social class has been operationalised for statistical analysis. Last, we discuss briefly our efforts to assess oral health from a Marxist framework, particularly from the Latin American Social Medicine tradition.

## Class structure in Latin America and Colombia: a brief synthesis

As a difference from the high levels of employment that characterised Europe during the second half of the twentieth century, Latin American countries maintained low levels of formal employment and high levels of informality and agricultural labour. The persistence of so-called 'traditional, backward, secondary, residual or marginal sectors of the economy' characterised what came to be known as underdeveloped economies (Petersen et al., 2005, p. 661). Assessing this level of 'economic development', however, requires an understanding of the consolidation of a class system in the region after independence. In Colombia, which has important resemblances to other countries in the region, the agroindustrial class became the dominant fraction of the bourgeoisie. During most of the nineteenth and twentieth century, industry owners entered into conflict and partnership with the other fractions of the capitalist sectors: landowners for agricultural and livestock businesses, commercial sectors, and financiers, all of whom were consolidating their economic and political power (Misas Arango, 2002; Ogliastri & Guerra, 1980; Ospina Vásquez, 1979; Safford & Palacios, 2001; Sáenz Rovner, 2007). Although with some changes in composition and regional differences, these capitalists class fractions have since maintained power, in part because the class struggles of the different fractions of the proletariat have been dominated by the bourgeoisie ideology. Also, leftist social movements and parties that have represented the interests of the proletariat have become political victims of the many cycles of civil and military violence (Cardenas, 2010; Misas Arango, 2002; Safford & Palacios, 2001; Sáenz Rovner, 2007).

As it happened in other countries in the region, during the mid-twentieth century, Colombia changed its economic policies towards a model known as 'import substitution and industrialisation', which transformed in important ways the regional class composition (Misas Arango, 2002). A rapid urbanisation process resulted in a significant, albeit partial, increase in formal employment. Indeed, by 1980, unemployment and underemployment (self-employed and unpaid family members) comprised around 40% of the economically active population (EAP) (Couriel, 1984; PREALC, 1991). The agricultural sector shrank to only 32% of the EAP (Couriel, 1984; PREALC, 1991). Only 47% of the EAP in non-agricultural sectors had formal employment and, consequently, paid taxes (PREALC, 1991), which meant both union protection and access of social security.

As a way to reduce informal labour and decrease unemployment rates, neoliberal ideologues pushed market-based reforms during the 1980s and 1990s in the whole region. Governments, responding to the needs of global capitalist sectors (Waitzkin & Jasso-Aguilar, 2015) attacked unions and union contracts in order to impose new labour regulations that made labour 'flexible' (E. De la Garza, 2000; N. Klein, 2007). Changes in bargaining agreements altered work-related entitlements, working conditions, and employment relations, allowing for a reduced work force and a deregulated labour context characterised by temporal, third-party, and informal labour (Benach, Muntaner, Solar, Santana, & Quinlan, 2014; Cruces & Ham, 2010). Against neoliberal predictions, unemployment rates remained at high levels (De la Garza, 2000; Portes & Hoffman, 2003).

As a way to increase social security coverage, neoliberal ideologues proposed privatisation. These reforms offered national and transnational insurance companies new markets for their pension funds and their health and work-disability policies (Benach et al., 2014; Iriart, Elías, & Waitzkin, 2001). For those who could not afford private insurance, state-sponsored subsidies signified the direct transfer of public funds to private insurance companies (Iriart et al., 2001).

## Social class and statistical analysis

While the historical situation in Colombia largely reflects the Latin American region, scholars high-light how the proximity of Colombian elites with International Financial Institutions, resulted in a deeper entrenchment of neoliberal logics around labour and social security (Garay, 1998; Restrepo, 2003). A challenge to analysis around social class and labour in the country originates in the ways in which labour-related indicators have been transformed under the new 'business and accountability' norms that regulate social life and state politics in neoliberalism (Centro de Investigaciones para el Desarrollo CID, 2006; Erikson, 2012). Indeed, the National Department of Statistics (NDS), and other public entities, have largely abandoned traditional work-related categories and replaced them with 'occupation-related' indicators. Official surveys define occupation as people who have worked at least one hour in the previous week, whether they received any economic compensation or not (DANE, 2014). Using some of the survey parameters, the NDS estimates that 47% of the occupied population are 'informal laborers' (DANE, 2018).

Scholars in economics and statistics have voiced their critiques with the new classification schemes, given their multiple technical and political problems. Not only has it become very difficult to trace working relationships, which impedes proper social analysis, but new classification schemes also obfuscate informality, underemployment, and unemployment (Centro de Investigaciones para el Desarrollo CID, 2006; Portes & Hoffman, 2003). Hence, updating the social class category needs to take into account: 1) the context of labour precarization and flexibilization previously described, 2) the rise of inequalities out of the concentration of capital in global elites (Robinson, 2004), and 3) the neoliberal disruption of national statistics that undermine labour as part of social class contradictions.

The most important challenge continues to be understanding the complexity and historical specificity of class relations within the shifting capitalist accumulation patterns. The other important challenge is to operationalise this conceptual framework (class relations within a class structure) into specific empirical studies, primarily those that are quantitative in origin. Portes and Hoffman (2003) attempted to develop a new category of social class attuned to the neoliberal transformation of labour in the Latin American region. Their neo-weberian framework, which emphasises the position of sub-jects within the market, is important in that it shows the heterogeneity of social classes in Latin America given the coexistence of multiple modes of production (Naveda, 2014; Wright, 2015). Nonetheless, this classification is produced with data coming from labour national statistical reports, which results in a partial picture given that the unemployed, reserved army of labour in a Marxian framework, and other people outside of the production process such as retirees and rentiers are not included. Furthermore, a risk of Porter and Hoffman's scheme is to conclude that people belonging to formal and informal labour have different class interests or that the neoliberal precarization of labour and informality has originated a class that is different from the proletariat (Elbert, 2015).

The issue of precariousness of labour and precariousness of material living conditions had been already presented by Engels and later conceptualised as part of Marx's understanding of the fluidity and interconnectedness between the working class (formal and informal) and the reserve army of labour (Antunes, 2018, p. 2; Jonna & Bellamy Foster, 2016). While the nature of class relations needs to remain central, this does not negate that a neo-marxist analysis can benefit from incorpor-ating other social science traditions. Wright (Wright, 2015), for example, proposes to integrate the Marxist analysis based on conflicts around the ownership of means of production with the Weberian analysis around rent distribution and market relationships, and with the other stratification schemes that highlight how individual levels of economic wellbeing and individual attributes are specific to different classes.

A recent neomarxist analysis in Colombia shows that the petite bourgeoisie in directorship pos-itions and independent workers in Colombia have increased substantially from 1994 to 2010, which might be the result of changes in classification surveys, modifications in the organisation of indus-tries or the new entrepreneurialism demanded of the professional class (Ó. Fresneda, 2016). They comprise as much as 36.6% of the EAP while the percentage farmers and workers without director-ship roles in all sectors of the economy have shrunk (Ó. Fresneda, 2016).

## Oral health and social class

Latin American Collective Health has long advocated for the importance of unveiling how capitalist social relationships influence the health-disease-treatment process of different population groups (Breilh, 2003; Laurell, 1982; López, 2013). Studies in Venezuela, Brazil, Argentina and Chile all indi-cate that health care outcomes in terms of prevention, health behaviour, or specific pathologies are influenced by social class (Benach et al., 2014; Muntaner et al., 2012; Rocha et al., 2013). Bronfman in México (1984) and Breilh in Ecuador (1989) respectively, operationalise Lenin's social class definition to differentiate population groups. For Lenin, classes are 'large groups of people distin-guished from one another by [1] their status in an historically-determined system of social pro-duction, [2] by the proportion of the means of wealth production they possess, [3] by the part they play in the social organisation of labour, and [4] by the kind and the quantity of socially pro-duced wealth they have at their disposal' (Lenin, 1919). For Bronfman and Breilh, each of these four distinguishing aspects result in dimensions, which can be assessed with one or more qualitative vari-ables (i.e. survey questions) and allow for conforming different class positions within the class struc-ture. A version of this operationalisation of social class was used for data collection of the National Survey as we will later explain.

While it is difficult to explain how higher or lower rates of labour exploitation influence oral health, it is possible to see how the living conditions of workers and families allow them to care for their oral health in a way that disease is prevented or treatment is accessed in a timely way. Importantly, the relationship between poorer oral health outcomes and higher consumption of sugars that we eluded to before, speaks not only to the conditions of production (i.e. labour exploita-tion as the centre of the labour theory of value) but, importantly, to the possibilities for social repro-duction (i.e. the reconstitution of worker's labour power via food, sheltering, rest, and care). As such, we see that health, understood both as developing diseases and caring for one's health, is at the core of the contradiction between production and social reproduction of the capitalist system (Fraser, 2016). On the one hand, profit depends on the exploitation of labour power and the conditions of workers' exploitation directly affect each worker's health (i.e. visual health, musculoskeletal health, environmental hazards, and so on). Furthermore, the rate of exploitation influences the progress of those diseases (i.e. amount of hours being exploited, higher productivity demands, and so on) (Breilh, 2003; Laurell, 1982). On the other hand, the social distribution of accumulated wealth influ-ences the living conditions of the working class and sets up the possibilities for social reproduction including enough rest, sufficient and good quality food, and, importantly, the possibility to recover from disease to reconstitute the physical strength needed for work. As we approached our interest in connecting a social class analysis with oral health, we argue that it is best to approach oral health through the contradictions between production and social reproduction of the capitalist system (Fra-ser, 2016).

Jaime Breilh, one of the most reputed Latin American Collective Health scholars by bridging social class analysis with epidemiology, served as advisor in the IV National Oral Health Survey (ENSAB IV) in Colombia. The ENSAB IV survey is an adaptation of his class position classification proposal to the Colombian context. The ENSAB IV survey contained 13 class positions, which equates to what Breilh calls 'social insertion' (Breilh, 1989) in his own studies in Ecuador. Most importantly, however, Breilh has clarified that a proper social class analysis only occurs through a historical interpretation of the data. Hence data are meant to reflect 'social insertion' or 'social pos-ition' and only a Marxist analysis of such classification produces adequate interpretations of social class. Thus, the debate should not be about the best technical parameters included in a given instru-ment exclusively, but how to best merge data with a critical political economy framework. Data may always be insufficient or limited given technical difficulties and the changing landscape of the contradictions that characterise social relationships in Capitalism. We aim to propose one way to analyze the relationship between social class and health in Colombia and explore its potentials and limitations when using oral health as an example.

For oral health, then, we reiterate that it is of outmost importance to think about the sphere of social reproduction, both in terms of the possibilities to care for one's oral health, the consumption patterns around healthy or unhealthy food, and the access to health care services which comprises prevention actions, treatment of oral disease (which also avoids further destruction of oral health tissues), and rehabilitation of already damaged tissues (Abadía-Barrero & Martínez-Parra, 2016). Our analysis made us realise that we needed an integrated approach in which social position based on class (sphere of production following Breilh's initial proposal) had to be paired with the living conditions that make the proletariat more or less vulnerable to developing oral disease (sphere of social reproduction). It is this proposal which we will now explain in more detail.

## Methods

### The ENSAB IV methodology

ENSAB IV is a cross sectional study with a stratified and multistage sampling design. The sample size of 20.533 people represented the six geographical regions most commonly used for official surveys. The sample included people belonging to the following age groups 1, 3, 5, 12, 15 and 18; adults between the ages of 20 and 79; and pregnant women between the ages of 20 and 49.

Data collection instruments included four modules: 1) Household information, 2) sociodemographic data, 3) social determination, and 4) clinical exam. Data were collected during 2013 and 2014. A detailed description of the survey and data collection parameters can be found in the official report (Ministerio de Salud y Protección social, 2014a).

### Population for this analysis

For the assessment of the influence of social class in oral health presented in this article we included the population between 20 and 79 years old only. The sample for this age group is 8040 people, which represents 29,444,964 Colombians (expanded sample). The sociodemographic characteristics of the population according to class position are included in Table 3.

### Statistical analysis

#### Class position

Following Lenin's definition of social class, Breilh proposes four variables to differentiate populations among different class positions. The ENSAB IV's social determination module contained these variables: Occupational Category (17 categories), Income Source (16 categories), Possession of Means of production (6 categories), and Labour-related Tasks (4 categories). The original proposed algorithm should have resulted in 13 class positions. Because of data collection errors and unforeseen characteristics of labour flexibilization, informality and underemployment, a significant number of people could not be classified in any of the 13 class positions. In order to address this data problem, we decided to use a statistical technique that guided by contemporary debates around social class (briefly sketched in the introduction) allowed us to reclassify the total sample into new categories of class position. The reclassification also allowed us to reduce the original number of categories for the Occupational Category variable (from 17 to 7) and Income Source variable (from 16 to 8).

We found particularly appealing Wright's integrated model to assess social class. We used hierarchical cluster analysis that included Breilh's four original variables (that follow a more classic Marxist framework) and added the income and educational level of the main breadwinner, which are used by Wright and Bronfman in some of their analyses (Bronfman & Tuirán, 1984; Wright, 1985). To locate family members in a given class position, we used the breadwinner's information.

We used hierarchical cluster analysis to reduce data dimensions, summarise data, and classify individuals into different groups. The main characteristic of the groups in a cluster analysis is their homogeneity (internal cohesion) and separation (external isolation) (Everitt, Landau, Leese, & Stahl, 2011; Johnson, 2000). For the hierarchical classification, data are split into a series of partitions, from 1 group with all individuals and to n number of groups with just one individual (Everitt et al., 2011). In order to assess the ideal number of clusters, we did a variance analysis among groups (F test). As dependent variables, we used all variables included in the clusters once they were standardised. We obtained the mean square error for different numbers of clusters and run a scree plot. (see Table 1). The driver of our cluster analysis was social class, meaning that we only allowed the conformation of clusters that made sense for the class structure of Colombia.

In addition to these class position clusters, we also wanted to include some 'living conditions' that could allow us to include a proxy for social reproduction into the analysis. Some Latin American Collective Health authors think of these differences as part of an 'intermediate sphere' that connects

**Table 1.** Description of class position clusters.

| Variable | Employee | Independent worker | Retired/rentier | Unskilled worker | Unemployed |
|---|---|---|---|---|---|
| n | 2543 | 745 | 614 | 3875 | 263 |
| N | 10,156,112 | 2,714,569 | 2,447,178 | 13,377,180 | 749,925 |
| % | 34.39 | 9.22 | 8.31 | 45.43 | 2.55 |
| Occupational category | Employee (public and private industry) | -Independent Professional or technician<br>-Small business merchant<br>-Owner of industrial, commercial or service company[1] | Retired/Rentier | Worker | Unemployed |
| Income source | Wage as employee | -Private business / street vending<br>-Honoraria[1] | Jubilee pension/ Property rental | -Wage as labourer (Most important)<br>-Salary as worker | -Donations / Subsidy / Alms<br>-None |
| Labour-related tasks | Directs and organises the work of others | Does and directs the work | Outside of the productive process | Does the work | Does the work[3] |
| Possession of means of production | Machinery<br>Nothing | Local Machinery Tools Commodities | Land Nothing | Land Tools | Nothing |
| Monthly income[2] | More than 1 MMW – Two MMW (>$589.501–$1.179.000)[1]<br>More than two MMW – less than 4 MMW (>$1.179.001–<$2.358.000)<br>More than 4 MMW (>$2.358.001[1]) | More than 4 MMW (>$2.358.001) | More than 1 MMW – less than four MMW (> $589.501–<$2.358.001) | Less than half MMW - one MMW (<294.750–589.500) | None - Less than half MMW (<$294.750) |
| Level of education | Technical/ Technological University Postgraduate[1] | University Postgraduate[1] | Primary University | None[1]<br>Primary<br>Does not know/ Not responding[1] | None Primary[1] |

[1]These categories characterise conglomerates with a weaker relation than the others.
[2]These are monthly minimum wage legal values (MMW) for Colombia in 2013.
[3]This reflects that even if unemployed the person does the main productive activity they describe.

class structure with individual life styles (Almeida-Filho, 2000; Blanco & Sáenz, 1994; Breilh, 2010; Samaja, 2004). Wright's integrated approach, in contrast, considers that living conditions (i.e. material conditions of existence, which include household characteristics and individual attributes) could also help define class positions (Wright, 2015). We also run a hierarchical cluster analysis of the following ENSAB's living conditions variables, included in the household module: area (urban vs rural), socioeconomic strata, monthly household income, lack of money during the previous week to buy food, housing tenure, type of housing, and water supply variables. (see Table 2, results section.) We think of these living condition clusters as reflecting, albeit partially, how the sphere of social reproduction influences oral health care and consumption patterns. Importantly, given the historical conformation of social classes in Colombia, we wanted to unveil the differences between the precarious living conditions of the agricultural labour force as compared with the living conditions of the labour force and petite bourgeoisie in the cities.

### Clinical indexes

In order to analyze clinical data we use 3 main indexes: 1) DMFT (Decayed Teeth + Missing Teeth + Filled Teeth), which is the index most frequently used and is recommended by the WHO to account for the severity of dental caries damage and treatment received (H. Klein, Palmer, & Knutson, 1938). 2) Treatment Needs Index (TNI = Decayed/decayed + filled). 3) Care Index (CI = filled teeth/ DMFT). Both treatment needs index and care index measure access and equity in health care (Agudelo Suárez & Martínez Herrera, 2009). Our social class analysis drove the search for these indexes given that we wanted to see clinical evidence of worse oral health and worse access to health care. While we hypothesised the DMFT index obfuscated inequalities, TNI and CI should make inequalities evident. Worse care and treatment indexes should indicate higher consumption of unhealthy foods, poorer prevention strategies, and poorer access to health care services.

### Variance analysis model

The effects of social position and living conditions clusters in oral health were assessed with variance analysis models for each categorical variable (social position with 5 categories and living condition with 3 categories) and a different variance analysis model with both categorical variables and their interaction. Given the importance of age in oral health, we added age (continuous variable) as a co-variable in all the models. We run one model per each clinical index as a dependent variable using the stata 13.0 function for complex surveys (svy). In cases in which the interactions were not statistically significant, we run Sheffé tests for each of the principal effects on the dependent variables to compare the means within groups of the same variable (StataCorp, 2013).

## Results

The cluster analysis in light of the theoretical debates around social class allowed us to group the sample in the following five class position clusters: Employee, Retired/Rentier, Unskilled Worker, Independent Worker, Unemployed. This National sample confirms what a review paper on social class and health found: it is almost impossible to include capitalist fractions in these samples, both because of their inaccessibility and also because of their small number as a percentage of the population (Muntaner et al., 2012). Hence, we are left with a range of fractions of the proletariat amidst a context of increasing precarization during neoliberalism and an increase in the 'intermediary class', meaning the petit bourgeoisie and independent workers (Ó. Fresneda, 2016). The characteristics of these clusters are presented in Table 1.

The sociodemographic characteristics of the population according to each class position are presented in Table 2.

Figure 1 shows the analytical correspondence between the social position clusters and social classes.

**Table 2.** Percentage frequency distributions of sociodemographic characteristics and means and standard errors of the oral health indexes by class position.

| | Employee | Independent worker | Retired/ rentier | Unskilled worker | Unemployed | Total |
|---|---|---|---|---|---|---|
| n | 2543 | 745 | 614 | 3875 | 263 | 8040 |
| N | 10,156,112 | 2,714,569 | 2,447,178 | 13,377,180 | 749,925 | 29,444,964 |
| *Age group* | | | | | | |
| 20–34 | 46.52 | 33.91 | 17.14 | 39.28 | 29.88 | 39.20 |
| 35–44 | 24.13 | 20.95 | 5.75 | 19.84 | 22.08 | 20.31 |
| 45–64 | 24.07 | 38.87 | 43.47 | 32.71 | 29.21 | 31.10 |
| 65–79 | 5.29 | 6.26 | 33.65 | 8.17 | 18.73 | 9.39 |
| *Sex* | | | | | | |
| Men | 49.23 | 45.52 | 45.27 | 49.63 | 40.42 | 48.51 |
| Women | 50.77 | 54.48 | 54.73 | 50.37 | 59.58 | 51.49 |
| *Ethnic group* | | | | | | |
| Indigenous | 3.33 | 5.61 | 2.31 | 6.73 | 1.95 | 4.97 |
| Black | 9.74 | 10.49 | 7.19 | 13.96 | 9.77 | 11.52 |
| White | 26.59 | 26.73 | 31.62 | 24.63 | 22.66 | 26.03 |
| Mixed | 46.70 | 42.68 | 45.39 | 39.48 | 46.25 | 42.93 |
| Other ethnic groups | 2.89 | 1.74 | 2.40 | 2.46 | 2.87 | 2.54 |
| Not defined | 3.71 | 8.46 | 2.62 | 5.96 | 5.50 | 5.13 |
| No sabe | 7.04 | 4.29 | 8.47 | 6.78 | 11.00 | 6.89 |
| *Marital status* | | | | | | |
| Married | 26.91 | 34.40 | 33.17 | 23.73 | 19.27 | 26.48 |
| Common law | 33.53 | 31.06 | 12.19 | 40.98 | 18.52 | 34.53 |
| Divorced | 0.77 | 1.02 | 1.17 | 0.30 | 0.15 | 0.59 |
| Separated | 8.24 | 6.96 | 9.56 | 10.34 | 17.31 | 9.42 |
| Widowed | 3.15 | 4.42 | 14.09 | 2.82 | 7.13 | 4.13 |
| Single | 27.40 | 22.14 | 29.82 | 21.83 | 37.63 | 24.85 |
| *Health care affiliation* | | | | | | |
| Contributive | 71.23 | 40.03 | 60.06 | 18.40 | 29.82 | 42.37 |
| Subsidized | 17.34 | 50.57 | 15.45 | 70.54 | 59.57 | 45.49 |
| Uninsured | 5.75 | 1.27 | 16.13 | 0.78 | 0.00 | 3.80 |
| Other regimens | 5.69 | 8.13 | 8.37 | 10.28 | 10.60 | 8.36 |
| *Education level* | | | | | | |
| None | 0.95 | 1.52 | 3.18 | 7.75 | 6.92 | 4.43 |
| Pre-primary | 0.03 | 0.00 | 0.00 | 0.05 | 0.00 | 0.03 |
| Primary | 12.89 | 25.52 | 28.63 | 42.42 | 41.76 | 29.51 |
| Secondary | 32.21 | 38.05 | 34.51 | 36.23 | 39.23 | 34.94 |
| Technical/technological | 20.13 | 13.53 | 13.95 | 8.02 | 4.56 | 13.11 |
| University | 27.66 | 14.83 | 17.80 | 3.52 | 5.35 | 14.12 |
| Postgraduate | 5.94 | 6.55 | 1.66 | 0.03 | 0.22 | 2.81 |
| Does not know/ Not responding | 0.19 | 0.00 | 0.29 | 1.98 | 1.96 | 1.04 |
| *Area/zone* | | | | | | |
| Urban | 88.46 | 89.10 | 96.53 | 64.10 | 80.77 | 77.93 |
| Rural | 11.54 | 10.90 | 3.47 | 35.90 | 19.23 | 22.07 |
| *Region* | | | | | | |
| Atlántica | 15.99 | 25.41 | 15.59 | 23.70 | 12.70 | 20.24 |
| Oriental | 13.33 | 18.26 | 14.13 | 19.73 | 32.68 | 17.25 |
| Central | 26.89 | 22.37 | 29.16 | 24.58 | 21.31 | 25.47 |
| Pacífica | 15.08 | 9.75 | 15.36 | 20.26 | 22.86 | 17.17 |
| Bogotá | 27.00 | 21.29 | 24.46 | 8.92 | 7.75 | 17.56 |
| Orinoquía-Amazonía | 1.71 | 2.91 | 1.31 | 2.82 | 2.69 | 2.32 |
| *Oral health indexes* | | | | | | |
| DMFT | 6.8 (0.34) | 6.9 (0.32) | 9.1 (0.54) | 7.2 (0.25) | 8.5 (0.80) | 7.2 (0.21) |
| Care index | 56.7 (3.09) | 48.1 (4.85) | 36.8 (4.50) | 30.6 (2.70) | 29.0 (5.81) | 41.7 (3.40) |
| Treatment need index | 16.1 (2.63) | 20.2 (4.51) | 20.3 (4.11) | 35.5 (3.84) | 33.0 (8.97) | 26.0 (3.60) |

Notes: Percentages were calculated per column for each variable.
Indexes are presented as means. Standard errors are provided in parentheses.

The additional cluster analysis for living conditions generated three groups: Urban Adequate, Urban Precarious, and Rural Precarious. The characteristics of these clusters are presented in Table 3.

Figure 2 shows the analytical correspondence between the living condition clusters and social classes.

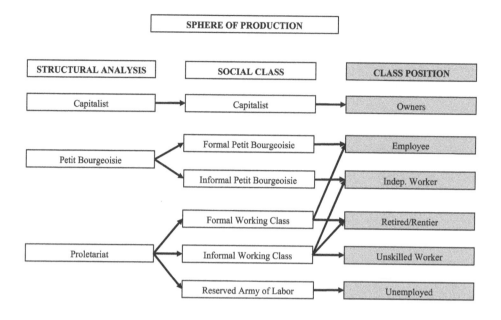

**Figure 1.** Class position as a proxy for social class.

Importantly, with our diagrams we wanted to show two different expressions of how social class influence oral health. While for statistical analysis the most adequate comparison would be between the proletariat and the capitalist, we are forced to use the petite bourgeoisie as the contrasting class.

**Table 3.** Description of the living conditions clusters.

|  | 1. Urban adequate | 2. Urban precarious | 3. Rural precarious |
|---|---|---|---|
| *n* | 352 | 4972 | 2716 |
| *N* | 1,955,546 | 19,404,691 | 8,084,727 |
| % | 4.38 | 61.84 | 33.78 |
| Area | Urban | Urban | Rural |
| Socioeconomic strata | High | Medium | Lower |
| Monthly household income* | More than four MMW (>$2.358.001) | More than one MMW – Less than three MMW (>$589.501– <$1.768.500) | Less than half MMW – one MMW (<$294.750)' – $589.500) |
| Lack of money during the previous week to buy food | Never | Never and almost never | Always |
| Housing tenure | -Owned outright -Owned with a mortgage | -Owned outright -Rented | -Untitled property -Usufruct |
| Type of housing | Apartment | Apartment | -Peasant shack -Improvised housing -Urban shack |
| Number of sleeping rooms in the house | Many | A few | ** |
| Water supply | Piped water with continuous supply | Piped water with continuous supply | -Piped water without continuous supply -Tube well pump -Dug well -Rain water -Surface water (river, spring, etc.) |

*Those are minimum legal wage (MMW) values for 2013 in Colombia.
**This is empty because it does not have any importance for this cluster.

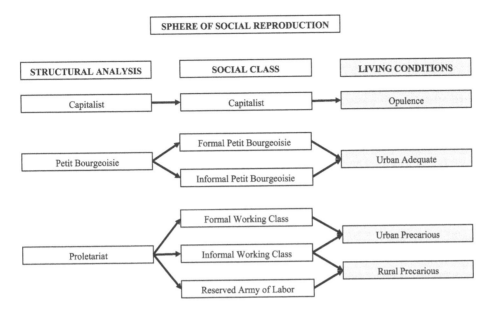

**Figure 2.** Living conditions as a proxy for social class.

The distribution of the population according to class positions and living conditions can be found in Table 4.

In order to assess oral health inequalities in relationship with class position and living conditions we did variance analysis models. In all of them we included age as a co-variable, given that it is well known that caries rates increase throughout the lifespan.

The variance analysis models for all oral health indicators (DMFT, TNI, and CI) including both class position and living conditions and their interaction resulted in models in which only living conditions was statistically significant for both TNI and CI. In order to assess if this result was due to a strong association between class position and living conditions, we conducted a correspondence analysis with a Pearson chi square test, which confirmed their association ($p < 0.001$). This result suggests that production (i.e. social position) and social reproduction (i.e. living conditions) are intimately related, which validates the importance of an integrated production/social reproduction approach. The correspondence between these two variables also prompted us to run separate variance analysis models, one for social position and another for living conditions, to assess their relationship with oral health.

### DMFT (decayed, missing, and filled teeth)

Our DMFT variance analysis model for class position was statistically significant ($p < 0.001$, R2 = 0.37), meaning that class position and age have an effect on DMFT. The assessment of the principal effect of each of these two variables (class position and age) showed that class position no longer had

**Table 4.** Distribution of living conditions by class position.

|  | Employee | Independent worker | Retired/ rentier | Unskilled worker | Unemployed | Total |
|---|---|---|---|---|---|---|
| n | 2543 | 3875 | 745 | 614 | 263 | 8040 |
| N | 10,156,112 | 13,377,180 | 2,714,569 | 2,447,178 | 749,925 | 29,444,964 |
| *Living conditions* |  |  |  |  |  |  |
| Urban 'adequate' | 13.05 | 9.51 | 9.18 | 1.10 | 0 | 6.64 |
| Urban precarious | 74.98 | 67.33 | 76.83 | 56.49 | 69.99 | 65.90 |
| Rural precarious | 11.97 | 23.16 | 13.99 | 42.41 | 30.01 | 27.46 |
| Total | 100.00 | 100.00 | 100.00 | 100.00 | 100.00 | 100.00 |

any effect. Age did have a statistically significant effect ($p < 0.01$) and the correlation coefficient showed that for each year of age the DMFT increases 17%.

The variance analysis model for living conditions was also statistically significant ($p < 0.01$, R2 = 0.36), meaning that living conditions and age have an effect on DMFT. Similarly, the assessment of the principal effects showed that age, but not living conditions, had a statistically significant effect on DMFT ($p < 0.01$). In this case, the correlation coefficient showed that each year of age represents an increase of 16% in the DMFT.

These results are not surprising and confirm that DMFT is not the best indicator to assess oral health inequalities (Broadbent & Thomson, 2005). While it is very likely that people from different class positions and living conditions do exhibit significant differences in terms of the presence of active disease or the ability to access health care, DMFT obscures these differences by lumping together teeth with active disease and treated and lost teeth.

### Treatment needs index (TNI)

The variance analysis model for TNI (Decayed teeth/decayed teeth + filled teeth), class position, and age was statistically significant ($p < 0.001$, R2 = 0.05). In this case, class position, rather than age, was the statistically significant principal effect ($p < 0.001$). We used Sheffé test to compare TNI means among class positions. Statistically significant differences were found between Unskilled Worker and Employee groups ($p < 0.001$) and between Unskilled Worker and Independent Worker groups ($p < 0.05$) (Figure 3).

For living conditions, the variance analysis model was also statistically significant ($p < 0.001$, R2 = 0.06) and, as in the class position model, living conditions rather than age was the statistically significant principal effect ($p < 0.001$). The Sheffé test that compared means between groups confirmed that differences between all living condition groups were statistically significant ($p < 0.001$) (Figure 4).

These results show that unskilled workers and the unemployed have more treatment needs than those who belong to the employee, independent worker, retired/rentier class positions. In addition, the results show that people belonging to urban precarious and rural precarious living condition groups have more treatment needs in comparison to those who belong to urban adequate living conditions.

### Care index (CI)

The variance analysis model for care index (filled teeth/DMFT), class position and age was statically significant ($p < 0.001$, R2 = 0.17). In this case both class position and age were statistically significant

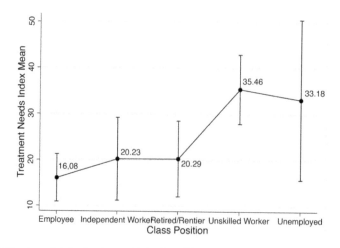

**Figure 3.** Average treatment needs index by class position adjusted by age.

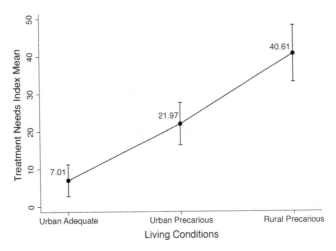

**Figure 4.** Average treatment needs index by living conditions adjusted by age.

principal effects ($p < 0.001$). The correlation coefficient showed that for each year of age the CI reduces by 7.6%, meaning that with age people have either more active caries lesions or more missing teeth. Another way to explain this result would be that with age the proportion of filled teeth reduces in comparison with the proportion of teeth with active caries or teeth that have been extracted. This means that there is longer time of exposure to the event. In order to compare means among class position groups we run a Sheffé test. Statistically significant differences were found between Unskilled Worker and Employee ($p < 0.001$), between Unemployed and Employee ($p < 0.01$), and between Unskilled Worker and Independent Worker ($p < 0.05$) (Figure 5).

For living conditions, the variance analysis model was statistically significant ($p < 0.001$ R2 = 0.17), and both age and class position were statistically significant principal effects ($p < 0.001$). Sheffé test showed statistically significant differences among all living condition groups: between Urban Precarious and Urban Adequate ($p < 0.05$); between Rural Precarious and Urban Adequate ($p < 0.001$); and between Rural Precarious vs Urban Precarious ($p < 0.001$) (Figure 6).

According to these results, people who belong to employee and independent worker class position groups have better care index than people who belong to unskilled worker and unemployed groups. This means that people in better class positions have more access to treatment, as measured in the

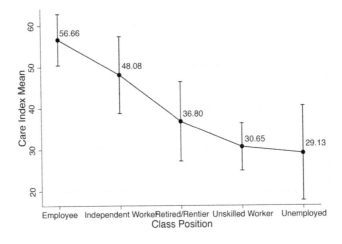

**Figure 5.** Average care index by class position adjusted by age.

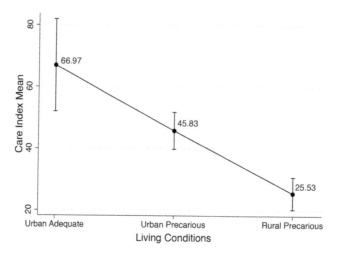

**Figure 6.** Average care index by living conditions adjusted by age.

percentage of filled teeth in comparison to active caries or missing teeth. In terms of living conditions, people with urban adequate living conditions have better care index in comparison to people with urban precarious and rural precarious living conditions. Figure 7 presents our final model that brings together the theoretical approach with the analyzed data.

Both Class Position and Living Conditions are proxies for social class. Conceptually, one social class can manifest in two or more class positions or living conditions, which also corresponds statistically to the range of each of these categories. The range in findings regarding class position and oral health (expressed in this diagram as different connecting arrows) indicates that besides being statistically significant one class position can have different oral health outcomes. Interestingly, the range is less prominent and the differences among all groups are statistically significant when testing for the relationship between living conditions and care index. This finding might indicate that the sphere of social reproduction is a stronger predictor of access to care.

## Discussion

The operationalisation of social class for statistical analysis brings many technical and conceptual challenges. It is very important to take into account the historical conditions of capital accumulation

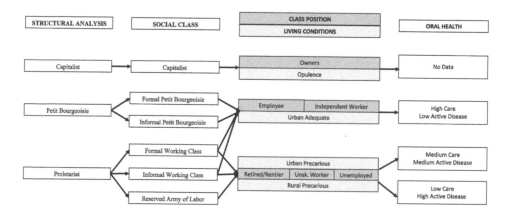

**Figure 7.** Final model. Social class (production and social reproduction) and oral health.

patterns, the transformation of labour dynamics, and the particularities of each country. As we mentioned in the introduction, the increasing rates of informal labour in Latin America as a result of neoliberalism come with an array of labour relationships in which lack of formal contracts, underemployment and self-employment are difficult to quantify in national statistics. Some authors recognise that the challenge to classify contemporary class positions resides in the difficulty to measure labour flexibility and informality. We experienced similar challenges classifying the population in different class position groups that allowed us to conduct a robust statistical analysis while maintaining a social class theoretical framework.

Portes and Hoffman (2003) propose to correct the overestimation of formal employment by considering social security contributions. In their analysis for Latin America, the largest social class is the 'informal proletariat', which comprises 47% of the economically active population (EAP) and corresponds to people without social security coverage. For the Colombian context, we could not apply their proposal because of the extend of neoliberal social security reforms, which forced both formal and informal workers to contribute to the market of pension funds, health insurance, and work-related insurance.

The Colombian National Health Observatory follows the social class structure proposed by Fresneda (2014) to assess the relationship between social class and health inequalities (Instituto Nacional de Salud & Observatorio Nacional de Salud, 2016). In their analysis, the 'petite bourgeoisie' represents around 30% of the EAP and corresponds to the largest social class in the country (Instituto Nacional de Salud & Observatorio Nacional de Salud, 2016). However, the authors of the reports of the observatory acknowledge that the petite bourgeoisie is a very heterogeneous group that includes different types of self-employment and other informal labour relationships. In addition, we believe that given the limitations of the national survey they use, they ended up including under 'petite bourgeoisie' different groups in terms of social position, income, rents and assets. Because of the framework of the ENSAB IV, we were able to include ownership of means of production. Furthermore, we considered that we could use Wright's insights and statistical tools to add additional variables and increase the level of specificity among class positions. We added income and education levels of the breadwinner to produce the five class positions.

While we also wanted to add some characteristics of the living conditions to produce a simpler version of Wright's integrated model (or to advance in the intermediate level according to the SDH proposal), the statistical analysis revealed collinearity between class position and living conditions. As such, we could not explain oral health inequalities as a result of an integrated class position and living conditions model. Two aspects are worth highlighting: 1) While this represents a setback in this kind of integrated proposal, we do not want to discourage further attempts to elaborate such integrated models. We think that thinking deeper about the interactions among the material conditions of labour, people's living conditions, and oral health parameters can shed light into new ways to measure these interactions. We are planning to go back to our data and make new attempts. 2) The separate class position and living conditions models of oral health inequalities did produce remarkable results.

Our objective was to assess the relationship between social class and oral health inequalities and, in fact, we found that class relationships do influence the ways in which Colombian populations experience oral disease and access to treatment. Noticeable, the ENSAB IV did not report any data that could represent the class position of capitalist sectors. Thus, all of our class position groups reflect the different configurations of the proletariat and the petite bourgeoisie that are more or less exploited and have better or worse standing within the class structure of Colombian society. Finding a relationship between social class and oral health, however, was not only a matter of using adequate social position and living conditions categories. In several analytical sessions, we tried to understand how social class in Colombia influence oral disease progression considering the added difficulty that caries disease increases throughout the lifespan. Hence, we concluded that the sphere of production had to be more clearly linked with the sphere of social reproduction as care and consumption patterns seemed fundamental for Marxists analysis in oral health (Abadía-Barrero & Martínez-Parra,

2016). We discussed how the widely accepted DMFT index had the problem of lumping together active caries, with treated teeth and missing teeth, obfuscating the differential impact of the relationship between social class and access to health care. TNI and CI seemed more promising in allowing to grasp that relationship (Agudelo Suárez & Martínez Herrera, 2009). The results in fact showed that people who belong to class positions with higher levels of labour exploitation or are altogether excluded from even the most precarious forms of labour (the unemployed) do experience higher levels of active disease and less access to treatment. Other studies use descriptive statistics to report this relationship for specific ethnic or age groups (A. M. Franco & Ochoa, 2012; Morón & Córdova, 2008). While the ENSAB IV did report some differences in terms of class positions and other inequality indicators (Ministerio de Salud y Protección Social, 2014b), we were able to operationalise better class position and offer more robust statistical and social class analysis.

While living conditions are not a direct class structure indicator, we do know that the transformation of labour in Colombia during the last 50 years have resulted in a further pauperisation of rural areas and growing urban inequalities. We also know that historical access to treatment inequalities due to the lack of health care networks in rural and urban poor areas have increased due to the neoliberal health reforms (Franco Agudelo, 2003; Hernández, 2002a, 2002b). Thus, our results might indicate that class-based oral health inequalities are the result of not only the precarization of labour during neoliberalism, but also of the transformation of the living conditions of fractions of the proletariat (flexible agricultural workers versus flexible workers in urban settings). While the privatisation of the country's health care infrastructure affected both of these class fractions of the proletariat, our data indicates that rural workers continue to exhibit more vulnerability to develop oral health and less access to treatment.

## Conclusions

Conducting a social class analysis for collective health is not merely a technical discussion. Researchers working under a critical framework need to combine a robust social class analysis that considers how capitalist accumulation patterns transforms labour relationships across the globe, with efforts to operationalise social class concepts (such as class positions and living conditions), and a careful reading of the given health condition that they aim to study. In our case, the relationship between social class and oral health was possible by selecting carefully the best clinical indicators and by proposing a combined production/social reproduction framework in which both the transformation of labour conditions reflected in class positions and the correspondent living conditions of the population indicate unequal oral health outcomes. Indeed, statistically significant differences were found in more exploited classes for higher oral health care needs and lower access to oral health care treatment.

Importantly, our analysis of social class in Colombia does not include upper classes and other capitalist sectors. Rather than an error in terms of social class sampling or analysis, we think that this is the result of the global reconfiguration of labour in the new financialized economy with a capitalist elite in the global north and proletariat classes in the global south. Hence, our analysis points to differences among proletariat fractions by using the petit bourgeoisie as the 'dominant' class.

In spite of the precarization of labour, a sound social class classification proposal built on the contradiction between production and social reproduction and an adequate reading of the specific health condition can unveil important health inequalities.

## Acknowledgements

We would like to thank Hanner Sánchez, Elizabeth Suarez, for their valuable contributions to understand technical issues from the ENSAB IV and Alejandra Moreno, Sergio López for their valuable contributions to think in oral health index and collective health. We also want to thank Jaime Breilh for his leadership role in advancing the understanding of how social class affect health and for his advisory role in the ENSAB.

## Disclosure statement

No potential conflict of interest was reported by the authors.

## Funding

Data collection of ENSAB IV was supported by Ministry of Health and Social Protection Government of Colombia by Contract 853 of 2012. Consejo Nacional de Ciencia y Tecnología - CONACYT, México, National Scholarship.

## ORCID

*César Ernesto Abadía-Barrero* http://orcid.org/0000-0001-7157-0842

## References

Abadía-Barrero, C. E., & Martínez-Parra, A. G. (2016). Care and consumption: A Latin American social medicine's conceptual framework to comprehend oral health inequalities. *Global Public Health*, 1–14. doi:10.1080/17441692.2016.1171377

Agudelo Suárez, A. A., & Martínez Herrera, E. (2009). La salud bucal colectiva y el contexto colombiano: un análisis crítico. *Revista Gerencia y Políticas de Salud*, 8, 91–105.

Almeida-Filho, N. (2000). *La ciencia tímida. Ensayos de Deconstrucción de la Epidemiología*. Buenos Aires: Lugar Editorial.

Antunes, R. (2018). The New service proletariat. *Monthly Review*, 69(11), 23. Retrieved from https://monthlyreview.org/2018/04/01/the-new-service-proletariat/

Benach, J., Muntaner, C., Solar, O., Santana, V., & Quinlan, M. (2014). *Employment, work and health inequalities: A global perspective*. Barcelona: Icaria Editorial.

Bernabe, E., & Hobdell, M. H. (2010). Is income inequality related to childhood dental caries in rich countries? *The Journal of the American Dental Association*, 141, 143–149.

Birn, A-E., Nervi, L., & Siqueira, E. (2016). Neoliberalism redux: The global health policy Agenda and the politics of cooptation in Latin America and beyond. *Development and Change*, 47(4), 734–759. doi:10.1111/dech.12247

Blanco, J., & Sáenz, O. (1994). *Espacio Urbano y Salud*. México: Universidad de Guadalajara.

Breilh, J. (1989). *Breve recopilación sobre operacionalización de la clase social para encuestas en la investigación social*. Quito: CEAS.

Breilh, J. (2003). *Epidemiología crítica. Ciencia emancipadora e interculturalidad*. Buenos Aires: Lugar Editorial.

Breilh, J. (2007). Nuevo modelo de acumulación y agroindustria: las implicaciones ecológicas y epidemiológicas de la floricultura en Ecuador. *Ciência & Saúde Coletiva*, 12, 91–104.

Breilh, J. (2010). La epidemiología crítica: una nueva forma de mirar la salud en el espacio urbano. *Salud Colectiva*, 6, 83–101.

Broadbent, J. M., & Thomson, W. M. (2005). For debate: Problems with the DMF index pertinent to dental caries data analysis. *Community Dentistry and Oral Epidemiology*, 33, 400–409. doi:10.1111/j.1600-0528.2005.00259.x

Bronfman, M., & Tuirán, R. A. (1984). La desigualdad social ante la muerte: Clases sociales y mortalidad en la niñez. *Cuadernos Médico Sociales*, 29/30, 53–75.

Cardenas, S. (2010). *Human rights in Latin America: A politics of terror and hope*. University of Pennsylvania Press. Retrieved from http://www.jstor.org/stable/j.ctt3fhm05

Centro de Investigaciones para el Desarrollo CID. (2006). *Bien-estar y Macroeconomía 2002–2006, Crecimiento insuficiente, inequitativo e insostenible* (p. 125). Bogotá: Universidad Nacional de Colombia.

Couriel, A. (1984). Pobreza y subempleo en América Latina. *Revista de La Cepal*, 24, 39–62.

Cruces, G., & Ham, A. (2010). *La flexibilidad laboral en América Latina: las reformas pasadas y las perspectivas futuras (Colección documentos de proyectos)* (p. 132). Santiago de Chile: CEPAL.

DANE. (2014). *Manual de recolección y conceptos básicos: Gran Encuesta Integrada de Hogares*.

DANE. (2018). *Principales indicadores del mercado laboral. Marzo de 2018* (Boletín Técnico Gran Encuesta Integrada de Hogares) (p. 27). Bogotá.

De la Garza, E. (2000). La flexibilidad del trabajo en América Latina. In E. (Coordinador) De la Garza (Ed.), *Tratado latinoamerica de sociología del trabajo* (1st ed.). México: COLMEX, FLACSO, UAM, Fondo de Cultura Económica.

Duque Naranjo, C., & Mora Díaz, II. (2012). La representación de la epidemiología de la caries en el mundo a través de mapas. *Universitas Odontológica*, 31(66), 39–48.

Elbert, R. (2015). Informalidad en la estructura de clases de Argentina: ¿Es el proletariado informal una nueva clase social? *Revisa Pilquen - Seccin Ciencias Sociales*, 18(3), 50–65.

Erikson, S. L. (2012). Global health business: The production and performativity of statistics in Sierra Leone and Germany. *Medical Anthropology, 31*, 367–384. doi:10.1080/01459740.2011.621908

Everitt, B., Landau, S., Leese, M., & Stahl, D. (2011). *Cluster analysis*. London: Wiley.

Franco Agudelo, S. (2003). Para que la salud sea pública: Algunas lecciones de la reforma de salud y seguridad social en Colombia. *Revista Gerencia y Políticas de Salud, 4*, 59–69.

Franco, A. M., & Ochoa, E. (2012). *Caries dental e inequidades sociales: resultados de un estudio exploratorio en escolares de la comuna tres de Medellin.*

Fraser, N. (2016). Contradictions of capital and care. *New Left Review, 100*, 99–117.

Fresneda, O. (2014). *Clases sociales, modo de desarrollo y desigualdad: lineamientos para su análisis.* Bogotá: Universidad Nacional de Colombia.

Fresneda, Ó. (2016). Regímenes de acumulación, estructura de clases sociales y desigualdad en Colombia-1810-2010. Tesis Doctoral. Facultad de Ciencias (Tesis doctoral). Facultad de Ciencias Económicas, Universidad Nacional de Colombia, Bogotá.

Garay, L. J. (1998). *Colombia: Estructura Industrial e Internacionalización 1967-1996.* Santafé de Bogotá: Departamento Nacional de Planeación y Colciencias.

Hernández, M. (2002a). El debate sobre la ley 100 de 1993: antes, durante y después. In S. Franco (Ed.), *La Salud Pública Hoy. Enfoques, y Dilemas Contemporáneos en Salud Pública. Memorias de la Cátedra Manuel Ancízar - I semestre 2002* (pp. 463–479). Bogotá: Universidad Nacional de Colombia.

Hernández, M. (2002b). Reforma sanitaria, equidad y derecho a la salud en Colombia. *Cadernos de Saúde Pública, 18* (4), 991–1001.

Instituto Nacional de Salud, & Observatorio Nacional de Salud. (2016). *Clase Social y Salud (Octavo Informe Técnico)* (p. 181). Bogotá: Observatorio Nacional de Salud.

Iriart, C., Elías, E., & Waitzkin, H. (2001). Managed care in Latin America: The new common sense in health policy reform. *Social Science and Medicine, 52*, 1243–1253.

Iriart, C., & Emerson-Elias, M. (2017). Disputas inter-capitalistas, biomedicalización y modelo médico hegemónico. *Interface - Comunicação, Saúde, Educação, 21*(63), 1005–1016. doi:10.1590/1807-57622016.0808

Johnson, D. E. (2000). *Métodos multivariados aplicados al análisis de datos.* México: International Thomson Editores.

Jonna, R. J., & Bellamy Foster, J. (2016). Marx's theory of working-class precariousness: Its relevance today. *Monthly Review, 67*(11), 1. Retrieved from https://monthlyreview.org/2016/04/01/marxs-theory-of-working-class-precariousness/

Klein, H., Palmer, C. E., & Knutson, J. W. (1938). Studies on dental caries: I. Dental status and dental needs of elementary school children. *Public Health Reports (1896–1970), 53*, 751–765. doi:10.2307/4582532.

Klein, N. (2007). *The shock doctrine. The rise of disaster capitalism.* New York: Metropolitan Books.

Laurell, A. C. (1982). La salud-enfermedad como proceso social. *Cuadernos Médico Sociales, 19*, 1–11.

Lenin, V. I. (1919). *The great initiative, including the story of "communist saturdays".* Glasgow: Socialist Labour Press.

López, O. (2013). Determinación social de la salud. Desafíos y agendas posibles. *Divulgação Em Saúde Para Debate, 49*, 144–150.

Medina-Solís, C. E., Maupomé, G., Pelcastre-Villafuerte, B., Avila-Burgos, L., Vallejos-Sánchez, A. A., & Casanova-Rosado, A. J. (2006). Desigualdades socioeconómicas en salud bucal: caries dental en niños de seis a 12 años de edad. *Revista de Investigación Clínica, 58*, 296–304.

Ministerio de Salud y Protección social. (2014a). *IV estudio Nacional de Salud Bucal - ENSAB IV: Metodología y Determinación Social de la Salud Bucal* (p. 195). Bogotá: Ministerio de Salud y Protección social.

Ministerio de Salud y Protección Social. (2014b). *IV estudio Nacional de Salud Bucal - ENSAB IV: Situación en Salud Bucal* (p. 381). Bogotá: Ministerio de Salud y Protección Social.

Mintz, S. W. (1985). *Sweetness and power: The place of sugar in modern history.* New York, NY: Viking.

Misas Arango, G. (2002). *La ruptura de los 90: del gradualismo al colapso.* Bogotá: Facultad de Ciencias Económicas, Universidad Nacional de Colombia.

Morón, A., & Córdova, M. (2008). Perfil epidemiológico bucal de las etnias venezolanas. Primer reporte nacional. *Ciencia Odontológica, 5*, 1–126.

Muntaner, C., Borrell, C., Vanroelen, C., Chung, H., Benach, J., Kim, I. H., & Ng, E. (2010). Employment relations, social class and health: A review and analysis of conceptual and measurement alternatives. *Social Science & Medicine, 71*, 2130–2140. doi:10.1016/j.socscimed.2010.09.038

Muntaner, C., Rocha, K. B., Borrell, C., Vallebuona, C., Ibáñez, C., Benach, J., & Sollar, O. (2012). Clase social y salud en América Latina. *Social Class and Health in Latin America, 31*, 166–175.

Navarro, V. (1976). *Medicine under capitalism* (1st ed.). New York: Prodist.

Navarro, V. (Ed.). (2007). *Neoliberalism, globalization, and inequalities: Consequences for health and quality of life.* Amityville, NY: Baywood Pub.

Naveda, A. (2014). Latinoamérica en el siglo XXI: clases y lucha de clases. *Theomai, 29*. Retrieved from http://www.redalyc.org/resumen.oa?id=12431432008

Ogliastri, E., & Guerra, E. (1980). Fracciones de clase en la burguesía de ciudades intermedias de Colombia: un estudio sociológico. *Revista Mexicana de Sociología, 42*(4), 1631–1661. doi:10.2307/3539964

Ospina Vásquez, L. (1979). *Industria y protección en Colombia, 1810–1930* (3ra ed.). Medellín: Biblioteca colombiana de ciencias sociales FAES.

Petersen, P. E., Bourgeois, D., Ogawa, H., Estupinan-Day, S., & Ndiaye, C. (2005). The global burden of oral diseases and risks to oral health. *Bulletin of the World Health Organization, 83*, 661–669.

Portes, A., & Hoffman, K. (2003). *Las estructuras de clase en América Latina: composición y cambios durante la época neoliberal (Políticas sociales)* (p. 51). Santiago de Chile: CEPAL.

PREALC. (1991). *Empleo y Equidad: El desafío de los 90*. Santiago: OIT, Programa Mundial del Empleo.

Restrepo, D. (2003). *La falacia neoliberal: crítica y alternativas*. Colombia: Universidad Nacional de Colombia.

Rocha, K. B., Muntaner, C., Rodríguez, G., José, M., Baksai, P. B., Vallebuona, C., … Solar, O. (2013). Clase social, desigualdades en salud y conductas relacionadas con la salud de la población trabajadora en chile. *Revista Panamericana de Salud Pública, 33*, 340–348. doi:10.1590/S1020-49892013000500005

Safford, F., & Palacios, M. (2001). *Colombia: Fragmented land, divided society*. Bogotá: Norma.

Samaja, J. (2004). *Epistemología de la salud*. Buenos Aires: Lugar Editorial.

Sáenz Rovner, E. (2007). *La ofensiva empresarial: industriales, políticos y violencia en los años 40 en Colombia*. Bogotá: Universidad Nacional de Colombia. CES.

StataCorp. (2013). *Stata 13 base reference manual*. College Station, TX: Stata Press.

Vettore, M. V., Marques, R. A. d. A., & Peres, M. A. (2013). Desigualdades sociais e doença periodontal no estudo SBBrasil 2010: Abordagem multinível. *Revista De Saúde Pública, 47*(Suppl. 3), 29–39. doi:10.1590/ S0034-8910. 2013047004422

Waitzkin, H. (2016). *Medicine and public health at the End of empire* (1st ed.). New York: Routledge.

Waitzkin, H., & Working Group for Health Beyond Capitalism. (2018). *Health care under the knife: Moving beyond capitalism for our health*. Monthly Review Press. Retrieved from https://monthlyreview.org/product/health_care_under_the_knife/

Waitzkin, H., & Jasso-Aguilar, R. (2015). Resisting the imperial order and building an alternative future in medicine and public health. *Monthly Review, 67*(3), Retrieved from https://monthlyreview.org/2015/07/01/resisting-the-imperial-order-and-building-an-alternative-future-in-medicine-and-public-health/

Wright, E. O. (1985). *Clases*. London: Verso.

Wright, E. O. (2000). *Class counts: Student edition*. Cambridge: Cambridge University Press.

Wright, E. O. (2015). *Understanding class*. London: Verso.

Zurriaga, O., Martínez-Beneito, M. A., Abellán, J. J., & Carda, C. (2004). Assessing the social class of children from parental information to study possible social inequalities in health outcomes. *Annals of Epidemiology, 14*(6), 378–384. doi:10.1016/j.annepidem.2003.06.001

# Struggles for the right to health at work in Colombia: The case of associations of workers with work-related illnesses

Mauricio Torres-Tovar ⓘ and Jairo Ernesto Luna-García ⓘ

**ABSTRACT**

The neoliberal reforms of the early 1990s in Colombia, mainly labour and social security reforms, transformed capital-labour relations and contributed to the erosion of working conditions and health protection at work, with devastating impacts on workers' health. In the context of these dramatic changes, Colombian workers mobilised around collective identities that have shaped new forms of workers' struggle and resistance. Since 2006, associations of workers suffering work-related illnesses have been active in Colombia. The associated workers engaged in collective actions have demanded from employers, the Ministry of Work, occupational risk administrators, disability rating boards and the judicial system the recognition of certain diseases as being of occupational origin and that these entities guarantee corresponding labour, economic and social security rights. This paper describes and analyses the dynamics of the struggle for the right to health at work undertaken by these associations in Colombia, adopting an analytical perspective inspired by collective action theory.

## Introduction

As an expression of collective action and struggles for the right to health and safety at work in Colombia, numerous associations of workers and ex-workers with work-related illnesses have been created since 2006 (Asolaborales, 2016; Torres-Tovar, Luna-García, & Ruiz-Vallejo, 2016). The creation of such associations is directly linked to the existence of workers with work-related injuries, disabilities and illnesses that have not been recognised or adequately treated and also relates to the recognition of the problem being of collective rather than individual nature.

Although the creation of associations of sick and disabled workers is not a new phenomenon and there are records of such associations, particularly of workers exposed to asbestos, since the 1970s at the international level (Barraza, Jansen, van Wendel de Joode, & Wesseling, 2013; Carrera, 2014; Fry, 2010, 2013; Hopkins, 2010; International Ban Asbestos Secretariat, 2017; Judkins, 1982, 1990, 1993; Knight, 1971; Silva & Ordúñez, 2014; Tello & Grau, 2015; Trabanino, Aguilar, Silva, Mercado, & Merino, 2002; Zavestoski, 2009), this constitutes a new phenomenon in Colombia.

We argue that this form of workers' mobilisation and social organisation is a consequence of changes related to neoliberal labour, health and social security reforms that have been undertaken since the early 1990s in Colombia as well as to technical and entrepreneurial changes in the production processes since the beginning of the nineteenth century (Davolos, 2012; Luna-García, Castro-Fraume, & Villamizar, 2016; Torres-Tovar, Luna-García, Parra, & Shell-Sparling, 2016). These changes had repercussions on work-related health and safety, particularly as they came along with a loss of decent and safe work due to the fragility of public policies and the lack of business strategies to protect workers' health. Several actors contributed to the deterioration of the workers' and their families' lives, including the tendency of the financial sector to assume an intermediary role in health and labour risk insurances; the absence or weakness of health services and the decay of health promotion and prevention at the workplace further contributed to the situation, as well as limitations in organisational processes and the participation of workers, as reflected in the difficulties faced by trade unions and workers' associations and none or only limited participation in business decisions (Corredor Jiménez, 2004; Luna-García, 2009; Muntaner, Benach, Quinlan, Solar, & Santana, 2010; Niño Chavarro & De Lafont De León, 2013; Schnall, Dobson, & Rosskam, 2011; Standing, 2011).

Yet another dimension of the problem is evident in the way labour risks have been characterised or 'qualified'. In this regard, the occupational origin of pathologies associated to working conditions is often has not been recognised and occupational risk administrators (ORA) as well as disability qualification boards have qualified work-related illnesses as being of common origin. As a result, many sick workers have been fired and lost labour and social protection rights (Torres-Tovar, Luna-García, Parra, et al., 2016).

This problem has been recognised by studies drawing attention to the suffering and negative consequences of unclear and prolonged routes of attention, recognition and rehabilitation of occupational diseases (Buitrago Echeverri, Abadía-Barrero, & Granja Palacios, 2017). These bureaucratic itineraries, that is, obligatory administrative, financial and judicial demands that the Colombian social security system has imposed on patients and their families to access health services or receive adequate medical attention have been found to cause suffering due to access and quality limitations and problems regarding integrity and timely attention (Abadía-Barrero & Oviedo, 2009). Furthermore, research suggests that despite labour stability regulations, which are constitutional guarantees that protect workers who have suffered a decline in their ability to work either by illness or accident, to avoid unemployment, many workers have been dismissed (Asolaborales, 2016; Buitrago Echeverri et al., 2017; Torres-Tovar & Torres-Echeverry, 2017).

This situation is compounded by the role played by the Ministry of Work, which is the governing entity of the general system of labour risks and by the Directorate of Labour Risks and the Territorial Labour Directorates is in charge of the inspection, supervision, and control of the system, yet has not played a relevant role in this problem. This situation viewed from the perspective of workers has allowed violations of labour, health and social security rights (Asolaborales, 2016; Buitrago Echeverri et al., 2017; Torres-Tovar, Luna-García, Parra, et al., 2016). Given this context, this article describes and analyses the Colombian workers' and ex-workers' struggles for the right to health at work, adopting an analytical perspective inspired by collective action theory.

## Methodology

We conducted multi-method participatory action research using quantitative and qualitative methods and directly engaging in the political-organisational dynamics of the workers' illness associations. The researchers' engagement with the organisations implied supporting the consolidation of the Federation of Associations and further entailed the organisation of workshops with several associations where the results of this research were presented to strengthen their action and respond to specific technical-political demands of the associations and the Federation.

The research involved a scoping review of national and international literature on the situation of associated workers and former workers with occupational diseases as well as a survey, semi-structured interviews and focus groups with members of the associations in all five macro-regions of Colombia (Caribbean, Northeast, Coffee Region, Center and South). All interview partners and participants of the focus groups gave their informed consent to use audio recordings of these activities for the purposes of this research. The data collection was carried out during the first semester of 2016 and the respective analysis and reports were elaborated during the second semester of the same year. Part of the results presented in this article were published in the Culture and Work Review of the National Trade Union School.

## Results

### Workers' Illness associations in Colombia

Since 2006, associations of workers suffering work-related illnesses, so called workers' illness associations, have emerged as an expression of collective action and the struggle for the right to health at work in Colombia (Asolaborales, 2016; Torres-Tovar, Luna-García, & Ruiz-Vallejo, 2016). This phenomenon is on the rise and today there are fourteen workers' illness associations (see Table 1). Apart from these associations, several trade unions have incorporated demands related to the recognition of illnesses as being of occupational origin and the guarantee of social security rights, as well as corresponding economic benefits. These associations operate in different regions of Colombia, including the Caribbean Coast (Santa Marta, Riohacha, Cartagena, as well as processes located in the departments of Córdoba and Cesar), Northeast (Santander and Arauca), Eje Cafetero, Centro (Cundinamarca and Bogotá) and the South (Huila and Meta).

### Characterisation of association members

A survey applied to 548 members of the workers' illness associations (Asolaborales, 2016), allowed for a characterisation of their sociodemographic characteristics, their epidemiological or morbidity profile, changes in the family structure and the process of affiliation to the association.

It was found that most of the associates are adult men with technical schooling and complete secondary education, belonging to economic strata 1 and 2, married or in common-law marriage, heads of household in charge of two or more people. Most of the associates work or primarily worked in the mining-energy, agro-food or construction sector, with at least five years of experience. The socio-demographic profile of the associates reflects a population group with economic limitations and precarious living conditions, which worsened upon falling sick and lacking labour, health and social security rights, with many families facing financial ruin.

Regarding the morbidity profile of the associates, the survey revealed a broad spectrum of pathologies related to working conditions. Associates that reported only one pathology represented 43%, while 57% reported multiple pathologies. Some even had eight work related conditions, simultaneously. The illnesses mainly involved the respiratory system, musculoskeletal system, auditory and cardiovascular systems. Furthermore, some associates suffered work accidents producing burns, sprains, fractures, spinal injuries and loss of corporal segments.

The association members indicated that the respective qualification boards qualified only 57% of these illnesses and recognise 79% of those qualified illnesses as being of occupational origin. Permanent disability was established in 53% of the cases and 47% of the workers were rated as temporarily disabled. Regarding the qualification percentage of the reduction in labour capacity, only 10% of the cases were rated with more than 50% of reduction and 28% of the pathologies were reclassified by the respective national boards establishing that only 62% of the pathologies were related to labour instead of originally 79%. The situation indicates that in the qualification or rating process a considerable number of cases lose their relation to work after requalification, which clearly complicates the conditions of the association members.

The survey results indicate that an important number of pathologies are associated with workplace hazards that cause permanent damages and disability. At the same time, the figures suggest that these health damages are often not recognised or qualified as disabilities and a significant percentage of pathologies originally recognised as being of occupational origin are later reclassified. According to the results of our survey, workers and former workers with work-related illnesses affiliate with two different types of association in order to protect their labour and health rights: the traditional ones led by trade unions and a new type of organisation that specifically brings together workers with work-related illnesses.

## Collective action undertaken by the associations

In Colombia, the rising phenomenon of demands and mobilizations of workers who have seen their health affected by labour diseases and/or accidents can be analysed from the theoretical perspective of collective action. This perspective highlights various aspects related to the configuration of organisational forms, from the establishment of collective identities, the repertoire of collective action, the set of demands and the proposals that define alliances and opponents.

### Organisational forms and collective identities

The situation of insecurity with regard to labour stability, health protection and social security, configured a collective social action framework to fight and enforce these rights and eventually led to the emergence of multiple expressions of social protests and organisation by workers and former workers with work-related illnesses, whose rights have not been granted by the responsible actors: corporations, governmental entities and occupational risk administrators (ORA). This situation forged closer social relations between the workers and generated organisational processes that culminated in the creation of Associations or the incorporation of the topic in the agendas of existing trade unions. This organisational dynamic is shaped by the construction of collective identities, which involves sharing experiences among workers with similar work-related pathologies, discussing the suffering inflicted by bureaucratic itineraries and feelings of pain, anger, frustration and injustice that are provoked by these conditions.

Some associations emerged due to the absence or inexistence of trade unions, as is the case for ASOTRADISNORT. In other cases, associations emerged although there were trade unions, as the topic did not receive adequate attention within them, as is the case for ASOTRECOL. Yet others emerged from trade unions, as is the case for Fundación Manos Muertas, and in some cases the trade union itself took up the problems, like Unión Sindical Obrera (USO). In this regard, different organisational modalities emerged: associations where there is no trade union, associations that emerged with the support of trade unions and finally modalities where the trade unions recognised the problem and no other association emerged.

According to our qualitative and quantitative data, the reasons for joining these associations are diverse, but are mostly related to the formation of collective identity, which allows workers to recognise that the guarantee of their rights depends on a collective and individual struggle, a process that is reinforced by psychological and moral support, solidarity, companionship, guidelines for treatment and rehabilitation, and legal advice, among other services offered to the members of the organisations. This is evident in the experiences of ASOTRECOL, ASORIESGOS, ASOTRADISCUNDINAMARCA and ASOTRADISNORT, which practically turned into support centres for workers whose rights have been violated (Asolaborales, 2016). Importantly, in Colombia, these organisational processes are novel and notable, considering the enormous difficulties trade unions and similar organisations have historically faced in the country.

The workers' illness associations are either organised around the economic sector to which the workers belong or a specific region in the country. What is found today in Colombia is that these workers' and former workers' organisations are mainly from the mining, energy, food, agro-industrial, construction, tobacco and services sectors, and are primarily found in the central, coastal and north-eastern regions of the country.

### Repertoire of collective actions

The repertoire of collective action refers to the types of protest used by social actors (Tilly, 2004). The collective action literature suggests that organised actors dispute social order through two different repertoires of action: so-called non-contentious collective action or legal action, referring to action that uses institutional channels to resolve their demands, which is the case of petitions and other legal

**Table 1.** Worker's associations with work-related illness 2006–2016.

| Name | Headquarter | Date of founded | Purpose | Non-contentious actions[a] | Contentious actions[a] | Adversaries[a] |
|---|---|---|---|---|---|---|
| Asociación de Trabajadores, ex trabajadores y Pensionados de la Empresa Colombit. Fundación Manos Muertas. | Manizales (Caldas) | April 15, 2006 | Organised to defend the health and social security rights of the workers | Administrative petitions directed at companies, the Ministry of Labour and Occupational Risk Administrators | Rallies  Marches  Occupation of buildings  Occupation of public space with tents  Hunger strikes (mouth is sewed)  Workers chain themselves to the entrance of companies or public institutions. | Companies  Occupational risk administrators  Regional qualification boards |
|  | Cartagena (Bolívar) | June 1, 2009 | Organised to defend health and labour rights and stand in for labour stability | Denunciation of the Ministry of Labour and the Public Ministry.  Criminal proceedings.  Public denunciation and national/ international incidence, using social media. |  | National qualification boards  Ministry of Labour |
| Asociación de Trabajadores Enfermos de Drummond Puerto – ASOTREDP.  Asociación de ex trabajadores enfermos y viudas de Drummond Puerto – ASOTRADEV. | Santa Marta (Magdalena) | March 10, 2010 | Emerged to manage negotiations with the Colombian state institutions, private companies of the mining sector, cooperatives, pension funds, national and foreign trade unions and economic resources allocated to promote activities directed at the health and well-being of the workers. | Participation in public audiences at the Colombian Parliament and at Parliaments of other countries to draw attention to the problem. |  |  |
| Asociación de Trabajadores Enfermos de General Motor Colombia – ASOTRECOL. | Bogotá, in a tent in front of United State Embassy per 6 years. | May 19, 2011 | Organised to protect the rights of the workers and former workers and denounce rights violations by the companies. | Support of draft bills directed at the protection of health rights of the workers. |  |  |
| Asociación Nacional de Usuarios del Sistema de Riesgos Laborales, Afiliados y Beneficiarios del Sistema de Seguridad Social – ASORIESGOS Colombia. | Girón (Santander) | September 9, 2012 | Organised as a response to the violation of labour and social security rights by companies located in the department of Santander. |  |  |  |
| Asociación de Trabajadores Discapacitados del Norte de Santander – ASOTRADISNORT. | Cúcuta (Norte de Santander) | March 15, 2013 | Emerged to defend the rights of workers that hold disabilities due to occupational accidents and illnesses. |  |  |  |
| Asociación de Trabajadores Discapacitados y Enfermos por la Industria Minero Energética – ASOTRADEIMENE in | Neiva (Huila) | November 1, 2013 | Organised to struggle for the rights that have been violated by the companies, by occupational risk administrators, health insurance companies and disability qualification boards. |  |  |  |
| Asociación de Trabajadores Discapacitados de Arauca – ASOTRADISARAUCA. | Arauca (Arauca) | November 3, 2014 | Organised to prevent occupational diseases and become a reference for the defence of workers' suffering occupational diseases. |  |  |  |

| Association | Location | Date | Description |
| --- | --- | --- | --- |
| Asociación de Trabajadores Discapacitados del Departamento de Cundinamarca – ASOTRADISCUNDINAMARCA | Ubaté (Cundinamarca). | July 27, 2015 | Organised to counter the violation of labour and social security rights in underground mining companies in the department of Cundinamarca. |
| Unión de *enfermos* de General Motors Colmotores – UNECOL | Bogotá | February 25, 2012 | Organised to protect the health and social security rights of the workers. |
| Asociación de Trabajadores Enfermos de la Floricultura. | Facatativa (Cundinamarca). | November, 2013 | As a response to the lack of protection of workers of the floriculture industry affected by occupational diseases. Formally employed and outsourced workers are affiliating to this association, despite the existence of a trade union. |
| Asociación de Trabajadores Enfermos del Carbón de La Jagua de Ibirico – ASOTRECAJ. | La Jagua de Ibirico (Cesar). | May 7, 2010 | Claim labour and social security rights in the context of the application of article 140 of the CST and the need to protect workers affected by occupational diseases that have been pursued by the mining companies. |
| Asociación de Trabajadores Discapacitados del Meta ASOTRADISMETA. | Acacias (Meta) | February 15, 2016 | Brings together workers with a physical disability in order to protect their common interests. |
| Federación Nacional de Trabajadores y ex Trabajadores Enfermos de Colombia-FENATRAECO. | Bogotá. | September 30, 2016 | Unification of forces to defend and claim better working conditions for workers affected by occupational diseases in Colombia. |

Source: Elaboration on the basis of information made available by Asolaborales (2016).
[a]These aspects apply to all Associations.

action, and what is referred to as contentious collective action or *de facto*, that is often used when non-contentious action is exhausted, including mass demonstrations, rallies, road closures, occupation of buildings and others.

Among the collective action that associations have taken to enforce their rights are a broad set of both individual and collective legal actions. Furthermore, the associations opted for traditional contentious collective action such as rallies, marches and the occupation of buildings and novel, more radical, action such as the indefinite occupation of public space with tents, hunger strikes (with sewed mouths), performance of burials and actions simulating crucifixion and with protesters tied up to recognised institutional buildings.

The demands ASOTREDP, UNECOL, ASOTRADISNORT and ASOTRADISMETA handed over to the Ministry of Work are an example of such forms of collective action, where the general situation and the workplace hazards are detailed and cases of individual workers who suffered injustice are outlined (Asolaborales, 2016; Saldarriaga, 2013). ASOTRECOL led more radical action including the performance of burials, hunger strikes and a simulation of crucifixions in front of the American Embassy in Bogotá (Torres-Tovar, Luna-García, Parra, et al., 2016), ASOTRADEI-MENE promoted the chaining of several workers at the entrance of the company and ASOTREDP protested with ropes around the workers' necks in front of the Ministry of Work (Asolaborales, 2016). The repertoire of collective action further includes international complaints and advocacy action, which seek to draw international attention to the problems the workers face in Colombia. These actions are mainly driven by workers and former workers from international companies.

When analysing the repertoire of these organisations, it can be observed that they replicate traditional repertories, both in contentious and non-contentious forms of action; but there are two facts that make a difference in the repertoire with respect to other mobilisation processes: First, the radical nature of non-contentious action, which reflects the enormous despair of the workers and former workers who found no answer to their problems in their interaction and negotiation with entrepreneurs, public institutions and social security institutions. Second, another distinctive feature constitutes the international perspective of several associations, that managed to put their demands on international agendas and thereby force national actors to attend and resolve their demands.

In relation to the cycle of protest, understood as a phase of intensification of conflicts and confrontation in the social system that includes a rapid diffusion of collective action from the most mobilised to less mobilised social sectors (Tarrow, 1997), in the case of these workers' and former workers' organisations with work-related illnesses, collective action has intensified since 2015. While this clearly reveals the lack of resolution of the workers' demands, the intensification of collective action also drew attention to the problem, being recognised by public institutions and mass media.

### *Demands and proposals*

The social dynamics driving the consolidation of organisations of workers and former workers with work-related illnesses is mainly a collective response to the repeated violation of labour, health and social security rights and reflect demands around the guarantee of these rights. In relation to the violation of their right to labour, the demands are aimed in two directions: one for those who kept their work and another for those who lost it. In the first case, demands focus on adequate processes of labour relocation that radically challenge the relocation of ill workers to marginal areas of work where they end up feeling useless. In the second case, the demands generally seek to achieve labour reincorporation with adequate rehabilitation processes, if required.

In relation to the violation of their right to health, the demands relate to the recognition of accidents and/or diseases, to adequate medical treatment and timely rehabilitation. Furthermore, the demands include re-adaptation measures that allow the worker to adequately perform his or her work, be and feel productive. In relation to the violation of their right to social security benefits due to illness or accidents, the demands focus on receiving adequate medical care for the health problems from both the employers and the social security institutions. It is demanded that work related illnesses are adequately qualified as such and that the percentage of impairment in working capacity is established in a reliable way, as the welfare and economic rights are calculated in accordance with these measures. Regarding the diagnostic and therapeutic itineraries that workers have to go through (Buitrago Echeverri et al., 2017), starting at the company and ending at the national disability qualification board, the central demand is that public institutions headed by the Ministry of Work, protect their occupational and health rights by intervening to oblige the companies to guarantee the rights. Furthermore, public institutions are called to protect the human rights of workers, forcing the Ministry of Work to assume leadership and push for appropriate action by companies, occupational risk administrators and disability rating boards.

These demands from workers' and former workers' organisations with work-related illnesses reflect structural problems related to the guarantee of labour, health, social security rights in Colombia and further evince impediments to the freedom of association that seriously hamper several organisations in Colombia (Escuela Nacional Sindical, 2017) and in this case, particularly obstruct the workers to organise themselves and participate in the transformation of norms and policies that define their situation. Furthermore, the demands of the workers' illness associations reflect the terrible impact on the quality and dignity of the population that generates the wealth of the nation.

In relation to the proposals that these organisations articulate, two types can be differentiated: some in relation to the previously discussed resolution of their demands and others of a rather organisational nature. As part of the organisational demands that are based on the understanding that a stronger organisation has a stronger capacity to influence and resolve their demands, workers and former workers created the Federación Nacional de Trabajadores y ex Trabajadores Enfermos de Colombia (FENATRAECO) in 2016. FENATRAECO aims to articulate current associations and increase the influence on companies, social security institutions, government, control agencies and judicial bodies. Demands include the creation of committees or associations in each occupational risk administration company to allow direct dialogue with insurers and promote the formation of new associations in companies with similar problems.

### Field of political contentions: between alliances and opponents

The political contentions in the field of health and security at work are primarily expressed in the conflictual interaction between two groups of actors. The first group is composed by those who are responsible for the guarantee of working conditions that do not damage the workers' health. Among them are the Ministry of Health and of Work (institutions representing the state), the entrepreneurs, the occupational risk administrators, and the disability qualification boards. The second group includes those who suffer the effects of the lack of protection at work, in other words the workers and former workers with work-related illnesses, their associations, and other social and academic actors that support demands for the guarantee and protection of the life and health of the worker. In this sense, the organisational processes of workers and former workers with work-related illnesses have defined the entrepreneurs, the occupational risk administration companies, the qualification boards and even the judicial system and state institutions represented by the Ministry of Work, as their opponents. At the same time, they have identified other workers, their families, some non-governmental organisations (NGO), other social and academic actors, and international social organisations as allies that support their claims. Political disputes in this field are currently won by the entrepreneurs and the occupational risk administration companies because they possess greater resources of power. The weakness of regulation and control by the Ministry of Work and the judicial system contributes to this result.

### Achievements and learning

Nonetheless, the workers' and former workers' illness associations have made several achievements and went through several significant learning processes. Among the achievements, we highlight the visibilization of their health problems and the violation of their rights; the dialogue established between several social, institutional and political actors to resolve their problems; the emotional support and counselling between the association members; and benefits that were gained by the associations such as medical treatment and economic compensation for those who qualify. Furthermore, several companies have had to take managerial and technological action to protect the health of the workers and the associations have clearly become a reference to other workers in similar conditions that seek solidarity and counselling and serve as an example for the struggle and resistance that can be replicated in other contexts.

As for key learning processes, we highlight the importance of documenting cases of illnesses related to working conditions in order to facilitate the enforceability of rights. Additionally, we highlight the important role of communication to disseminate the allegations and complaints and also the work that is being carried out by the associations. Finally, we highlight the importance of lobbying national and international actors to become involved in workers' struggles and we recognise persistence as a transcendental factor in the context of the wear and tear this type of collective action can generate.

ASOTRECOL offers an example of the achievements accomplished by associations to date. This association became a reference due to its persistent struggle symbolised by a tent in front of the American embassy in Bogotá over the course of 6 years. The online communication of the association has been decisive as it allowed for wide dissemination of the workers' struggle. Furthermore, the associated workers and former workers recognise that the company saw itself in the need to provide medical treatment to the workers who had fallen ill and were further obliged to manage rehabilitation and relocalization of the affected workers as a direct result of international pressure. As a result, the company did not manage to lay off the workers and was forced to adopt technological changes with an ergonomic perspective to prevent illness in workers (Torres-Tovar, Luna-García, Parra, et al., 2016).

Another example constitutes the international incidence and lobby work of the Asociación de Trabajadores, ex trabajadores y pensionados de la empresa Colombit, ASOTRECOL, Fundación Manos Muertas and ASOTREDP, who managed to draw international attention to the problem and mobilise political actors such as the Congress of the United States and the European Union, that eventually supported the activities and protected the organisational processes (Torres-Tovar, Luna-García, & Villamizar, 2016; Torres-Tovar, Luna-García, Parra, et al., 2016).

## Conclusions

The deterioration of working conditions in the context of the labour and social security reforms of the 1990s created a field of political contention which generated social unrest and set the stage for the consolidation of associations demanding the protection of workers in hazardous working conditions and the guarantee of labour, health and social security rights as part of broader political demands related to health and social security policies in Colombia.

Our analysis here and previous publications on similar issues reveal a set of barriers that delay the recognition and guarantee of labour and health rights of workers who suffer work-related diseases and forced the workers to organise and act collectively to demand the guarantee of their rights. In this context, novel forms of collective action have developed in more traditional associations like trade unions and new collective actors, namely, workers' and former workers' illness associations emerged. The emergence of these new associations can be interpreted as an expression of the traditional trade union movement's weakness in the context of neoliberal labour reforms (Isaza Castro, 2003; Niño Chavarro & De Lafont De León, 2013; Schnall et al., 2011), but also as a response to the fact that many trade unions were slow or did not incorporate the topic in their agenda (Luna-García, 2017).

The epidemic of work-related pathologies is an expression of neoliberal labour regimes characterised by overexploitation and flexibilization, which have exacerbated the contradictions between capital and labour, accumulation and accident, and between profit and lack of social protection (Abadía-Barrera, Pinilla, Ariza, & Ruíz, 2012). At the same time, they reflect the defeat of a health protection model at the workplace, which was subordinated by an emphasis on productivity and capital accumulation to the benefit of employers and occupational risk administration companies that have focused on the insurance business. Public institutions headed by the Ministry of Work have not properly fulfilled their regulation and inspection functions and the disability qualification boards have mostly failed to adequately assess the health situation of workers and assume neutrality, which eventually exacerbated a compensational or indemnity-oriented perspective rather than a preventive perspective.

The collective action undertaken by workers' and former workers' associations with work-related illnesses could lead to the configuration of a new political subject capable of transforming the poor working conditions and the lack of social protection that led to this type of social mobilisation. Nonetheless, this requires strengthening organisational processes, alliances between associations, trade unions and other allies, and further requires gaining space in society by raising awareness on the unacceptability of the violation of the workers' rights.

As a direct result of the work done by the associations of workers and trade unions, workplace health issues are now on the public agenda and strategic demands regarding the establishment of a health protection system in multiple work scenarios in Colombia have been formulated, where the Ministry of Health and the financial superintendence assume their function and oblige companies and occupational risk administrators to grant the workers' rights and involve all actors in the decision making processes, radically challenging business models and labour regimes that promote the accumulation of capital at the expense of the suffering, sickness and death of male and female workers.

## ORCID

*Mauricio Torres-Tovar* http://orcid.org/0000-0002-6232-6706
*Jairo Ernesto Luna-García* http://orcid.org/0000-0002-0885-7223

## Acknowledgments

We are grateful to the group of associations of workers with work-related illnesses who opened their spaces to be able to inquire about their collective processes. Likewise, we thank the People's Health Movement that contributed with resources of the project "The contribution of civil society to achievement of health for all" to did this research and to carry out the translation of this paper.

## Disclosure statement

No potential conflict of interest was reported by the authors.

## References

Abadía-Barrera, C., Pinilla, M., Ariza, K., & Ruíz, H. (2012). Neoliberalismo en salud: La tortura de trabajadoras y trabajadores del Instituto Materno Infantil de Bogotá. *Revista de salud pública, 14*(1), 18–31. doi:10.1590/S0124-00642012000700003.
Abadía-Barrero, C. E., & Oviedo, D. G. (2009). Bureaucratic itineraries in Colombia. A theoretical and methodological tool to assess managed-care health care systems. *Social Science & Medicine, 68*, 1153–1160. doi:10.1016/j.socscimed. 2008.12.049
Asolaborales. (2016). *Caracterización de los trabajadores y extrabajadores enfermos asociados en Colombia.* Bogotá: Asociación de Abogados Laboralistas de los Trabajadores – Asolaborales. Unpublished.
Barraza, D., Jansen, K., van Wendel de Joode, B., & Wesseling, C. (2013). Social movements and risk perception: Unions, churches, pesticides and bananas in Costa Rica. *International Journal of Occupational and Environmental Health, 19*(1), 11–21. doi:10.1179/2049396712Y.0000000018
Buitrago Echeverri, M. T., Abadía-Barrero, C. E., & Granja Palacios, C. (2017). Work-related illness, work-related accidents, and lack of social security in Colombia. *Social Science & Medicine, 187*, 118–125. doi:0.1016/j.socscimed. 2017.06.030

Carrera, J. E. (2014). Meio Ambiente, classe e trabalho no capitalismo global: uma análise das novas formas de resistência a partir da experiência da ACPO. Retrieved from http://fboms.org.br/wp-content/uploads/2014/10/Anexo-Avalia%C3%A7%C3%A3o-FBOMS-2014.pdf

Corredor Jiménez, C. (2004). Papel del trabajo en el contexto de la globalización. *Porik An, 9*(1), 131–160. Retrieved from http://www.unicauca.edu.co/porik_an/imagenes_3noanteriores/No.9porikan/porikan_5.pdf

Davolos, P. (2012). Nuevas tendencias en el mundo del trabajo: las huellas de más de una década de reformas estructurales. In M. J. Soul et al. (Ed.), *El mundo del trabajo en América Latina: Tendencias y resistencias* (pp. 11–37). Buenos Aires: CLACSO.

Escuela Nacional Sindical. (2017). *Informe de Coyuntura Laboral y Sindical 2017. Objetivos de Desarrollo Sostenible estratégicos para la consecución de Trabajo Decente.* Medellín: ENS. Recover from http://www.ens.org.co/wp-content/uploads/2017/05/Resumen-informe-nacional-coyuntura-laboral-y-sindical-2017.pdf

Fry, R. (2010). *Fighting for survival: Coal miners and the struggle over health and safety in the United States, 1968–1988* (*Thesis for the degree of Doctor of Philosophy*). Wayne State University, Detroit, MI. Recover from http://digitalcommons.wayne.edu/cgi/viewcontent.cgi?article=1087&context=oa_dissertations

Fry, R. (2013). Making amends: Coal miners, the black lung association, and federal compensation reform, 1969–1972. *Federal History Journal, 5*, 35–56. Retrieved from http://shfg.org/shfg/wp-content/uploads/2013/12/Fry.pdf

Hopkins, G. W. (2010). Union reform and labor law: Miners for democracy and the use of the Landrum-Griffin Act. *Journal of Labor Research, 31*, 348–364. doi:10.1007/s12122-010-9097

International Ban Asbestos Secretariat. (2017). *Groups.* Retrieved from http://www.ibasecretariat.org

Isaza Castro, J. G. (2003). Flexibilización laboral: un análisis de sus efectos sociales para el caso colombiano. *Revista Equidad y Desarrollo, 1*, 10–40. Retrieved from https://revistas.lasalle.edu.co/index.php/ed/article/view/398/327

Judkins, B. M. (1982). Occupational health and the developing class consciousness of southern textile workers: The case of the brown lung association. *The Maryland Historian, 13*, 55–71.

Judkins, B. M. (1990). Workplace democracy and occupational health. *Humanity & Society, 14*(1), 34–54.

Judkins, B. M. (1993). The people's respirator: Coalition building and the black lung association. In S. L. Fisher (Ed.), *Fighting back in Appalachia: Traditions of resistance and change* (pp. 120–122). Philadelphia: Temple University Press.

Knight, R. M. (1971). Compensation for black lung at the federal level: A precedent for nationalized workmen's compensation. *Virginia Law Review, 57*(1), 97–127. doi:10.2307/1072079

Luna-García, J. E. (2009). Globalización y salud de los trabajadores. *Boletín del Observatorio de Salud, 2*(5), 2–11. Retrieved from http://revistas.unal.edu.co/index.php/bos/article/view/10978/11665

Luna-García, J. E. (2017). *Contribución a la construcción de lineamientos estratégicos para el desarrollo de la protección de la vida y la salud en el trabajo, a través de la negociación colectiva.* Bogotá: Organización Internacional del Trabajo. Retrieved from http://embargo.ilo.org/wcmsp5/groups/public/—americas/—ro-lima/—sro-lima/documents/genericdocument/wcms_564500.pdf

Luna-García, J. E., Castro-Fraume C. J., & Villamizar, G. (2016). COLOMBIT: A case of social responsibility towards the withdrawal of asbestos? In O. Gallo & E. Castaño (Ed.), *Occupational health in the 20th and 21st centuries. On the denial of the right to health and freedom from sickness* (pp. 443–472). Medellín: Escuela Nacional Sindical.

Muntaner, C., Benach, J., Quinlan, M., Solar, O., & Santana, V. (2010). *Empleo, trabajo y desigualdades en salud: una visión global.* Barcelona: Icaria editorial.

Niño Chavarro, L., & De Lafont De León, F. (2013). El mundo del trabajo en Colombia: incidencia de la globalización y el neoliberalismo en las relaciones de trabajo y en la jurisprudencia. *Revista Republicana, 14*, 61–82. Retrieved from file:///C:/Users/Usuario/Downloads/47-177-1-PB.pdf

Saldarriaga, J. (2013, March 23). Sobrevivir del carbón los tiene enfermos y en oscuro drama. *El Colombiano.* Retrieved from http://www.elcolombiano.com/historico/sobrevivir_del_carbon_los_tiene_enfermos_y_en_oscuro_drama-PEEC_234784

Schnall, P., Dobson, M., & Rosskam, E. (2011). *Trabajo no saludable. Causas, consecuencias, curas.* Bogotá: Universidad de los Andes.

Silva, L. C., & Ordúñez, P. (2014). Chronic kidney disease in central American agricultural communities: Challenges for epidemiology and public health. *MEDICC Review, 16*(2), 66–71.

Standing, G. (2011). *The precariat: The new dangerous class.* London: Bloomsbury Academic.

Tarrow, S. (1997). *El poder en movimiento. Los movimientos sociales, la acción colectiva y la política.* Madrid: Alianza Universidad.

Tello, L. M., & Grau, D. (2015). Towards a sustainable and healthy work environment –lessons learned from the unprevented exposure of miners to coal dust. *Procedia Engineering, 118*, 457–464. doi:10.1016/j.proeng.2015.08.447

Tilly, C. (2004). *Social movements, 1768–2004.* Boulder, CO: Paradigm.

Torres-Tovar, M., Luna-García, J. E., Parra, J., & Shell-Sparling, P. (2016). Acción colectiva por el derecho a la salud en el trabajo: el caso de ASOTRECOL. In O. Gallo (Ed.), *La salud laboral en el siglo XX y el XXI: De la negación al derecho* (pp. 413–442). Medellín: Escuela Nacional Sindical.

Torres-Tovar, M., Luna-García, J. E., & Ruiz-Vallejo, R. (2016). Asociaciones de trabajadores y extrabajadores enfermos. Derrota de la protección y la prevención de la salud en el mundo del trabajo. *Revista Cultura y Trabajo, 92*, 82–91.

Torres-Tovar, M., & Torres-Echeverry, N. (2017). Trabajo y salud: La Corte Constitucional frente a la tutela por accidentes y enfermedades laborales. *Revista de Salud Pública, 19*(6), 772–779.

Trabanino, R. G., Aguilar, R., Silva, C. R., Mercado, M. O., & Merino, R. L. (2002). Nefropatía terminal en pacientes de un hospital de referencia en El Salvador. *Revista Panamericana de Salud Pública, 12*(3), 202–206.

Zavestoski, S. (2009). The struggle for justice in Bhopal. A new/old breed of transnational social movement. *Global Social Policy: An Interdisciplinary Journal of Public Policy and Social Development, 9*, 383–407. doi:10.1177/1468018109343643

# The mental health users' movement in Argentina from the perspective of Latin American Collective Health

Sara Ardila-Gómez ⓘ , Martín Agrest ⓘ , Marina A. Fernández ⓘ , Melina Rosales ⓘ ,
Lucila López , Alberto Rodolfo Velzi Díaz ⓘ , Santiago Javier Vivas ⓘ , Guadalupe Ares
Lavalle ⓘ , Eduardo Basz , Pamela Scorza ⓘ  and Alicia Stolkiner ⓘ

**ABSTRACT**
The mental health users' movement is a worldwide phenomenon that seeks to resist disempowerment and marginalisation of people living with mental illness. The Latin American Collective Health movement sees the mental health users' movement as an opportunity for power redistribution and for autonomous participation. The present paper aims to analyze the users' movement in Argentina from a Collective Health perspective, by tracing the history of users' movement in the Country. A heterogeneous research team used a qualitative approach to study mental health users' associations in Argentina. The local impact of the Convention on the Rights of Persons with Disabilities and the regulations of Argentina's National Mental Health Law are taken as fundamental milestones. A strong tradition of social activism in Argentina ensured that the mental health care reforms included users' involvement. However, the resulting growth of users' associations after 2006, mainly to promote their participation through institutional channels, has not been followed by a more radical power distribution. Associations dedicated to the self-advocacy include a combination of actors with different motives. Despite the need for users to form alliances with other actors to gain ground, professional power struggles and the historical disempowerment of 'patients' stand as obstacles for users' autonomous participation.

## Introduction

The mental health users' movement is about human rights, power distribution, recovery and also making profound changes to mental health services. A worldwide phenomenon, the movement seeks to resist the impact of disempowerment and marginalisation that people living with mental illness have historically experienced (Crane-Ross, Lutz, & Roth, 2006).

The mental health users' movement has received attention in both high income and low and middle-income countries (Chamberlin, 1978; Kleintjes, Lund, & Swartz, 2013; Yaro & de Menil,

2010; Zinman, 2009). Though it has adopted heterogeneous characteristics and assumed varied pathways across countries and cultures, the users' movement has consistently struggled to actuate a redistribution of power. Studies from high-income countries have shown that users' participation in care and treatment, and in service and policy planning, has not been followed by an increase in decision making and, due to their mental diagnosis, their opinions have not been equally valued as those of professionals (Campbell, 2006; Carr, 2007; Connor & Wilson, 2006; Hodge, 2005; Lewis, 2009; Rose, 2001; Rutter, Manley, Weaver, Crawford, & Fulop, 2004; Wallcraft, Read, & Sweeney, 2003; Webb, Clifford, Fowler, Morgan, & Hanson, 2000). For example, a National Survey of Mental Health Services from Australia found that 46% of mental health services included users in their advisory committees, but only 8% had users in their management committees (Honey, 1999). In this sense, users' participation is limited because professionals still control the process and the result of such participation (Broer, Nieboer, & Bal, 2014; Milewa, Dowswell, & Harrison, 2002).

The ethos of human rights, social inclusion, and power distribution inherent in the mental health users' movement resonates with the Latin American Collective Health movement. Argentina, one of the countries where the Collective Health tradition has developed, has a long tradition of social activism and social participation from local grass-root movements (Retamozo, 2011; Waitzkin, Iriart, Estrada, & Lamadrid, 2001). Following scholars from the Collective Health tradition, we understand social participation as the process through which people take part in the development of actions that aim toward collective goals (Fassin, 2006; Menéndez, 2006). In this sense, social participation is seen as a psychosocial process where the personal level is articulated with the collective level, mutually constructing each other. Social activism and collective action are key to offering persons 'the possibility of a joyful discovery of free action' and, thus, constituting 'the finest human experience' (Hilb, 2013, pp. 30–31). This specific type of participation ranks high in order to attain full personhood in Argentina.

Particularly in the health field, social participation has been conceived simultaneously as a method --or a means-- and as a goal, a way to achieving health objectives and an indicator of health and citizenship (Menéndez, 2006). In addition, social participation is usually related to democracy as a system of political organisation, since it is through participation that power can be redistributed, transforming the social world, including mental health services and systems (Ferullo de Parajón, 2006; Rovere, 1999).

In the specific case of mental health services users, and under the framework of the Convention on the Rights of People with Disabilities (United Nations, 2006), social participation has been considered as a fundamental right, as a way to gain social inclusion and to exercise full citizenship, and also as a way to challenge and transform the traditional psychiatric model of care. Social participation is key to the 'dignity of risk' --the dignity in making one's own decisions and being responsible for their consequences (Basz, 2014), and has been conceptualised as the opposite of social exclusion (Burchardt, Le Grand, & Piachaud, 2002). Given the importance placed on social participation in the Collective Health movement in Argentina, autonomous participation by mental health service users defines a successful mental health service users' movement from this perspective.

### Context: mental health reforms in Argentina

Argentina is an upper-middle income country (World Bank, 2017), with significant social and health inequities and almost a third of its population under the poverty line.

The mental health system's development has not been linear in Argentina. The first mental institutions were created in the second part of the nineteenth century. Several unconnected psychiatric reforms were attempted after 1950, some of them interrupted by military governments and neoliberal reforms, but also by disputes that have interfered with a nationwide mental health reform (e.g. trade unions resisting the closing of asylums because of a threatening loss of working opportunities for administrative and other support staff, power disputes between psychiatrists and psychologists, etc.) (Chiarvetti, 2008).

Currently, at a national level, the mental health system is heterogeneous. Psychiatric hospitals still prevail in terms of the distribution of beds for people with mental problems. An overwhelming majority of psychiatric beds (81.5%) are located in psychiatric hospitals (Di Nella et al., 2011). Most primary health care facilities include psychologists among their professional staff, and in the specific case of Buenos Aires, Argentina's capital city, the highest psychologist to population ratio in the world can be found: one in 90 inhabitants is a psychologist (Alonso & Klinar, 2013).

A national mental health law was enacted in 2010, in the context of other important laws regarding vulnerable populations that were passed around the same time (e.g. gender identity, migrants, etc.). The success in passing this law has been attributed to a post-neoliberal government that was in power (Grugel & Riggirozzi, 2012) and the newly re-empowered social movements from the previous decades.

This 2010 national law followed a rights-based approach and, among other key aspects, mandated that users' associations participate in psychiatric reform through institutional channels (Honorable Cámara del Senado de la Nación, 2010a). Those institutional channels for users' participation were the *Organo de Revisión* (OR) or 'Review Body', responsible for monitoring how the law is being executed, and the *Consejo Consultivo Honorario* (CCH) or 'Honorary Consulting Council', charged with designing new mental health policy proposals. Both groups, the OR and the CHH, were explicitly required to have among their members a certain number of representatives of users' associations (Ministerio de Salud, 2013). Thereafter, from the moment of the implementation of the law, several organisations self-defined as users' associations developed.

The aim of this work is to describe and analyze from a Collective Health framework the recent history of the mental health users' movement in Argentina, mapping key associations and their role in the movement. Specifically, we seek to analyze the extent to which the users' movement fulfils the Collective Health ideal of users advocating for their own rights—i.e. people with similar experiences advocating for their own needs, collectively strengthening their voice (Mind, 2015; Walmsley, 2002).

## Methods

The research team was composed of one clinician, eight researchers, and two activists.[1] The research design followed a qualitative approach and included: literature review, document analysis, grey literature review, interviews, and participatory observation.

(1) A literature review regarding the users' participation, users' perspectives, users' movement and users' associations in Argentina was conducted. The term 'user' was selected, in line with how these associations have chosen to name themselves in Argentina and how these social actors were named by the 2010 national mental health law (# 26.657). A Pubmed search was conducted using the terms 'mental health', 'user' and 'Argentina'. Lilacs, Redalyc and Scielo databases were used with 'salud mental', 'usuario' and 'Argentina' in January 2017.

(2) The analysis of documents included: The national mental health law (# 26.657) and its regulations (Ministerio de Salud, 2013), the verbatim transcriptions of the Senate's debates during 2009 and 2010 in the preparation of the law, National Mental Health Direction's documents and recommendations, and the human rights report -and its repercussions- on the state of inpatient units of people with mental illness living in several psychiatric hospitals, produced by human rights NGOs (MDRI/CELS, 2007). Sections regarding users' participation were prioritised in search of activists and associations that could be key players in the field of users' associations. Content analysis was also performed looking into themes relevant to users participating in advocacy activities.

(3) Twenty-five newspapers (three with nationwide circulation and twenty-two local) were reviewed for articles on users' associations participating in the reviewing body (OR). To be included, users' associations had to fulfil two criteria: (a) They are composed of mental health services

users and, (b) They are doing rights' advocacy tasks and/or participating from the OR at any level.

(4) Interviews were performed with key informants from the *Asamblea de Usuarios/as de Salud Mental por Nuestros Derechos*, or 'Assembly of Mental Health Users for Our Rights' (Santa Fe Province), from the *Usuarios, Familiares y Amigos de los Servicios de Salud Mental*, or 'Users, Family Members and Friends of the Mental Health Services' (Córdoba Province), and from the *Asociación Manos Abiertas y Solidarias* (AMAS), or 'Association of Open Hands in Solidarity' (Río Negro Province). Topics addressed covered their origins, composition, aims, activities, relationships with other associations, and barriers and facilitators for their daily work and for their intended objectives. A secondary analysis was performed based on a previous study conducted in *Asamblea Permanente de Usuarios de los Servicios de Salud Mental* (APUS-SAM), or "Permanent Assembly of Mental Health Service Users" (Rosales, 2014) and with *Red de Familiares, Usuarios y Voluntarios por los Derechos de las Personas con Padecimiento Mental* (Red FUV), or 'Network of Family Members, Users and Volunteers for the Rights of People with Mental Suffering' (López Cirio, Bugoslawski, & Zucchelli, 2015). AMAS, APUSSAM and Red FUV participated as representatives of users' associations in the OR and the CCH. The APUS-SAM study analyzed the participation process in the assembly from the participants' perspective, and the changes attributed to such participation. The Red FUV study focused on the participation of such association in the OR.

(5) Grey literature of users' associations (e.g. web pages, Facebook and blogs) was analyzed. Based on a previous search (Rosales, Fernández, Agrest, Ardila-Gómez, & Stolkiner, 2015), where 18 users' associations had been identified, the Facebook, web pages and blogs of these associations were reviewed during 2016 in search of the activities performed by the associations. Their composition and links with other associations were integral to the analysis.

(6) Five members of the research team participated in 2016 from the First National Meeting of Mental Health Service Users and acted as participant observers taking field notes and adopting different roles: One was part of the organising committee, two were activists and two others were non-user attendants.

The analysis was based on two broad categories: Historical and current dynamics of users' associations. The material was analyzed in groups by different members of the research team between 2015 and 2017. A first round of analysis was held in sub-groups. Findings were triangulated in large group meetings.

## Results

The literature review and secondary citation search identified eight papers focusing on user participation and perspective in Argentina (Agrest, 2011; Agrest et al., 2017; Ardila, 2011; Ceriani, Obiols, & Stolkiner, 2010; Michalewicz, Obiols, Ceriani, & Stolkiner, 2012; Rosales et al., 2015; Stolkiner, 2012; Tisera & Lohigorry, 2015).

Through these articles, as well as the newspapers reviewed and the key informant interviews, we identified 26 users' associations in Argentina distributed along 13 of 24 provinces that met the inclusion criteria by the time of the research (See Figure 1). None of the association had a national presence and many of them lacked a communication platform (e.g. Facebook, web page or blog) or had considerable delays updating them. Only two of the associations (Red FUV and APEF) have presence in more than one province and only Río Negro province has more than three associations in its territory.

The results are organised according to the two broad categories of analysis above mentioned:

(1) For a historical analysis, two crucial events were considered: (a) The adoption of the Convention on the Rights of Persons with Disabilities (CRPD) (UN, 2006), and (b) the regulations of the

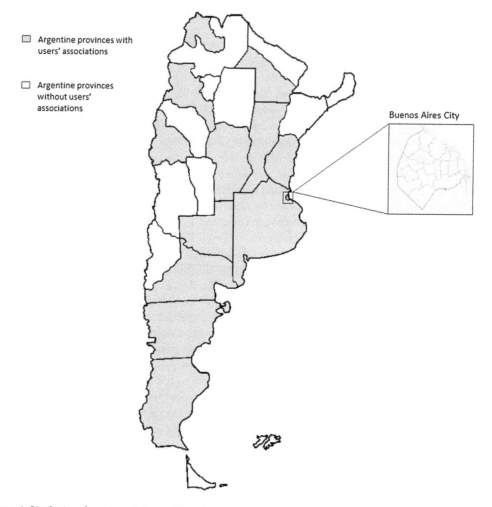

**Figure 1.** Distribution of users' associations in Argentina.

national mental health law in 2013 (Ministerio de Salud, 2013). These two milestones were selected because the CRPD is an international convention acknowledging the rights of people with disabilities that, at an international level, legitimatises Argentina's later decision to adopt a rights-based mental health reform law. In addition, the regulations of the mental health law establish concrete areas for users to participate in public policies related to mental health in Argentina, and such regulations have implicitly defined *users' associations* as those advocating or promoting users' civil rights.

(2) For the analysis of the current situation, we considered two major factors: a) How relationships are established among users participating in the associations and, b) how relationships are established between users and other actors (e.g. mental health professionals and family members). These relationships are integral to understanding the degree of users' autonomous participation in Argentina.

Despite restricting our study to associations centred on users advocating for their own rights, fuzzy borders of these associations were the rule and not the exemption. Associations were sometimes formed by one single participant, fluctuated in number of members in short periods of time, composed mostly by mental health professionals, carried out activities very partially related to advocacy, existed at some point of time and then faded or disappeared, or progressively incorporated advocacy activities after years of existing with other purposes.

## Historical analysis of mental health users' associations in Argentina

### Early users' associations

Based on the information analyzed, it was possible to establish that users' associations existed before the CRPD, totalling six by 2006. The first associations of mental health services users were created between late 1980s and early 1990s. They were created around specific mental conditions, as indicated by their names, and they were organised based on mental health professionals' recommendations or by users' family members' initiative. *Fundación Bipolares Argentina* (FUBIPA), or 'Bipolar Foundation Argentina', and *Asociación Argentina de Ayuda a la Persona que Padece Esquizofrenia y su Familia* (APEF), or 'Argentinean Association for Helping People with Schizophrenia and their Family', were described as direct predecessors of users' associations (Agrest, 2011) but did not primarily consist of users advocating for their own rights (Ceriani et al., 2010). FUBIPA was created by a psychiatrist in 1989. APEF was created by family members of people diagnosed with schizophrenia in 1994. Their main impetuses when they were formed were: psychiatrists seeking treatment compliance, and family members seeking resources and information that could improve patients' quality of life, respectively.

AMAS was founded in 1995 in the province of Río Negro. As described by one of its members, AMAS was born in connection to the local psychiatric reform process that culminated with the enactment of provincial mental health law in 1991, and was strongly promoted and supported by one psychiatrist in particular. Following the model of social entrepreneurships, a type of organisation developed by the Italian psychiatric reform (de Leonardis, Mauri, & Rotelli, 1995), it aimed for social inclusion through work.

Compared with other associations, AMAS has some features that align well with the Collective Health ideal of users' rights: Unlike some other associations, it is legally and formally constituted, and rights are addressed in a 'practical' fashion, i.c. while other associations offer a more 'theoretical' approach to advocacy, AMAS centres its activities around offering working opportunities to people with mental illness through social entrepreneurships associated and dependent on it. AMAS has a formal board which is composed of twelve members: Nine of them are mental health professionals, two are family members of persons with mental illness and one is identified as a mental health service user.

### Users organisations involved in the passage of the mental health reform law

The Red FUV association was created in July of 2006, and it is currently formed by relatives, mental health services' users, volunteers, students and mental health professionals. Red FUV actively participated in the debates surrounding the enactment of the national mental health law (Honorable Cámara de Senadores de la Nación, 2010b).

After the enactment of the mental health law, jointly with the Panamerican Health Organization (PAHO), Red FUV convened in 2011 the 'First National Meeting of Latin American Relatives, Users and Volunteers advocating for Human Rights in Mental Health', supported by the National Direction of Mental Health and Substance Abuse. A Latin American network of users, relatives and volunteers for the Human Rights in Mental Health was also created during that meeting (PAHO, 2011). Two years later, in 2013, Red FUV participated in PAHO's 'First Regional Meeting of Mental Health Services' users and their relatives' (PAHO, 2013).

The *Asamblea Permanente de Usuarios de Servicios de Salud Mental* (APUSSAM) was created in 2007 in Buenos Aires City with a close collaboration from the *Centro de Estudios Legales y Sociales* (CELS), or Center of Legal and Social Studies, an emblematic human rights organisation. According to a former participant from APUSSAM, this association did not emerge from users' activities but from CELS' interest in generating a space where the rights of persons with psychosocial disabilities could be discussed --specifically, their rights to be involved in the planning and execution of mental health policies centred on the CRPD. After ten years of uninterrupted work, APUSSAM still meets at the CELS' offices, on a fortnightly basis. APUSSAM is centred on raising awareness regarding the rights of mental health service users so other users can acknowledge their own rights and can advocate for themselves. Members of APUSSAM participated in the editing of the national mental health law drafts and, after it was passed, APUSSAM had representatives in the CCH and the provincial OR of Buenos Aires Province.

### Users' organisations arising after the mental health reform law

After the passage of the national mental health law, users' association blossomed across the country in direct response to the creation of local ORs and their legal mandate to include users. Seven associations, included in our list of 26 existing associations, were created between 2013 and 2016. However, despite the rapid rise of users' organisations, a national or articulated users' movement was not clearly seen.

Participants from two users' associations that were created after 2013 were interviewed for this study: (1) The *Asamblea de Usuarios/as de Salud Mental por Nuestros Derechos*, was created in the city of Rosario, Santa Fe Province, in 2013. This association started as an extension programme from the university. An initial group composed of faculty members, students and other mental health professionals convened users from several mental health services. This new group, the majority of members being users, began to function as an assembly. (2) The association *Usuarios, Familiares y Amigos de los Servicios de Salud Mental*, was created in the city of Córdoba, Córdoba Province, in 2014. This association was initiated by one user and university faculty members who were also part of the staff of an asylum but just a few months later this user continued on his own and constituted a 'one-participant association'.

For a two-year period, starting in 2013, Red FUV was the users' association taking part in the national OR. Their representatives noted several benefits from participating in the OR: Sharing their experiences of living with mental suffering and their struggle finding appropriate care from different health care providers, identifying and disputing stigmatising or degrading daily practices that had become naturalised by mental health professionals, and producing/receiving materials created by mental health service users rather than the medico-legal community (López Cirio et al., 2015).

The other body in which users' associations participated was the CCH. For APUSSAM's and for AMAS' members, participating in the CHH was considered important. According to AMAS participants, being part of the CHH gave them the opportunity to interact with other users across the country and mutually share their experiences. For APUSSAM's participants it was more about 'conquering' their right to participate in the development of mental health policies in concordance with the CRPD and with the national mental health law. APUSSAM's members mentioned that they felt as if they were 'regarded as citizens and not only as mental health services users' (Rosales & Ardila-Gómez, 2017).

In 2016 the National Mental Health and Substance Abuse Direction withdrew most of the support to users' participation it had been given by the previous administration. Nevertheless, it is interesting to note that users continue their organisation and a first national meeting of users was held in 2016.

### Current analysis of users participating in associations dedicated to advocacy tasks

Participants from APUSSAM who were interviewed and had been involved in the 2010 mental health law preparation expressed that they had felt 'excited to become members of the Consulting Honorary Council' and acknowledged several benefits drawing from their participation: '[Having a] more positive way of seeing reality and themselves' and 'making recovery a reality through helping others'. 'Greater consciousness of achieved rights and others pending to be achieved', 'an evolving identity linked to activism instead of patienthood' and 'configuring a new sense of citizenship' were integral to this transformation (Rosales & Ardila-Gómez, 2017).

One user, as an indicator of successful participation and activism, mentioned that he had been 'able to reach out to thousands of people, sharing ideas and news regarding mental health treatment, and even to debate with a prestigious mental health professional.' Taking note of this remark, an activist expressed the challenge of users needing to organise themselves when everyone around is denying them full citizenship.

The mental health law has changed, but patronising attitudes by professionals have not. Closing down the asylums and moving to a community care approach, on behalf of mental health professionals, have been the central aspects of mental health rights' fight. Despite users' recognition of the importance of this fight, some of the interviewed users expressed that other needs--and infringed rights--would go 'beyond psychiatric hospital walls' and should be addressed. Demanding full citizenship is a much broader request than demanding better mental health services or human rights being respected during hospitalisations.

### 'By' users or 'for' users

Family members, mental health professionals, academic institutions, non-government organisations, and state organisms, had a decisive role at the beginning of every users' association. As presented above, in many occasions these actors' participation was crucial in supporting or maintaining users' associations. In some cases, the leadership roles were adopted by non-users--despite users having the original initiative. An association located in Entre Ríos Province is representative of this situation: A user convened other users, but it was a mental health professional who ultimately remained as the head of the organisation.

Even if from the perspective of the CRPD it may be understandable that users' associations may have needed non-users acting as collaborators, it remains unanswered why and how these supports remained as a necessity. In a comparison between building houses and building users' associations, a mental health activist told us:

> When you build a house, engineers and architects may be needed. But once the house is ready they don't stay living in the house. In the case of users' associations, professionals do stay.

The Collective Health movement has influenced Argentine scholars and activists to see a crucial difference between associations *of/by* users, from associations *with* users or *for* users (Rosales et al., 2015). A users' association, from this perspective, would be defined by the roles that users have when the association is operative. In line with this, a users' association would be conducted by users, whose objectives and actions are decided and executed according to their interests.

Although financial support was considered to be necessary, and support as defined by the CRPD was welcome, paternalism and interference by mental health professionals were criticised. Rather than wanting greater support from professionals, activists complained about the existence of too much interference from professional organisms and mental health professionals posing barriers to mental health users to organise by themselves.

According to a participant from the 'First National Meeting of Mental Health Services Users, for a society without asylums,' in 2016, in Rosario, Santa Fe Province, 'a few users attending the reunion were still hospitalised in asylums, and some others were coming with their relatives or with mental health professionals.' (…) 'Not many users/activists were there on their own.' Dependency on relatives or professionals and the existence of asylums were considered as barriers for a full activism.

Nevertheless, some steps have also been taken to move away from paternalism. The 2016 users' national meeting was convened and organised by the local assembly of users, and funding was provided by the extension programme at the university. Some activities and debates were for users only--and non-users were invited to stay outside. As an activist said, sustaining such differences and excluding non-users from specific activities or decisions may be necessary for the users' movement to strengthen.

## Battleground for professional power

Users' associations striving for self-advocacy had to navigate an ongoing professional battle between psychologists and psychiatrists. The national mental health law had a profound effect and divided the mental health professionals: Most psychiatrists stood against several of its principles (e.g. closing down the asylums, allowing other mental health professionals to be the head of mental health units, etc.) while a majority of psychologists advocated for passing the law. In the passage and implementation of the mental health law, ample participation of mental health service users was mandated, however registered users' associations were scarce by the time the mental health law was enacted, and participation from users was fraught with the challenges described above. Therefore, mental health professionals saw a role as 'mental health user advocate' --also influencing the mental health reform in their favour.

On some occasions, users reported suspicion of mental health professionals having a different agenda. An activist told us:

> "I fight to promote users' rights and users' mental health, but the professionals are there for a political fight that has nothing to do with mental health" (...) "There are no mental health professionals working in the association right now ... And I would look sideways at them if there were."

It is important to mention that every social movement conveys conflicts and that social dynamics cannot exist without conflicts (Testa, 2007). However, participants from users' associations repeatedly mentioned that users who stood up against mental health professionals and family members, ultimately confronting the mental health system, ended up leaving the local associations and a few of them joined international networks or networks from other countries.

## Discussion

From the analysis of data on the mental health service users' movement in Argentina, we see both great potential for, as well as challenges to power redistribution and users' self-advocacy. Mental health professionals and users' families have a central role in the history and current activities of many associations, casting doubt on the potential of these associations to contribute to power redistribution. A similar doubt arises for the institutional channels offered by the State to guarantee the users' participation (e.g. OR and CCH) and whether through these initiatives the users' movement will be strengthened or, instead, appeased or co-opted. It is yet to be determined if mental health service users, who have historically been disempowered, can actually benefit from these alliances or if they are succumbing to these greater powers.

On the other hand, in its current form, the users' movement in Argentina may not be able to oppose psychiatrists and other mental health professionals who have been historically empowered. It remains to be determined which actors could help users become an independent and strong counter-power. By establishing an alliance with human rights advocacy associations, users have tended to be seen as 'survivors of human rights violations perpetrated mostly by mental health workers.' By establishing an alliance with psychologists, users have tended to be seen as 'patients'. And when establishing alliances with people from the academia, users' identity tended to be as 'object of study.' This oversimplification should take into consideration that each of these potential allies may present a wide range of alternatives: Psychologists can centre their approach on disabilities or can have a recovery orientation, people from the academia can have a radical positivist stance or can base their work on critical theory. Overall, such necessary alliances may pose specific challenges and opportunities for the users' movement.

Our diverse team reflected the differences in the data analysis between a professional and a users' perspective. While mental health professionals highlighted the disputes regarding the national mental health law, activists perceived the whole professional field as having an overprotective attitude towards them and a neglecting attitude towards the CRPD.

In Argentina, as in other parts of the globe, the users' movement has not entirely gained autonomy from other actors and powers. It remains unanswered how mental health service users could create associations and organise themselves in order to claim the unrestricted fulfilment of the CRPD when they are not acknowledged by their communities with full legal capacities.

Ultimately, the Argentine Collective Health perspective sees the users' movement as a social actor that intends to go beyond making mental health services more 'humane' and, instead, to fully actualize their human rights. Whilst many mental health professionals tend to see it as 'domestic' problem, activists consider it a much broader and general problem.

In conclusion, embracing the right to self-determination and autonomy may be revolutionary, but it is the goal of Argentinean activists participating from users' movements, who believe, taking the perspective of Latin American Collective Health, that users should be listened to in terms of persons fighting for rights instead of patients claiming services.

## Note

1. In the text the term 'activist' refers exclusively to social activists who simultaneously or previously self-defined as service users and who have chosen to name themselves as 'activists'.

## Disclosure statement

No potential conflict of interest was reported by the authors.

## Funding

This work was supported by Universidad de Buenos Aires, UBACyT # 20020130100543BA

## ORCID

*Sara Ardila-Gómez* http://orcid.org/0000-0002-0022-7438
*Martín Agrest* http://orcid.org/0000-0003-3756-2229
*Marina A. Fernández* http://orcid.org/0000-0001-5767-4047
*Melina Rosales* http://orcid.org/0000-0001-5707-9467
*Alberto Rodolfo Velzi Díaz* http://orcid.org/0000-0001-6304-2150
*Santiago Javier Vivas* http://orcid.org/0000-0003-0119-6685
*Guadalupe Ares Lavalle* http://orcid.org/0000-0003-0027-1540
*Pamela Scorza* http://orcid.org/0000-0001-8895-8675
*Alicia Stolkiner* http://orcid.org/0000-0001-9372-7556

## References

Agrest, M. (2011). La participación de los usuarios en los servicios de salud mental. *Vertex, Revista Argentina de Psiquiatría, 22*(100), 409–418.

Agrest, M., Barruti, S., Gabriel, R., Zalazar, V., Wikinski, S., & Ardila-Gómez, S. (2017). Day hospital treatment for people with severe mental illness according to users' perspectives: What helps and what hinders recovery? *Journal of Mental Health, 13,* 1–7.

Alonso, M., & Klinar, D. (2013). *Los Psicólogos en Argentina. Relevamiento Cuantitativo* 2012. Congreso internacional de investigación y práctica profesional en Psicología. Noviembre, Ciudad Autónoma de Buenos Aires, Argentina.

Ardila, S. (2011). La inclusión de la perspectiva de los usuarios en los servicios de Salud Mental. *Vertex, Revista Argentina de Psiquiatría, 22*(95), 49–55.

Basz, E. (2014). La dignidad del riesgo como antídoto al estigma. Retrieved from https://www.linkedin.com/pulse/20140703134507-15416747-la-dignidad-del-riesgo-como-antidoto-al-estigma

Broer, T., Nieboer, A. P., & Bal, R. (2014). Mutual powerlessness in client participation practices in mental health care. *Health Expectations, 17*(2), 208–219. doi:10.1111/j.1369-7625.2011.00748.x

Burchardt, T., Le Grand, J., & Piachaud, D. (2002). Degrees of exclusion: Developing a dynamic,multidimensional measure. In J. Hills, J. LeGrand, & D. Piachaud (Eds.), *Understanding social exclusion* (pp. 30–43). New York: Oxford University Press.

Campbell, P. (2006). Changing the mental health system – a survivor's view. *Journal of Psychiatric and Mental Health Nursing, 13*, 578–580.

Carr, S. (2007). Participation, power, conflict and change: Theorising dynamics of service user participation in the social care system of England and Wales. *Critical Social Policy, 27*(2), 266–276.

Ceriani, L., Obiols, J., & Stolkiner, A. (2010). *Potencialidades y obstáculos en la construcción de un nuevo actor social: Las organizaciones de usuarios*. Memorias del II Congreso Internacional de Investigación y práctica profesional en Psicología. XVII Jornadas de Investigación y Sexto Encuentro de Investigadores en Psicología del Mercosur. Facultad de Psicología, Universidad de Buenos Aires.

Chamberlin, J. (1978). *On our own: Patient controlled alternatives to the mental health system*. Michigan: Haworth Press.

Chiarvetti, S. (2008). La reforma en salud mental en Argentina: una asignatura pendiente. Sobre el artículo: hacia la construcción de una política en salud mental. *Revista Argentina de Clínica Psicológica, 17*, 173–183.

Connor, S. L., & Wilson, R. (2006). It's important that they learn from us for mental health to progress. *Journal of Mental Health, 15*(4), 461–474.

Crane-Ross, D., Lutz, W. J., & Roth, D. (2006). Consumer and case manage perspectives of service empowerment: Relationship to mental health recovery. *Journal of Behavioral Health Services & Research, 33*, 142–155.

de Leonardis, O., Mauri, D., & Rotelli, F. (1995). *La Empresa Social*. Buenos Aires: Nueva Visión.

Di Nella, Y., Sola, M., Calvillo, L., Negro, L., Paz, A., & Venesio, S. (2011). Las camas del sector público como indicador del proceso de cambio hacia el nuevo paradigma, mayo 2010-mayo 2011. *Revista Argentina de Salud Pública, 2*(8), 43–46.

Fassin, D. (2006). Entre ideología y pragmatismo. Ambigüedades y contradicciones de la participación comunitaria en salud. In E. L. Menéndez y H. Spinelli (Eds.), *Participación Social. ¿Para qué?* (pp. 117–143). Buenos Aires: Lugar Editorial.

Ferullo de Parajón, A. (2006). *El triángulo de las tres p: Psicología, participación y poder*. Santiago del Estero: Paidós Tramas Sociales.

Grugel, J., & Riggirozzi, P. (2012). Post-neoliberalism in Latin America: Rebuilding and reclaiming the state after crisis. *Development and Change, 43*(1), 1–21.

Hilb, C. (2013). *Usos del pasado. Qué hacemos hoy con los setenta*. Buenos Aires: Ed. Siglo XXI.

Hodge, S. (2005). Participation, discourse and power: A case study in service user involvement. *Critical Social Policy, 25* (2), 164–179. doi:10.1177/0261018305051324

Honey, A. (1999). Empowerment versus power: Consumer participation in mental health services. *Occupational Therapy International, 6*(4), 257–276.

Honorable Cámara de Senadores de la Nación. (2010a). Sesión plenaria de la Legislación General, Justicia y Asuntos penales, Salud y Deporte, y Presupuesto y Hacienda. Versión taquigráfica. 23 de Noviembre, Buenos Aires, Argentina.

Honorable Cámara de Senadores de la Nación. (2010b). Ley #26.657. Ley Nacional de Salud Mental.

Kleintjes, S., Lund, C., & Swartz, L. (2013). Organising for self-advocacy in mental health: Experiences from seven African countries. *African Journal of Psychiatry, 16*, 187–195.

Lewis, L. (2009). Politics of recognition: What can a human rights perspective contribute to understanding users' experiences of involvement in mental health services? *Social Policy and Society, 8*(2), 257–274. doi:10.1017/S1474746408004776

López Cirio, L., Bugoslawski, T., & Zucchelli, J. (2015). *Análisis del trabajo conjunto entre el Órgano de Revisión Nacional de la Ley de Salud Mental # 26657 y la Red FUV, durante el primer período de acción (2014/2015): potencialidades y obstáculos*. Final work. Presented in the Professional Practice on Research (code 818). Facultad de Psicología, Universidad de Buenos Aires, Argentina.

Menéndez, E. (2006). Las múltiples trayectorias de la participación social. In E. L. Menéndez y H. Spinelli (Eds.), *Participación Social. ¿Para qué?* (pp. 51–80). Buenos Aires: Lugar Editorial.

Mental Disability Rights International & Centro de Estudios Legales y Sociales (MDRI & CELS). (2007). *Vidas arrasadas. La segregación de las personas en los asilos psiquiátricos argentinos*. Retrieved from http://www.cels.org.ar/common/documentos/mdri_cels.pdf

Michalewicz, A., Obiols, J., Ceriani, L., & Stolkiner, A. (2012). *Usuarios de servicios de salud mental: del estigma de la internación psiquiátrica a la posibilidad de hablar en nombre propio*. IV Congreso Internacional de Investigación y práctica profesional en Psicología. XIX Jornadas de Investigación y VIII Encuentro de Investigadores en Psicología del Mercosur. Ediciones de la Facultad de Psicología, Universidad de Buenos Aires.

Milewa, T., Dowswell, G., & Harrison, S. (2002). Partnerships, power and the "new" politics of community participation in British health care. *Social Policy and Administration, 36*(7), 796–809. doi:10.1111/1467-9515.00318

Mind, National Association for Mental Health. (2015). *Guide to advocacy*. London: Mind.

Ministerio de Salud de la Nación. (2013). Reglamentación de la ley de salud mental # 26.657. Act 603/13. Retrieved from http://servicios.infoleg.gob.ar/infolegInternet/anexos/215000-219999/215485/norma.htm

Pan American Health Organization (PAHO). (2011). *Buenos Aires Consensus*. Retrieved from http://www.paho.org/arg/index.php?option=com_content&view=article&id=778&Itemid=269

Pan American Health Organization (PAHO). (2013). *Brasilia Consensus (Newsletter)*. Retrieved from http://www.paho.org/bulletins/index.php?option=com_content&view=article&id=1689:brasilia-consensus-&Itemid=0&lang=en

Retamozo, M. (2011). Movimientos sociales, política y hegemonía en Argentina. *Polis, Revista de la Universidad Bolivariana, 10*(28), 243–227.

Rosales, M. (2014). *Análisis de la Relación entre la Participación en Asociaciones de Usuarios de Servicios de Salud Mental y el Ejercicio de Derechos: Perspectiva de los Usuarios. Estudio de Caso en una Asociación de Usuarios en la Ciudad de Buenos Aires*, 2014. Retrieved from: http://www.psi.uba.ar/investigaciones.php?var=investigaciones/ubacyt/becarios/finalizados/estimulo/rosales.php

Rosales, M., & Ardila-Gómez, S. (2017). *El proceso de implementación de la Ley Nacional de Salud Mental: obstáculos y desafíos: ¿Qué dicen los usuarios de servicios de salud mental?* I Congreso Provincial de Salud Mental y Adicciones. Ciudad de Tandil, Buenos Aires, Argentina.

Rosales, M., Fernández, M., Agrest, M., Ardila-Gómez, S., y Stolkiner, A. (2015). *Asociaciones para, con y de usuarios de servicios de salud mental: elementos para su conceptualización y desarrollo.* I Congreso Latinoamericano de Salud Mental: "Los rostros actuales del malestar", Salta, Argentina.

Rose, D. (2001). *Users' voices: The perspectives of mental health service users on community and hospital care*. London: The Sainsbury Centre for Mental Health.

Rovere, M. (1999). Planificación estratégica en salud: Acompañando la democratización de un sector en crisis. *Cuadernos Médico Sociales, 75*, 31–63.

Rutter, D., Manley, C., Weaver, T., Crawford, M., & Fulop, N. (2004). Patients or partners? Case studies of user involvement in the planning and delivery of adult mental health services in London. *Social Science and Medicine, 58*, 1973–1984.

Stolkiner, A. (2012). Subjetividad y derechos: las organizaciones de usuarios y familiares como nuevos actores del campo de la salud mental. *Revista Intersecciones Psi. Revista Virtual de la Facultad de Psicología de la UBA, 2*(4). Retrieved from http://intersecciones.psi.uba.ar/index.php?option=com_content&view=article&id=134:las-organizaciones-de-usuarios-y-familiares-como-nuevos-actores-del-campo-de-la-salud-mental&catid=17:investigaciones&Itemid=1

Testa, M. (2007). *Pensamiento estratégico y lógica de programación*. Buenos Aires: Lugar Editorial.

Tisera, A., & Lohigorry, J. (2015). Sentido y significados sobre servicios de salud mental desde la perspectiva de usuarios/as, en la Ciudad Autónoma de Buenos Aires. *Anuario de Investigaciones, 22*, 263–271.

The United Nations (UN). (2006). *Convention on the Rights of Persons with Disabilities*. Retrieved from https://www.un.org/development/desa/disabilities/convention-on-the-rights-of-persons-with-disabilities.html

Waitzkin, H., Iriart, C., Estrada, A., & Lamadrid, S. (2001). Social medicine then and now: Lessons from Latin America. *American Journal of Public Health, 91*(10), 1592–1601.

Wallcraft, J., Read, J., & Sweeney, A. (2003). *On our own terms: Users and survivors of mental health services working together for support and change*. London: The Sainsbury Centre for Mental Health.

Walmsley, J. (2002). Principles and types of advocacy. In B. Gray, & R. Jackson (Eds.), *Advocacy and learning disability* (pp. 24–37). London: Jessica Kingsley Publishers.

Webb, Y., Clifford, P., Fowler, V., Morgan, C., & Hanson, M. (2000). "Comparing patients" experience of mental health services in England: A five-trust survey. *International Journal of Health Care Quality Assurance, 13*(6), 273–281.

World Bank. (2017). *World Bank Country and Lending Groups*. Retrieved from: https://datahelpdesk.worldbank.org/knowledgebase/articles/906519-world-bank-country-and-lending-groups

Yaro, P., & de Menil, V. (2010). Lessons from the African user movement: The case of Ghana. Retrieved from https://www.researchgate.net/publication/291577383_Lessons_from_the_African_user_movement_the_case_of_Ghana

Zinman, S. (2009). *History of the consumer/survivor movement*. Bethesda: SAMHSA, ADS Center.

# Global frameworks, local strategies: Women's rights, health, and the tobacco control movement in Argentina

Hepzibah Muñoz Martínez and Ann Pederson

**ABSTRACT**

The article examines how civil society organisations in Argentina used the United Nations Convention on the Elimination of All Forms of Discrimination Against Women (CEDAW) to frame the country's failure to enact strong national tobacco control legislation as a violation of women's rights in the late 2000s. We analyze this case study through the politics of scale, namely the social processes that produce, reproduce, and contest the boundaries of policies and socio-economic relations. This approach understands how multiple scales overlap and connect to obstruct or enhance the right to health in Latin America. In Argentina, the global organisation of tobacco companies, the reach of international financial institutions and the national dynamics of economic austerity and export-orientation promoted the local production and use of tobacco (leaf and cigarettes) and reproduced health inequalities in the country throughout the 1990s and the early 2000s. Yet, the visible legacy of local and national human rights struggles in the adoption of international human rights treaties into Argentina's national constitution allowed the tobacco control movement to link the scale of women's bodies to the right to health through the use of CEDAW to change national legislation, tackling the social determinants of the tobacco epidemic.

This article explores how Argentina's tobacco control movement used a global legal framework, namely international human rights law, to mobilise around local health issues in the late 2000s. Using the framework of the United Nations Convention on the Elimination of All Forms of Discrimination Against Women (CEDAW), which Argentina ratified in 1985, civil society organisations successfully framed the country's failure to enact strong national tobacco control legislation as a violation of women's rights. Social mobilisation on health issues in Latin America are often viewed as part of the concerns within women's, environmental justice and indigenous movements. This is particularly the case of reproductive rights and access to health services in women's movements in this region (Jelin, Zammit, & Thomson, 1990; Lebon, 2010; Molyneux, 2001). Analyses of Latin American environmental justice and indigenous movements address the ways in which the effects of environmental degradation caused by state and non-state actors affect the health of communities, which triggers mobilisation around the defense of the environment and the territories of indigenous communities (Carruthers, 2008; Dwivedi & Díez, 2008; Urkidi & Walter, 2011). Such mobilisations as well as the analyses that accompany them have been crucial to understand health as the outcome of social processes rather than as an individual condition independent of social context. It also remains important to locate social mobilisation around the social determinants of health in Latin America, such as the tobacco control movement.

The latter has been addressed in descriptive examinations of the tobacco control movement in Latin America (Champagne, Sebrié, & Schoj, 2010). Yet, an understanding of how the tobacco control movement has been able to reformulate the meanings of tobacco consumption and distribution to define locations of power and the strategic scale of action is central to address the structures of health inequalities in the region. For that reason, the article examines the use of international human rights treaties by the tobacco control movement in Argentina through the politics of scale, an approach that has been suggested as long overdue in the literature on the tobacco epidemic (Barnett, Moon, Pearce, Thompson, & Twigg, 2017). Politics of scale refer to the social processes that produce, reproduce and contest the boundaries of particular practices, policies and socio-economic relations (Keil & Mahon, 2009). Scales therefore become spatial arrangements that organise and secure interests to deal with political conflict which can be challenged and transformed (Wissen & Brand, 2011, p. 6). Because political scales are historical and social processes, a particular scale does not necessarily have priority or dominance over others. Such an approach allows an understanding of how spatial arrangements in the form of jurisdictional hierarchies are significant in reproducing health inequalities as well as in social mobilising around the right to health. Politics of scale also include the way in which actors define a social issue around a particular scale is also central to effecting change (Delaney & Leitner, 1997; Kurtz, 2003; Van Lieshout, Dewulf, Aarts, & Termeer, 2011). This process of scale framing also has concrete consequences shaping social practices (Conway, 2009, p. 284).

Approaches to social movements examine how cultural meanings and practices of domination are confronted by redefining relations of power through new identities and counterhegenomic discourses (Alvarez, Dagnino, & Escobar, 1998; Escobar & Alvarez, 1992). Also, the literature on social movements provides insights into the organisation of contestation through networks, access of resources and identification of political opportunities, which allows local contentious politics to become a transnational movement (Dufour, Masson, & Caouette, 2010; McAdam, Mccarthy, & Zald, 1996; Tarrow, 2005). Global legal frameworks then become part of the array of resources and political opportunities that create new discourses to redefine power relations. The international relations literature on global governance also acknowledge how social mobilisation in the form of transnational networks have assisted in shaping global norms and its local implementation (Kardam, 2004).

While the article acknowledges the valuable insights of these approaches, spatial hierarchies are seen as one more element influencing political opportunities, resource mobilisation or the creation of international norms and counterhegemoic discourses. In other words, spatial arrangements are depicted as a container of social interactions rather than the product of materially and discursively constituted relationships (Radcliffe, 2007). The latter is crucial for analysing mobilisation around the right to health in Latin America because spatial hierarchies shape social conditions for mobilisation, which can be contested to produce new scalar arrangements (Conway, 2009; Leitner & Sheppard, 2009).

When approaches on social mobilisations consider politics of scale, the emphasis is on 'scale jumping,' namely the capacity of social groups to move to higher hierarchical levels of state and global legal regulations, to fulfil their social demands (Masson, 2010). These analyses focus on how social groups undertake forum shopping, that is the selection of a human right tribunal to have a favourable decision, to produce a 'boomerang strategy' of pressuring on states via international organisations encourages local change (Keck & Sikkink, 1998). Here, the global scale of international human rights treaties is considered as the most effective hierarchy of action, giving ontological priority to this scale over others. Such an understanding depicts broader scales as 'structures mechanically determining the possibilities of local scales' (Leitner & Sheppard, 2009, p. 235). Thus, the social processes and the structures of power behind the constructions of scales producing and reproducing health inequalities, and the way these scalar arrangements are contested, are overlooked.

Thus, we argue that a politics of scale approach to the right to health, particularly in the case of the use and health effects of tobacco, is useful in understanding how multiple scales, and their constitutive social processes and structures of power and contestation, overlap and connect to obstruct or enhance the right to health in Latin America. On the one hand, the global organisation of tobacco companies and the global reach of international financial institutions connected with national dynamics of economic austerity and export-orientation, promoting the local production and use of tobacco in Argentina and reproducing the social inequalities in the country throughout the 1990s and early 2000s. On the other hand, the visible legacy of local and national human rights struggles in the adoption of international human rights treaties into Argentina's national constitution allowed the tobacco control movement to link the scale of women's bodies to the right to health through the use of CEDAW to change national legislation, tackling the social determinants of the tobacco epidemic in the late 2000s. As such, this approach does not emphasise the effectiveness of the global scale for mobilisation but rather focuses on the socio-spatial processes behind the production of health inequalities and their contestation.

The article also acknowledges the contribution of the study of women's and feminist movements in Latin America, particularly their analyses on their organisation through transnationalised networks (Alvarez, 2014; Dufour et al., 2010; Lopreite, 2010). While the article focuses on how a gender undertanding of tobacco use and distribution has allowed the tobacco control movement in Argentina to access CEDAW mechanisms to transform the national and local social determinants of health, this article does not focus on this movement as a women's or feminist movement. Although the tobacco control movement does consider women a group that needs mobilised and has developed political strategies around women's issues (DiMarco, 2010, p. 165; Dufour et al., 2010), the article examines the framing of tobacco use and distribution through a gendered understanding as a scalar strategy.

The article begins by briefly describing the ways in which the integration of Argentina into the global economy led to the intensification of tobacco production, manufacturing, and commercialisation in the country and its effects on women's health. This informs our understanding of the obstacles faced by the tobacco control movement in Argentina. Second, we examine the strategies civil society organisations used to establish the connections between gender and health in the CEDAW monitoring processes to advance and legitimise their struggle to establish (and enact) national tobacco control legislation. Third, the article discusses how civil society in Argentina continues to link multiple scalar frames to enact action to push for tobacco regulations and enforcement.

## The global and national scales of power in the tobacco epidemic

As mentioned above, political scales are manifestations of the strategies of social groups to extend their control by creating social spatial regulations and arrangements in which scale is actively produced (Swyngedouw, 1997). Scalar arrangements have been influential in the tobacco epidemic in Argentina, particularly in its detrimental effects on the right to health in general and women's health in particular. First, higher political scales in the form of the International Monetary Fund's (IMF) structural adjustment policies of the 1980s and 1990s favoured global tobacco companies. Second, the national scale of state policy has been crucial in internalising global economic imperatives.

The global integration of Argentina's economy in the 1980s and 1990s favoured the production and commercialisation of tobacco products, as well as the concentration of the industry in two global companies. Hit by a debt crisis in 1982, Argentina underwent a series of structural reforms in order to obtain loans from the IMF and the World Bank (WB) to repay its international debt throughout the 1980s and 1990s. Through the imposition of structural adjustment programs (SAPs), the WB and the IMF encouraged the Argentine state to support large farms growing crops for export, including tobacco (Felder & Patroni, 2016). For instance, the liberalisation of trade included in SAPs promoted agricultural exports, including tobacco among large producers (Cao, 2007). Export promotion, also part of SAPs, was also encouraged through tax exemptions to acquire large areas of land and invest in agricultural enterprises, particularly in poor regions such as the northern region of Argentina, characterised by tobacco production (Aráoz, 2007, p. 285). This practice reinforced earlier government support to tobacco growers through the Special Tobacco Fund (STF) started in 1972. The STF is financed by a tax on tobacco use and the funds are redistributed to the tobacco-growing provinces to promote cheap tobacco production and keep the price of cigarettes low (Mejia & Perez-Stable, 2006, p. 53). During the 1990s, there was a large investment flow into the tobacco sector and trade liberalisation and de-regulation also increased market access opportunities for global tobacco companies. Between 1993 and 2000, for example, direct foreign investment in food and tobacco production increased 40%, representing 29% of the Argentinean total GDP in manufacturing, compared to a 28% and 19% of chemical and auto industries respectively (Ernst, 2005, p. 18). This trend was also reflected in the increase of tobacco leaf production and leaf exports by 27% between 1980 and 1995 and 133% between 1980 and 1990 respectively. Cigarette production rose 10.63% between 1980 and 1995 while the volume of cigarette exports in million sticks grew from 11 to 724 between 1980s and 1990 and to 2452 in 1995 (WHO, 2002).

The reliance of the state's export-oriented strategy on tobacco production and commercialisation was further intensified by the financial crisis of 2001. The Argentine government further promoted an economic model based on the export of agricultural commodities, including tobacco, to increase the flow of foreign exchange into the country. The opening of markets and the financial crisis also triggered a process of acquisitions of Argentine tobacco companies by global corporations. In the 2000s, the two major tobacco companies in Argentina, Massaline Particulares S.A., and Nobleza Piccardo, were fully acquired by the global corporations Philip Morris (PM) and British American Tobacco (BAT), which control 70% and 30% of the Argentine tobacco market respectively (Alderete, 2014). Accordingly, the subsidiaries of PM and BAT became the main destination for the tobacco produced in the northern provinces of Argentina (Bercovich, 2004). These provinces produced 80% of tobacco leaf production during the 1990s and early 2000s (Corradini et al., 2005).

The concentration of the tobacco industry as well as Argentina's reliance on producing and exporting agricultural commodities such as tobacco increased the political influence of global tobacco corporations as well as tobacco growers and tobacco leaf buyers in domestic policy who have lobbied the government to avoid the imposition of regulations on the tobacco industry (Sebrie, Barnoya, Perez-Stable, & Glantz, 2005, pp. 53–5). An example of this is the Argentine Senate's lack of ratification of the World Health Organisation (WHO) Framework Convention on Tobacco Control (FCTC), despite its signing by Argentina's Executive branch in 2003, as the FCTC identifies mechanisms to reduce the health, social, and economic damage caused by tobacco production, consumption and distribution. These mechanisms include bans on tobacco advertising and marketing, place warnings on packages, implement measures to protect exposure to second-hand smoking, and promote higher taxes on tobacco products as well as government support for alternatives to tobacco-related economic activities (WHO FCTC, 2009). Overall, the tobacco control movement in Argentina confronted several economic actors at different political scales which had connections to each other. While the WB and the IMF indirectly set the conditions for the growth of the tobacco industry in Argentina throughout the 1980s and 1990s, it was the national state that internalised the structural adjustment policies with the support of sectors of the Ministry of Agriculture, Congress representatives and local legislatures of tobacco growing regions, global tobacco companies (BAT and PM), the Argentinean Tobacco Growers Association (Mejia, Schoj, Barnoya, Flores, & Pérez-Stable, 2008; Ministerio de Agricultura, Ganadería y Pesca de la Nación, 2011). The latter, global companies and the growers' association, are also connected through the International Tobacco Growers Association. The links between the national state and domestic tobacco growers is also evident in cases such as that of Ramon Puerta, Senator and who owned a tobacco-producing farm in northern Argentina the ratification of the FCTC was obstructed in the mid-2000s (Mejia et al., 2008).

The politics of scale of tobacco production and commercialisation have become part of the social determinants of health of non-communicable diseases associated to tobacco use in Argentina. The country has had one of the highest smoking rates in Latin America since the 1990s. By 2014, one in four adults in Argentina smoke (Alderete, 2014). Tobacco production and consumption in the country affected women's health in particular. In the 1990s women accounted for a higher relative proportion of smoking related diseases and mortality than men (Corrao, Guindon, Sharma, & Shookohi, 2000, p. 27). As of 2006, 47% of women and 20% of children were exposed to second-hand smoke (Wipfli et al., 2008, p. 674). In a 2008 study in Buenos Aires, 10% of women continued smoking during pregnancy while an estimated 50% of women were exposed to second-hand smoking during pregnancy (Althabe, Colomar, Gibbons, Belizan, & Buekens, 2008).

The decline in the provision of public health services, which was another product of structural adjustment of the 1980s and 1990s policies and austerity measures implemented in the aftermath of the 2001 crisis, also impacted women as public health care users and unpaid caregivers (Cavagnero, 2008; Lloyd-Sherlock, 2005). Argentine women who smoke or suffer from tobacco-related non-communicable diseases remained vulnerable during the 1990s and 2000s (Batthyanny & Correa, 2010, p. 138; Durand, 2000), particularly as women's access to health care declined. In 2001, for example, only 59% of women were covered by some form of health care insurance (Hernandez Bello, 2004, p. 12). The direct of costs for health care in Argentina related to diseases attributable to tobacco use reached 14% of the GDP in 2006 (Carbajal, 2006). This placed heavier demands on women as unpaid caregivers for children, seniors, and the sick or disabled (Budlender, 2008, p. 9; Durand, 2000). This domestic context prompted the tobacco control movement to contest the existing politics of scale of tobacco production and use in Argentina through the connection of multiple scales, namely international human rights treaties, women's bodies and their health and the household in order to push for an agenda similar to that of the FCTC.

## The multiple scales of human rights

This section explores the ways in the tobacco control movement connected multiple scales to frame the right to health around tobacco-related non-communicable diseases through the lens of women's rights. This, however, is not new in Argentina. During the military dictatorship of the 1970s and early 1980s, mothers of the disappeared, namely the Mothers of the Plaza de Mayo, mobilised around human rights issues in Argentina by linking the personal, that is the scale of the household, to national politics, and later on to international human rights treaties. The movement politicised the scale of the family household by stressing how the individual suffering of mothers was connected to larger structures of power at the national level to make demands to the state (DiMarco, 2010, p. 161). The legacy of this movement is the internalisation of the international human rights treaties into the national constitution.

Constitutional reforms in 1994 (article 75.22) incorporated nine international human rights treaties into the constitution, including the UN CEDAW (Shelton, 2011). CEDAW requires states to guarantee women's rights, support education that contributes to their health, and eliminate all forms of discrimination of women in health care. Conventions such as CEDAW also includes monitoring mechanisms and request regular updates from state parties to track progress against priorities. In addition, the Supreme Court of Argentina has recognised other human rights treaties ratified by Argentina such as the International Covenant on Economic, Social and Cultural Rights (CESR) as having constitutional hierarchy (Council of Europe, 2014, pp. 11–12) and reports to human rights committees are considered relevant to the interpretation of domestic law. This legal context set the stage for the tobacco control movement to connect the scale of women's bodies to national politics and the global scale of international human rights treaties to contest the existing politics of tobacco production and consumption in Argentina.

Argentine Smoke-Free Alliance (ALIAR) and the Inter American Heart Foundation, based in the United States, which has an affiliate in FIC-A (Fundación Interamericana del Corazón Argentina), have led the tobacco control movement in Argentina. ALIAR was established in 2007 and represents an alliance of more than 100 civil society organisations committed to tobacco control which include human rights advocates, health workers and researchers, professional medical associations and environmental organisations (Champagne et al., 2010). FIC-A serves as the secretariat for ALIAR (Champagne et al., 2010). The mandate of the FIC-A is to address the contributors to cardiovascular disease, for which tobacco use is a prominent risk factor. In partnership with the O'Neill Institute for National and Global Health Law, ALIAR and FIC-A mobilised to counter the influence of global tobacco corporations and domestic tobacco growers in Argentina's health policy through shadow reports to the CEDAW Committee. Shadow reports are formal mechanisms that UN bodies use which permit civil society to participate in monitoring the implementation of UN international human rights treaties. These shadow reports provide an alternative account to formal national reports on of the implementation of treaties (Cabrera & Gostin, 2013). The partnership with the O'Neil Institute also shows how challenges to political economic structures behind health inequalities struggles do not have to cover larger political scales but rather about connecting local spaces (Gibson-Graham, 2002, p. 32).

In a 2010 shadow report presented to the CEDAW Committee, ALIAR and FIC-A demonstrated that Argentina was not complying with Articles 3, 10, and 12, which respectively address the state party's obligation to guarantee women's rights, facilitate access to information to guarantee women's and their families' well-being, and eliminate discrimination against women in health care (ALIAR et al., 2010, p. 6). The report argued that the lack of compliance arose from the absence of a national policy regulating tobacco advertising (which heavily targeted women) and a failure to promote smoke-free spaces, thereby increasing women's and children's exposure to secondhand smoke. The shadow report also indicated that state policies promote the tobacco industry such as the STF, which undermine efforts to protect women's health from targeting tobacco industry marketing. The submission highlighted the need to approach tobacco control through a gender lens (ALIAR et al., 2010, p. 15). In the same way, the report cites CEDAW's Committee's commentaries and reports that call for a gender perspective in understanding the social determinants of health and the gendered effects of tobacco smoking. Finally, the report called for the adoption of national tobacco control legislation and the ratification of FCTC to uphold country's international commitments (Cabrera & Carballo, 2014, p. 238). ALIAR and FIC-A also argued that women's vulnerability to secondhand smoke exposure increases with more extreme poverty.

The shadow reports show the framing of the right to health through the connections of multiple scales in order transform the social and political determinants of the tobacco epidemic in Argentina. The national and the global scale of international human rights treaties are implicated through Argentina's constitution, which allows for the use of international human rights treaties as a tool to enforce the human right to health domestically. The consequences of tobacco use and exposure among women encouraged ALIAR and FIC-A to view this epidemic through the scale of women's bodies, the household and the locality. The multiscale framing of the right to health offered the tobacco control movement a route to engage with the CEDAW monitoring mechanisms. These organisations focused on consumption rates and exposure to secondhand smoke in the household, workplace, and public spaces, highlighting the marginalisation of women's health in everyday interactions and settings at multiple political scales. The coalition also highlighted the role of national structures of political power in the form of STF, economic austerity and declining health services in undermining women's health.

The CEDAW Shadow report, in addition to the coalition's mobilisation at the national level, influenced the approval of a national tobacco control law in Argentina's Congress in 2011. The Law 26.687 on Advertising and Promotion and Tobacco Product Consumption bans tobacco advertising and sponsorship, forces manufacturers to put public health warnings on cigarette packets and prohibits smoking in enclosed spaces such as bars, restaurants, covered stadiums, schools, hospitals, and workplaces. It also makes it illegal to sell cigarettes to under-aged youth and ends the practice of selling single cigarettes. The law imposes fines of those who fail to comply. Yet, there are several loopholes and exceptions within this law. For instance, advertising can take place at the point of sale and smoking is permitted in parks, public squares, and open-air stadiums, and clubs of smokers (Presidencia de la Nacion Argentina, 2011).

Also, lack of regulations to limit the various exceptions in the law has allowed tobacco companies avenues to continue to circumvent the law. For instance, tobacco companies could turn any space such as a nightclub or a bar into a point of sale in order to advertise. In lieu of sponsorships, tobacco companies implemented corporate social responsibility (CSR) programmes as a way of promote their cigarettes. For instance, tobacco companies have financed anti-poverty campaigns in the form of road pavement in poor neighbourhoods in order to include the logo and name of the company in these CSR programmes (Lipcovich, 2012). In the same way, any enclosed space could be turned into a smokers' club (FIC-A et al., 2012; Hecha la Ley, 2013).

For these reasons, FIC-A, along its international partners, employed other international human rights treaties in a similar manner to the way they had engaged with CEDAW. For example, they presented the shadow report presented by the same coalition to the CESR committee in 2011. In their report, the coalition placed emphasis on article 7 and 12 of the CESR, which refers to the right to safe and healthy working conditions and improvements in environmental and industrial hygiene (FIC-A et al., 2011, p. 9). In this way, the report connected the threat of second-hand smoking to economic rights, as in the right to a healthy environment in the workplace. By doing so, it pointed out the weaknesses and legal gaps in Argentine's tobacco control legislation and indicated how these gaps reflect the lack of implementation of the FCTC as the legislation does not comply with the maximum international standard set by the WHO convention (2011, p. 11, 18). In its account to the CESR committee, FIC-A introduced taxation and pricing as new issues, which is particularly important in Argentina as cigarettes in the country are the cheapest in the region (Pan American Health Organization [PAHO], 2013, p. 20). The report refers to article 2 of the CESR which indicates the state parties' obligation to allocate the maximum available resources to realise and protect economic, social and cultural rights to justify the need of state intervention to increase taxes and prices on cigarettes in Argentina to reduce tobacco consumption (2011, p. 16). Thus, this shadow report framed the right to health through the scale of the workplace with the enforcement of this economic right in national and international law.

Subsequently, the continued mobilisation of ALIAR and FIC-A prompted the enactment of specific regulatory legislation in 2013, prohibiting direct and indirect promotion and advertising, including the use of non-traditional advertising such as television screens and movable and luminous signs. The only form of advertising allowed is the use of banners at the point of sale (Ministerio de Salud Argentina, 2013). The regulations specify the characteristics of open and enclosed spaces as well as the characteristics required to turn a site into a retail location or a smokers' club. For instance, the regulations indicate that a smokers' club cannot have employees and must not have a commercial activity (Hecha la Ley, 2013). This latter measure aims to prevent tobacco companies from changing any location into commercial site or a smokers' club.

In the aftermath of challenging the scalar arrangements of the tobacco industry, the tobacco control movement constructed new scales of national regulation, including the integration of some stipulations of the FCTC into national legislation such as the banning of advertising and the promotion of smoke-free environments. This has been influential in setting a context where smoking rates among adult women in Argentina decreased from 34% in 2000 to 18.4% in 2015 (World Bank, 2017). In 2005, 52% of people in Argentina were exposed to second-hand smoking. This percentage decreased to 40.2% in 2009 and 36.3% in 2013 (Secretaría de Programación para la Prevención de la Drogadicción y Lucha contra el Narcotráfico [SPPDLN], 2016, p. 30).

It is worth noting that such changes in legislation took place during the presidential administration of Cristina Fernandez de Kirchner (2007–2015), who is considered part of the Latin American Pink Tide movement. The Pink Tide refers to the rise of left-wing governments in South America opposing the market liberalisation and austerity measures promoted by IMF and WB from 2000 to 2014 (Spronk, 2014). While a change in policy direction could have provided the tobacco control movement in Argentina political opportunities to push for its agenda, this was not necessarily central to the coalition as the administration of Fernandez de Kirchner was reliant on taxes on agricultural exports for revenues to fund social programmes. This included the continued reliance on agricultural exports of tobacco (Gruss, 2014).

The ALIAR and FIC-A coalition has focused most of its reporting and advocacy on tobacco consumption and second-hand exposure. Other social processes behind tobacco consumption and distribution and women's right to health continue to be overlooked. For instance, limited attention has been placed on women as tobacco producers. This is particularly significant in Argentina because it is the sixth largest worldwide producer of tobacco leaf (Tovar, 2012). The Argentine tobacco industry employs nearly half a million people, including significant numbers of women and children (Tovar, 2012). Tobacco cultivation introduces specific health risks as a result of transdermal nicotine absorption (Schmitt, Schmitt, Kouimintzis, & Kirch, 2007). These health hazards affect women and children mostly who work in this industry under precarious conditions (Soto Baquero & Klein, 2012). A focus on women as tobacco producers might allow ALIAR and FIC-A to build support for the ratification of the FCTC among female workers in the producing tobacco provinces of the north of Argentina, especially since the FCTC also includes economic support to alternative livelihoods for tobacco farmers and farm workers in Article 17. Nevertheless, the strategy used by ALIAR and FIC-A based on human rights treaties paved the way to address this issue through their work in the shadow report in the CESR Committee.

## Conclusions

This article employed a scalar analysis to explore recent tobacco control movement activities in Argentina. Such an approach recognises that changes in scale offer different possibilities for how an issue is framed, what actions can be envisioned to address it, and who are the stakeholders involved thereby changing the conditions, opportunities and structures for action. The tobacco control movement in Argentina is fundamentally engaged in a struggle of relations of power that range from the intimate, embodied level of the individual to the supranational level of the FCTC. By examining scales, we are able to illustrate how the tobacco control movement in Argentina employed policy discourses and frames at varying scales to argue that the women's right to health was being violated.

The Argentine case illustrates how international human rights frameworks do not automatically or mechanically protect the right to health at the local level. Rather, the contestation of existing political scales that obstruct the right to health and the framing of tobacco-related diseases through different scales are central to bringing about more concrete legislation that materialises international treaties domestically and addresses the particular needs of citizens, especially women. Such a strategy has been effective in changing national and local socio-political determinants of health related to the tobacco epidemic to the extent that the same coalition has created a guide for the elaboration of shadow reports to be presented at UN bodies in relation to the implementation of tobacco controls for other civil society organisations (FIC-A and O'Neil Institute, 2012). In this case study, the tobacco control movement in Argentina connected the effects on global and national scales of tobacco production and commercialisation on women's bodies and their position in the household, related them to the obligation of the Argentine state to protect, respect and fulfil the right to health contained in the national constitution and international human rights treaties through the lens of women's rights, and later one through an approach to economic rights. In this sense, the framing through women's rights has been key to make these scalar connections. For instance, indigenous women in Chiapas, Mexico, have addressed their subordinate position in their households and local villages as well as the political autonomy of their indigenous community through the language of women's rights in international human rights law (Speed, 2008). Still, mobilisation around women's rights also depends on the historical legacies of concrete forms of contestation by feminist and women's movements at the national level, as reflected in the case of Argentina.

A scalar approach to the right to health in Latin America shows how a solution to the global tobacco epidemic needs to go beyond a focus on individual tobacco use and health in order to consider sources of inequality, and the structures at the global and national level that create them, which impair women's health and promote the profits of tobacco companies. This in turn opens spaces for institutions and civil society organisations that are pushing not only for tobacco control policies but also for gender-specific health and social agendas at different political scales.

## Acknowledgements

We would like to thank Dr. Lorraine Greaves and the Canadian Institutes of Health Research (Project GGH-84622) for their support in 2008 of our initial work on gender, globalization and tobacco control in Argentina. We thank the reviewers for their thoughtful feedback throughout the manuscript development process.

## Disclosure statement

No potential conflict of interest was reported by the author(s).

## References

Alderete, M. (2014). *Health is not negotiable: Civil society against the tobacco industry's strategies in Latin America. Case studies* (F. Casciaro, Trans.). Buenos Aires: Fundaciö Interamericana del Corazön Argentina (FIC Argentina).

Althabe, F., Colomar, M., Gibbons, L., Belizan, J. M., & Buekens, P. (2008). Tabaquismo durante el embarazo en Argentina y Uruguay. *Medicina, 68*, 48–54.

Alvarez, S. E. (2014). Ambivalent engagements, paradoxical effects: Latin American feminist and women's movements and/in/against development. In C. Verschuur, I. Guérin, & H. Guétat-Bernard (Eds.), *Under development: Gender. Gender, development and social change* (pp. 211–235). London: Palgrave Macmillan.

Alvarez, S. E., Dagnino, E., & Escobar, A. (1998). *Cultures of politics/politics of cultures: Re-visioning Latin American social movements*. Boulder, CO: Westview Press.

Aráoz, H. M. (2007). *Economía politica del clientelismo. Democracia y capitalismo en los márgenes*. Cordoba: Editorial Brujas.

Argentine Smoke-Free Alliance (ALIAR), FIC-A, Argentine Cardiology Foundation, Centre for the Study of State and Society, Foundation for Women's Study and Research, Argentine Cardiology Society, the Foundation for the Development of Sustainable Policy, the O'Neill Institute for National and Global Health Law and the Campaign for Tobacco-Free Kids. (2010, July). *Shadow report to the sixth periodic report by the government of Argentina.* Prepared for the UN committee on the elimination of discrimination against women.

Barnett, R., Moon, G., Pearce, J., Thompson, L., & Twigg, L. (2017). *Smoking geographies: Space, place and tobacco.* Chichester: John Wiley and Sons.

Batthyanny, K., & Correa, S. (2010). Gender, health and poverty in Latin America. In G. Sen & P. Ostlin (Eds.), *Gender equity in health* (pp. 126–160). New York: Routledge.

Bercovich, A. (2004, July 25). El Camino. *Pagina 12*. Retrieved from https://www.pagina12.com.ar/diario/suplementos/cash/17-1425-2004-07-26.html

Budlender, D. (2008). *The statistical evidence on care and non-care work across six countries.* UNRISD Gender and Development Programme Paper, 4.

Cabrera, O. A, & Carballo, J. (2014). Chapter 13: Tobacco control in Latin America. In A. Mitchell & T. Voon (Eds.), *The global tobacco epidemic and the law* (pp. 235–257). Cheltenham: Edward Elgar. doi:10.4337/9781783471522.00021

Cabrera, O., & Gostin, L. (2013). Global tobacco control: A vital component of the right to health. In J. Zuniga, S. Marks, & L. Gostin (Eds.), *Advancing the right to human health* (pp. 261–274). Oxford: Oxford University Press.

Cao, H. (2007). Las políticas regionales en la Argentina de los '90. *Documentos y aportes en administración pública y gestión estatal, 8*, 27–51.

Carbajal, M. (2006, November 5). El Costo de las Muertes por Tabaco. *Pagina 12*.

Carruthers, D. V. (2008). Popular environmentalism and social justice in Latin America. In D. V. Carruthers (Ed.), *Environmental justice in Latin America. Problems, promise, and practice* (pp. 1–22). Cambridge, MA: MIT.

Cavagnero, E. (2008). Health sector reforms in Argentina and the performance of the health financing system. *Health Policy, 88*, 88–99.

Champagne, B. M., Sebrié, E., & Schoj, V. (2010). The role of organized civil society in tobacco control in Latin American and the Caribbean. *Salud pública de México, 52*(Suppl. 2), S330–S339.

Conway, J. (2009). The empire, the movement and the politics of scale: Considering the world social forum. In R. Keil & R. Mahon (Eds.), *Leviathan undone? Towards a political economy of scale* (pp. 281–300). Vancouver: UBC Press.

Corradini, E., Zilocchi, H., Cuesta, R., Segesso, R., Jiménez, M. L., & Musco, J. M. (2005). *Caracterización Del Sector Productor Tabacalero En La Republica Argentina*. Buenos Aires: Universidad Catolica Argentina Santa Maria de los

Buenos Aires. Retrieved from http://www.minagri.gob.ar/sitio/areas/tabaco/informes/publicaciones/_archivos// 000002-Estudios/000002-Caracterizaci%C3%B3n%20del%20Sector%20Tabacalero%20Argentino/000001-Informe %203%C2%BA%20Versi%C3%B3n%20-%20Junio%202005.pdf

Corrao, M. A., Guindon, E., Sharma, N., Shookohi, D.F. (2000). *Tobacco control country profile*. Atlanta: American Cancer Society.

Council of Europe. (2014). *Report on the implementation of international human rights treaties into domestic law and the role of courts*. Study 690/2012, Rome.

Delaney, D., & Leitner, H. (1997). The political construction of scale. *Political Geography, 16,* 93–97.

DiMarco, G. (2010). Women's movements in Argentina. Tensions and articulations. In E. Maier & N. Lebon (Eds.), *Women's activism in Latin America and the Caribbean: Engendering social justice, democratizing citizenship* (pp. 159–174). New Brunswick, NJ: Rutgers University Press.

Dufour, P., Masson, D., & Caouette, D. (2010). Introduction. In P. Dufour, D. Masson, & D. Caouette (Eds.), *Solidarities beyond borders: Transnationalizing women's movements* (pp. 1–34). Vancouver: UBC Press.

Durand, T. (2000). *Flexibilizando cuerpos:(in) equidad de género en trabajo y salud. publicación: Informe final del concurso: Democracia, derechos sociales y equidad; y Estado, política y conflictos sociales*. Buenos Aires: Programa Regional de Becas CLACSO.

Dwivedi, O. P., & Díez, J. (2008). *Global environmental challenges: Perspectives from the South*. Peterborough, ON: Broadview Press.

Ernst, C. (2005). *The FDI – employment link in a globalizing world: The case of Argentina, Brazil and Mexico*. ILO Employment Strategy Papers, 2005/17.

Escobar, A., & Alvarez, S. E. (1992). *The making of social movements in Latin America: Identity, strategy, and democracy*. Boulder, CO: Westview Press.

Felder, R., & Patroni, V. (2016). Precarious work in recession and growth: A new structural feature of labor markets in Argentina? *Review of Radical Political Economics*, 1–22. doi:10.1177/0486613416635053

Fundacion Interamericana del Corazon Argentina (FIC-A), Centre for the Study of State and Society, the O'Neill Institute for National and Global Health Law. (2011, November). *Shadow report to the periodic report by the government of Argentina*. Presented to the UN Committee on Economic, Social and Cultural Rights. Retrieved from http://www2.ohchr.org/english/bodies/cescr/docs/ngos/ONeill_FIC_Fundeps_Argentina47_en.pdf.

Fundacion Interamericana del Corazon Argentina (FIC-A), Fundacion Interamericana del Corazon Mexico, Aliança de Controle do Tabagismo, Corporate Accountability International. (2012). *Health is non-negotiable. Civil society against the tobacco industry's strategies in Latin America*. Buenos Aires. Retrieved from http://www.ficargentina. org/images/stories/Documentos/reportes_de_casos_lsns_ingles.pdf

Fundacion Interamericana del Corazon Argentina (FIC-A) and O'Neill Institute for National and Global Health Law at Georgetown University. (2012). *Guía para la elaboración y presentación de reportes sombra sobre tabaco ante organismos de derechos humanos de las Naciones Unidas*. Retrieved from http://ficargentina.org/index.php? option=com_content&view=article&id=248:guia-para-la-elaboracion-y-presentacion-de-reportes-sombra&catid= 92:publicaciones&Itemid=84&lang=es

Gibson-Graham, J. K. (2002). Beyond global vs. local: Economic politics outside the binary frame. In A. Herod & M. Wright (Eds.), *Geographies of power: Placing scale* (pp. 25–60). Oxford: Blackwell Publishers.

Gruss, B. (2014). *After the boom: Commodity prices and economic growth in Latin America and the Caribbean*. IMF Working Paper, 14/154.

Hecha la ley, hecha la forma de evitar la trampa. (2013, May 30). *Pagina 12*. Retrieved from https://www.pagina12.com. ar/diario/sociedad/3-221139-2013-05-30.html

Hernandez Bello, A. (2004, April 29–30). *Equidad de Género y Reforma del Sector Salud en América Latina. Situación y Perspectivas*. Paper for the International Seminar Gender Equity in Health Sector Reform: Opportunities and Challenges, Washington.

Jelin, E., Zammit, J. A., & Thomson, M. (1990). *Women and social change in Latin America*. Geneva: United Nations Research Institute for Social Development.

Kardam, N. (2004). The emerging global gender equality regime from neoliberal and constructivist perspectives in international relations. *International Feminist Journal of Politics, 6,* 85–109.

Keck, E., & Sikkink, K. (1998). *Activists beyond borders: Advocacy networks in international politics*. Ithaca, NY: Cornell University Press.

Keil, R., & Mahon, R. (2009). Introduction. In R. Keil & R. Mahon (Eds.), *Leviathan undone? Towards a political economy of scale* (pp. 3–26). Vancouver: UBC Press.

Kurtz, H. E. (2003). Scale frames and counter-scale frames: Constructing the problem of environmental injustice. *Political Geography, 22,* 887–916.

Lebon, N. (2010). Introduction. Women building plural democracy in Latin America and the Caribbean. In E. Maier & N. Lebon (Eds.), *Women's activism in Latin America and the Caribbean: Engendering social justice, democratizing citizenship* (pp. 3–25). New Brunswick, NJ: Rutgers University Press.

Leitner, H., & Sheppard, E. (2009). The spatiality of contentious politics. More than politics of scale. In R. Keil & R. Mahon (Eds.), *Leviathan undone? Towards a political economy of scale* (pp. 231–246). Vancouver: UBC Press.

Lipcovich, P. (2012, June 11). El Lobby Tabacalero. *Pagina 12*. Retrieved from https://www.pagina12.com.ar/diario/elpais/subnotas/1-59311-2012-06-11.html

Lloyd-Sherlock, P. (2005). Health sector reform in Argentina: A cautionary tale. *Social Science and Medicine*, 60, 1893–1903.

Lopreite, D. (2010). Transnational activism and the Argentine women's movement. In P. Dufour, D. Masson, & D. Caouette (Eds.), *Solidarities beyond borders: Transnationalizing women's movements* (pp. 127–148). Vancouver: UBC Press.

Masson, D. (2010). Transnationalizing feminist and women's movements. A scalar approach. In P. Dufour, D. Masson, & D. Caouette (Eds.), *Solidarities beyond borders: Transnationalizing women's movements* (pp. 35–55). Vancouver: UBC Press.

McAdam, D., Mccarthy, J. D., & Zald, M. N. (1996). *Comparative perspectives on social movements: Political opportunities, mobilizing structures, and cultural framings*. Cambridge: Cambridge University Press.

Mejia, R., & Perez-Stable, E. J. (2006). Tobacco epidemic in Argentina: The cutting edge of Latin America. *Prevention and Control*, 2(1), 49–55.

Mejia, R., Schoj, V., Barnoya, J., Flores, M. L., & Pérez-Stable, E. J. (2008). Tobacco industry strategies to obstruct the FCTC in Argentina. *CVD Prevention and Control*, 3(4), 173–179.

Ministerio de Agricultura, Ganadería y Pesca de la Nación. (2011). *Regional impact of the framework agreement of tobacoo control*. Buenos Aires: Ministerio de Agricultura, Ganadería y Pesca de la Nación.

Ministerio de Salud Argentina. (2013). *Se reglamentó la ley que prohíbe la promoción del consumo de tabaco*. Programa Nacional de Control de Tabaco. Retrieved from http://www.msal.gob.ar/tabaco/index.php/component/content/article/4-destacados-slide/333-se-reglamento-la-ley-que-prohibe-la-promocion-del-consumo-de-tabaco

Molyneux, M. (2001). *Women's movements in international perspective: Latin America and beyond*. New York: Palgrave.

Pan American Health Organization (PAHO). (2013). *Tobacco control report for the region of the Americas*. Washington, DC. Retrieved from http://www2.paho.org/hq/index.php?option=com_docman&task=doc_view&gid=24768&itemid&Itemid=270

Presidencia de la Nacion Argentina. (2011, June 13). Ley 26687. *Boletín Oficial*.

Radcliffe, S. A. (2007). FORUM: Latin American indigenous geographies of fear: Living in the shadow of racism, lack of development, and antiterror measures. *Annals of the Association of American Geographers*, 97(2), 385–397.

Schmitt, N. M., Schmitt, J., Kouimintzis, D. J., & Kirch, W. (2007). Health risks in tobacco farm workers—a review of the literature. *Journal of Public Health*, 15(4), 255–264.

Sebrie, E. M., Barnoya, J., Perez-Stable, E., & Glantz, S. (2005). *Tobacco industry dominating national tobacco policy making in Argentina, 1966–2005*. San Francisco: Center for Tobacco Control Research and Education. Tobacco Control Policy Making: International.

Secretaría de Programación para la Prevención de la Drogadicción y Lucha contra el Narcotráfico (SPPDLN). (2016). *Informe epidemiológico sobre el Consumo de Tabaco en la Argentina*. Buenos Aires: SPPDLN.

Shelton, D. (2011). Introduction. In D. Shelton (Ed.), *International law and domestic legal systems* (pp. 1–22). Oxford: Oxford University Press.

Soto Baquero, F., & Klein, E. (2012). *Empleo y condiciones de Trabajo De Mujeres Temporeras Agricolas*. Roma: OIT, CEPAL, FAO.

Speed, S. (2008). *Rights in rebellion: Indigenous struggle and human rights in Chiapas*. Stanford, CA: Stanford University Press.

Spronk, S. (2014). Pink tide? Neoliberalism and its alternatives in Latin America. *Canadian Journal of Latin American and Caribbean Studies*, 33(65), 173–186.

Swyngedouw, E. (1997). Neither global nor local: Glocalisation and the politics of scale. In K. Cox (Ed.), *Spaces of globalisation: Reasserting the power of the local* (pp. 133–166). New York: Guilford Press.

Tarrow, S. G. (2005). *The new transnational activism*. New York: Cambridge University Press.

Tovar, J. (2012). *Tobacco cultivation in Latin America*. Bogota: Universidad de los Andes-Facultad de Economia-CEDE.

Urkidi, L., & Walter, M. (2011). Dimensions of environmental justice in anti-gold mining movements in Latin America. *Geoforum*, 42, 683–695.

Van Lieshout, M., Dewulf, A., Aarts, N., & Termeer, C. (2011). Do scale frames matter? Scale frame mismatches in the decision making process about a "mega farm" in a small Dutch village. *Ecology and Society*, 16(1), 1–38.

Wipfli, H., Avila-Tang, E., Navas-Acien, A., Kim, S., Onicescu, G., Yuan, J., ... Samet, J. M. (2008). Secondhand smoke exposure among women and children: Evidence from 31 countries. *American Journal of Public Health*, 98(4), 672–679.

Wissen, M., & Brand, U. (2011). Approaching the internationalization of the state: An introduction. *Antipode*, 43(1), 1–11.

World Bank. (2017). Smoking prevalence, females (% of adults) Argentina. *Databank*. Retrieved from http://data.worldbank.org/indicator/SH.PRV.SMOK.FE?locations=AR&page=6

World Health Organization (WHO). (2002). *Argentina. Smoking prevalence. Tobacco economy*. Retrieved from http://www.who.int/tobacco/media/en/Argentina.pdf

World Health Organisation Framework Convention on Tobacco Control (WHO FCTC). (2009). *History of the WHO framework convention on tobacco control*. Geneva: World Health Organization.

# The decriminalisation of abortion in Colombia as cautionary tale. Social movements, numbers and socio-technical struggles in the promotion of health as a right

Oscar Javier Maldonado ⓘ

**ABSTRACT**

This paper discusses the complexity of contemporary struggles for collective health in Colombia, by analysing the efforts of different actors to inscribe abortion as a matter of public health and as a human right. In 2006 the Colombian Constitutional Court (Sentence C 355 of 2006) partially decriminalised abortion in specific circumstances. Such a change in regulation was the result of the strategic coordination of international organisations, researchers and women's social movements. These groups produced a powerful network of international regulation and epidemiological data about abortion's mortality and burden of disease in order to move the discussion from the moral field to public health and international law. Despite the significance of the sentence in terms of civil rights, ten years after the regulation there is no clarity about its impact. Conservative sectors within the government have limited the operation of the regulation, through eliciting convoluted rules for hospitals and care providers. On the other hand, data about safe abortions are weak and precarious. Recently groups opposed of abortion have exploited such weakness to undermine the impact of the decriminalisation and to criticise the justification of legalising abortion as a matter of public health.

## Abortion and sexual and reproductive rights in Colombia

In Latin America, the decriminalisation of abortion and the promotion of other reproductive rights have been the result of the work of civil society (Baer, 2002). Women's organisations and international public health authorities have promoted a public debate about the consequences of unsafe abortion and, in general, about reproductive rights in universities, media and civil courts. In the case of Colombia such work has been framed into the civil rights protected by the National Constitution of 1991. Different social movements have used the mechanisms of political participation opened up by this constitution.

The decriminalisation of abortion in specific circumstances in Colombia was the result of the work of feminist scholars and women's organisations. In addition to their local work in media, street demonstrations and courts, they recruited international healthcare authorities and sexual and reproductive health organisations such as Planned Parenthood and the Alan Guttmacher Institute (AGI). They strategically situated the discussion about abortion as a matter of public health and human rights, moving the debate from the traditional moral and philosophical confrontations.

The controversy about abortion in Colombia has its origins in the decade of the 1970s with the introduction of reproductive technologies, birth control policies, second-wave feminism and the international impact of US legalisation (Roe vs Wade, 1973). These elements triggered a fight for the social and medical control of sexuality and reproduction between the state – influenced by the Catholic Church and social groups – and international networks promoting women and sexual and reproductive rights (Maldonado, 2014; Ruibal, 2015; Viveros, 1996, 2003; Viveros & Gil, 2006). Since then, many bills tried to change regulation through parliamentary mechanisms. Since the 2000s the strategy changed and women groups focused their actions on influencing High Courts, specifically the Constitutional Court (Jaramillo & Alonso, 2008). Such strategy has been successful in decriminalising abortion in the region and in the promotion of other sexual and reproductive rights such as the same-sex right to adoption and civil union.

In the last five decades, eight bills and four Constitutional lawsuits were presented to decriminalise abortion in Colombia. The latest request was presented by the Colombian lawyer Monica Roa, representative of the organisation Womeńs Link Worldwide. This lawsuit lifted the total ban by allowing the 'voluntary interruption of pregnancy' in the following cases: (i) when a doctor certifies that the life or health of the pregnant woman is threatened; (ii) when a doctor certifies that the foetus has an abnormality incompatible with life; (iii) when a pregnancy results from rape, incest or unconsented embryo transplant (Sentence C 355 of 2006, p. 301).[1]

Although in many ways Roe v. Wade (1973) set the rhetoric of those groups advocating for a change in legislation regarding abortion in Colombia, in terms of legal strategy such groups constructed abortion as a matter of public health and human rights, rather than a matter of individual choice. Accordingly, the decriminalisation of abortion has been promoted as a public health intervention, intended to reduce mortality rates of women forced to use risky and unregulated practices (Maldonado, 2014).

This paper discusses the complexity of contemporary struggles for collective health in Colombia, by analysing the efforts of different actors to inscribe abortion as a matter of public health and as a human right. The decriminalisation of abortion was the result of the strategic coordination of international organisations, researchers and women's social movements. These groups produced a powerful network of international regulation and epidemiological data about abortion's mortality and burden of disease in order to move the discussion from the moral field to public health and international law.

In what follows, this article describes the efforts of women organisations and other interest groups to transform the debate about abortion in Colombia into a matter of International Law and Public Health. Firstly, it provides an analysis of the role of statistics and quantification in the success of the prolife strategic litigation. Numbers and a sociology of quantification contributes to understand the development of the controversy after the decriminalisation of abortion and the justification strategies elicited by both parts. Secondly, it describes the bureaucratic obstacles and difficulties in the enforcement of the Court decision. The opposition of high officials and the lack of data infrastructure have made extremely difficult the access to safe abortion in the country. Finally, this article reflects on the power and fragility of numbers. It shows the changing strategies of conservative groups that oppose sexual and reproductive rights. These groups have contested 'official' statistics to undermine the definition of abortion as a public health concern.

Despite the significance of the decision in terms of civil rights, ten years after the regulation there is no clarity about its impact. Conservative sectors within the government have limited the operation of the regulation, through eliciting convoluted rules for hospitals and care providers. On the other hand, data about safe abortions are weak and precarious. Recently, groups against abortion have exploited such weakness to undermine the impact of the decriminalisation and to criticise the justification of legalising abortion as a matter of public health.

This story provides an interesting case for analysing the political, legal and technical challenges that social movements face in tackling social and gender inequalities in healthcare. A socio-technical approach to the development of this controversy shows the importance of data infrastructures in the attainment of political objectives, and the entanglements between knowledge, regulation and grass-root processes.

## Civil society, evidence and strategic litigation

The study of abortion in Colombia has been from diverse political approaches and disciplines, from theological and philosophical perspectives (Cotes, 2005), public health and medicine (Alan Guttmacher Institute [AGI], 2006, 2011), economics and sociology (Faúndes & Barzelatto, 2005; González, 2005; Gómez, 2006; Viveros, 1996; Viveros & Gil, 2006; Zamudio, 2000), to legal studies (Hoyos, 2005; Jaramillo & Alonso, 2008; Velazquez, 2006), among others. Within this scholarship gender studies have explored in detail the social dimensions of this debate and its implications in terms of gender politics. These works have understood the debate as a cultural and political fight between traditionalist and modern conceptions of the state and society (Viveros, 1996; Jaramillo & Alonso, 2008; La Mesa por la Vida y la Salud de las Mujeres [MVSM], 2009; Dalén, 2011). From this perspective, some works have analysed the discourses and rhetoric of the groups in debate (Dalén, 2011; Viveros, 1996), others have analysed the role of experts (Maldonado, 2014; Viveros, 1996) and the role of women's social movements (Jaramillo & Alonso, 2008; MVSM, 2009).

Other academic works have studied the legal frame used to build the decision C 355 of 2006. Jaramillo and Alonso (2008) trace the two strategies developed by the organisation involved in the lawsuit, access to the mass media and the process of the lawsuit. By doing so, they argue, there is transformation in the conceptual apparatus that the decision introduced to the National Constitutional tradition. The C 355, according to the authors, makes a distinction between 'life as a good' and 'life as a right'.

Although engagement and concern with women's health of this scholarship is shared by many, these works have a tendency to approach only the groups in favour of legalising abortion, ignoring some of civil society's other expressions of civil and political mobilisation. Social movements have had increasing impact on the relationships between knowledge and politics, specifically between biomedical knowledge, regulation and healthcare provision (Brown & Zavestoski, 2004; Epstein, 1996; Murphy, 2012). These movements have learnt about the importance of strategically influencing the state's decision making. Recent work (Ruibal, 2015) has addressed the organisation of a counter-reformation in Colombia that has gone beyond traditional actors such as the Catholic Church, involving highly placed officers in government and religious grass-roots movements.

This paper focuses on the political use of numbers, specifically the quantification of the burden of abortion in the discussion about sexual and reproductive rights in Colombia and in Latin America. During litigation and discussion in the Constitutional Court, the production of figures about the death and illness caused by unsafe abortion was a key argument in favour of decriminalisation. However, once the change of regulation had taken place, health authorities noted the difficulties of keeping a reliable register of legal and illegal voluntary interruptions to pregnancy. This lack of statistics and clinical register have contributed to the misinformation and confusion about the limits of the legality of abortion in Colombia. This is partially orchestrated by conservative officers within public institutions and the government, such as the former General Prosecutor Alejando Ordoñez (Ruibal, 2015).

Figures and statistics have become the centre of discussions about abortion in the country and the region. The effort to decriminalise abortion in Chile and Mexico has triggered a discussion about the reliability of the data produced by national governments and international organisations about mortality and burden of disease related to unsafe abortion. In 2012 the Chilean epidemiologist Elard Koch published a series of papers questioning the methodology used by the AGI to estimate unsafe abortion in Mexico and Colombia. This opened a controversy about the reliability of the statistics about abortion and most importantly about the impact of the decriminalisation of abortion in the reduction of maternal mortality (MMR) and post-abortion emergencies. Religious universities and anti-abortion[2] groups have embraced this critique to reopen the discussions about decriminalisation and the status of abortion as a matter of public health.

Social movements and patients' organisations have been key actors in the shaping of contemporary healthcare. Their work has transformed standards of care, advocating for the inclusion of new technologies and treatments and for the establishment of new relations between health professionals and particular groups of patients (Brown & Zavestoski, 2004; Epstein, 1996). Their advocacy has involved in many cases a deep engagement with the production of biomedical and technical knowledge. These groups have contested the design of medical trials, supported and encouraged research on specific drugs and have raised some issues as matters of concern through the production and communication of statistics and other forms of evidence (Adams, 2016; Akrich, Leaneb, Roberts, & Arriscado, 2014; Epstein, 1996; Murphy, 2012). The importance of the production of evidence in the governance of contemporary healthcare has been recognised by patients' organisations and some of them have critically appropriated this framework to enhance their own claims (Akrich et al., 2014; Moreira, 2012).

Drawing on sociology of quantification this paper explores the strategic role of statistics and indicators in the contemporary struggles for sexual and reproductive rights in Colombia. Science and technology studies (STS) and sociology have shown an increasing interest in studying the numbers and effects of quantification in policy, public affairs (Desrosières, 1998) and healthcare (Epstein, 1996; Murphy, 2012). The sociological analysis of quantification has focused on numbers' practical uses and the ways in which these are related to wider networks of practices (Desrosières, 1998; Espeland & Stevens, 2009; Fourcade, 2011). Through a discursive analysis of technical literature, regulation and press, this research provides an account of the tensions between evidence, reproductive rights, and the social movements that converge in the debate about abortion. These stories provide an interesting case for analysing the political, legal and technical challenges that face social movements and confrontations inside civil society when values and goals are contradictory. Finally, this paper wishes to open a discussion about the importance of numbers and statistics in public arenas and highly divisive political debates.

The methodological strategy used in this work is a discursive analysis of Colombian regulation, technical studies, newspapers and websites that document the debate about abortion in Colombia over the last decade. Specifically, I present a detailed analysis of decision C 355 of the National Constitution of Colombia and the regulation formulated by the National Ministry for Social Protection regarding IVE (voluntary interruption of pregnancy) from 2006 to 2010. Finally, to the extent that international organisations and groups have been engaged with the national discussion, I explore additional connections that complement the Colombian sources. I include in this discursive analysis AGI reports about abortion and the controversies that have grown around these reports and statistics.

### Numbers and matters of concern: Making abortion a question of public health

Since the decade of the 1970s different social organisations have escalated around the idea of sexual and reproductive health and rights (Viveros, 2003; Viveros & Gil, 2006). This movement has taken as its flagship the decriminalisation of abortion. One of the most visible organisations within the movement is La Mesa. In 2004 leaders of this organisation discussed the possibility of decriminalising abortion through litigation in the Constitutional Court.

La Mesa has worked in the promotion of sexual and reproductive health since 1993. This organisation is a good example of the use of medical and technical expertise as instrument in wider political strategies. Different activists, women's organisations, universities and think tanks converged in the agenda set by this board. The strategy was to open a public debate about the criminalisation of abortion as a human rights violation in parallel with discussion about the constitutionality of the current regulation. While some works (Jaramillo & Alonso, 2008) have understood the decriminalisation as the result of the work of experts and a highly trained circle of activists with experience in international law and lawsuits, La Mesa (board for the health and lives of women) highlights the role of a grass-rooted women's social movement as the main actor in the transformation of abortion restrictions in reaching a consensus and coordinated mobilisation between the diverse social groups promoting gender equity. However, in terms of strategy, the focus of the group was to present abortion decriminalisation to the court as a matter of human and international right and as a problem of public health for national healthcare authorities.

The Colombian government, particularly, the Ministry of Health, embraced the last argument. In the deliberations of the Constitutional Court the ministry presented 'evidence' and figures to show the impact on public health of unsafe abortion in the country (C 355 of 2006) quoting a study developed by the AGI in 2006 about unsafe abortion in Colombia and the National Health Survey developed by Profamilia, a Colombian sexual and reproductive health organisation. AGI's (2006) study calculated that in 2004 in Colombia around 30.000 unsafe abortions were performed. Additionally these studies established a connection between unsafe abortion and poverty, portraying the decriminalisation as an issue of social justice.

An understanding of abortion in terms of public health was key in the Constitutional Court's discussions. The ruling is full of references to the burden of illegal abortion in terms of women's mortality and morbidity. In many cases the sources of the figures are not quoted. However the main source of data about abortion in Colombia, at the time of the debate, was the study developed by the AGI (2006) about unsafe abortion. In other articles (Maldonado, 2014) I have shown the impact of this study in influencing court decisions by presenting the citation network that supports judges' reasoning and argumentation. The Guttmacher study is assumed by the court to be evidence of the public health character of abortion in the country.

These numbers and the relations that they assume are the result of calculating fecundity rates, maternal mortality and actual number of births in specific populations. The court adopts this reasoning, as it is noted in the decision C 355 of 2006.

> Therefore, in the poorest towns of the country converge high fecundity rates, high unemployment, unmet basic needs, precarious access to education and a poor performance in other healthcare indicators such as child and maternal mortality. This reflects inequalities and gaps in the social development of these communities. (C 355 of 2006, p. 1020)

Despite accepting the importance of this argument, at the time of the debate the court complained about the lack of epidemiological studies about abortion in the country. *The Lancet*, three years after the ruling, notes still the lack of reliable figures about legal and unsafe abortion in the country (*The Lancet*, 23 February 2009).

The production of statistics about abortion is a complex and contested matter. Abortion is still a taboo subject in many countries and an illegal practice prosecuted in some nations. Although figures about legal abortion should be produced in the same manner as other medical statistics through hospitals' medical registers, in practice they tend to be under-reported (Brack & Rochat, 2016. On the other hand, estimations about unsafe abortion are very complex. Most of them are inferred from a wide and diverse set of sources such as hospitalisation for abortion, maternal mortality associated with unsafe abortion, and by contrasting the difference between estimated pregnancies and actual number of births in the population.

These data are complemented by information from the Ministry of Health and the National Institute of Legal Medicine. However none of these sources captured abortion. An indirect estimation of abortion had to rely on the identification of population at risk. High fecundity and poverty became key relations in the estimation of abortion figures. Such a way of estimating those figures highlights the vulnerability of specific populations, for example adolescents and rural immigrants. For instance, the National Survey of Demography and Health (ENDS) has shown a steady increase in adolescent pregnancy, growing from 19% in 2000 to 21% in 2005. These data are some of the elements for guessing the burden of abortion in the country.

In Colombia the main source of epidemiological data about sexual and reproductive health is ENDS. This is part of the international survey (DHS+) produced by Macro International and supported by the US Agency for International Development (USAID) and the United Nations Population Fund (UNFPA). Since the 1990s this survey has been not only a tool to provide decision makers with information about sexual and reproductive health but also a mechanism to open discussions in the media and public arenas about the importance of these issues. The statistics about abortion in Colombia have shared in this. They have reported matters of fact in order to produce matters of concern (Latour, 2004) in Colombian society.

Healthcare data and statistics in many regions of the country are mostly precarious. In the case of sexual and reproductive health most data are produced by independent organisations such as Profamilia and the Centre of Social Dynamics at Universidad Externado. The Ministry of Health manages the main epidemiological data with the National Health Institute. However in matters of social and reproductive health the main technical source is the DHS (ENDS).

At the time of the debate another important figure was related to the number of illegal abortion in Bogotá. The city's Health Department calculated that 37,000 unsafe abortions are performed every year in Bogotá (Secretaria de Salud de Bogotá, 2006). This number supported the AGI's estimates and contributed to the understanding of decriminalisation as a matter of public health. However, a year after the Constitutional Court's ruling, a new debate arose about the impact of decriminalisation.

The figures about legal and illegal abortion in Colombia remain deeply confusing and a matter of intense debate. A year after the Constitutional Court's decision, local media asked public authorities about the impact of decriminalisation in terms of numbers of performed abortions. One of the earliest attempts to estimate the impact of abortion decriminalisation was published in a Colombian newspaper *El Tiempo* in 2007. According to data provided by Bogotá's Health Department, during the first year ten legal abortions were performed in hospitals in Bogotá, seven related to interruption of pregnancy as a result of rape (*El Tiempo*, 2007). However, the Secretary of Health noted that possibly many private clinics were not reporting the procedure.

### A bureaucratic counter-reform and conservative social movements

Ruibal (2015) has identified two main phases in the process of implementation of Decision C-355 in Colombia. The first one (2006-09) was marked by the active role of government agencies, in particular the Ministry of Health, in enacting regulations to implement the decision and to provide abortion services through the public health system. The second phase (2010-15) has been marked by a strong reaction led by powerful conservative actors in key positions within the state, who have systematically attempted to obstruct the implementation of Decision C-355 and the development of demographic and epidemiological data to diminish the impact of decriminalisation. In response, feminist organisations have developed creative litigation strategies to demand the right to information about abortion services and organisations such as the AGI have continued their work in providing data about the impact of abortion in Latin America and in Colombia, stating that the problem remains a problem of public health in the region.

The process of regulation and implementation of the ruling was slow and strongly contested. The Ministry of Health enacted Decree 4444 of 2006 and produced technical guidelines for the voluntary interruption of pregnancy. However, the lack of adequate information and the resistance of many practitioners, and hospitals arguing conscientious objection and refusing to treat cases were the biggest obstacles to the implementation of the ruling. As a consequence many women had to go to the courts again asking practitioners to obey the law. This created additional rulings (T 714 of 2007, T 209 of 2008 and T 388 of 2009) declaring that hospitals and organisations cannot argue conscientious objection to deny medical attention and interruption of pregnancy. In cases in which practitioners refuse to deliver these services, the hospital should guarantee that other professionals are available to provide the healthcare being sought.

The Catholic Church has historically led the opposition to abortion. However, in the last decade, this movement has been transformed by a coalition of Christian churches. Catholic bishops and Christian preachers have been representatives of the anti-abortion movement in the country both in media and in courts. Additionally religious universities and national and international anti-abortion organisations have submitted *amici curiae* presenting arguments in favour of their position to the Constitutional Court at different times in the debate.

Both parts of the controversy made intensive use of *amici curiae* during the debate in the Constitutional Court (Maldonado, 2014). At that time the anti-abortion groups adapted their own discourse. moving their arguments from an ethical and theological framework to a jargon based on demography. The Population Research Institute was particularly visible (PRI, 2005). Anti-abortion organisations have attempted to appropriate the language of research organisations which they have perceived as biased. The PRI presents itself as a non-profit organisation whose goal is to criticise the overpopulation myth, expose human rights violations related to population control and promote people as the biggest natural resource. However, most of its work is focused on fighting abortion and its decriminalisation. One of *amicus curiae* of this organisation notes:

> A comparative analysis of maternal mortality rates and decriminalization of abortion between countries shows that there is not significant co-relation or evidence to argue that the decriminalisation (liberalisation) of abortion has an impact in reducing maternal mortality. (PRI, 2005)

Through *amici curiae* different interest groups presented legal and scientific evidence that they considered may influence the decisions of the court. In the ruling that decriminalised abortion – decision C 355 of 2006 – the Constitutional Court presented a register of the different *amici curiae* and citizens' declarations. These elements constitute a rhetoric device to show that the court's ruling was based on listening carefully to the different voices of society.

However, during discussions in the Constitutional Court the *amici curiae* of the PRI failed to be recognised as a legitimate source of scientific data and the court did not recognise its expertise. A citation analysis of the court's ruling shows that while the Guttmacher reports are repeatedly used as a source of information, the PRI is not quoted once (see Maldonado, 2014). The PRI could not obtain the same legitimacy as AGI. The institute has a well-established reputation as a non-profit organisation devoted to the study and analysis of policy in sexual and reproductive health. It works closely with the World Health Organization (WHO) and other international organisations such as the UNFPA. However, as I will show in the last section the anti-abortion movement has improved its technical skills, producing improved engagement with statistics and numbers to legitimise their political agenda.

In the last ten years, different conservative groups in Colombia have transformed the rhetoric and methods adopting the strategies of other social movements to oppose the advancement of sexual and reproductive rights claims. As Ruibal notes they have appropriated the 'language of rights, mobilisation based on civil society organisations, legislative lobbying and strategic litigation' (Ruibal, 2015, p. 19). This has been displayed in recent attempts to make referenda about abortion, the right of lesbian, gay, bisexual and transgender (LGBT) couples to adopt and be married.

At first, these groups' actions were relatively uncoordinated without a clear leadership. However, the appointment of conservative activists at key state institutions triggered a big counter-mobilisation against sexual and reproductive health and rights and specifically against the decriminalisation of abortion. In 2009, a prominent conservative public official, Alejandro Ordoñez, was appointed as General Prosecutor, head of the *Procuraduría General de la Nación*. This institution was created by the 1991 Constitution to cover the duties of both Inspector General and Attorney General. This institution should enforce the Constitution, general laws, judicial decisions and administrative acts.

Ordoñez led different actions in order to sabotage the court's decision on abortion. First he appointed as prosecutor for issues related to childhood and family to the conservative activist Ilva Myriam Hoyos, leader of the opposition to the decriminalisation of abortion. Second, he opened an enquiry into the use of misoprostol in hospitals. He argued that such a drug was unsafe and expensive in comparison with other methods. Ordoñez told public officials in charge of the implementation of abortion services that they could go to jail for reducing public finances by purchasing misoprostol.[3] In addition in 2009, the prosecutor ordered the investigation and suspension of the construction of the *Clínica de la Mujer* (Women's Clinic) in the city of Medellín, intended to provide sexual and reproductive health services (*La Silla Vacía*, 11 July 2012).

However the most serious action, in terms of obstacles to the delivery of healthcare services related to abortion and post-abortion events, was a lawsuit led by the prosecutor in 2009 demanding Decree 4444. Such a decree regulates the organisation of these services, giving guidelines for the implementation of the court's decision. 'The State Council upheld the claim, immediately suspended the Decree, and declared it null in March 2013' (Ruibal, 2015).

These actions encouraged the coordinated resistance of different actors in the country to defend the decriminalisation. New lawsuits were presented to the Constitutional Court. This court kept the support of its ruling, extending the health exception. New decisions included a more comprehensive definition of health, introducing mental health as a criterion in making abortion legal. Finally, in 2016 the Council of State removed Ordoñez from his position as prosecutor after an enquiry that found serious offences in his election. Ordoñez responded by claiming that such a decision was politically motivated and that it was a request from the far-left guerrillas to sign a peace agreement. He joined the campaign of the elected President of Colombia Iván Duque in the 2018 Presidential Election.

The current General Prosecutor Fernando Carrillo has shown a more favourable stand regarding sexual and reproductive health, closing the debate within state institutions about the implementation of the Constitutional Court ruling. However, the debate about abortion in Colombia is not over. The presidential election (2018) has offered an opportunity for the mobilisation of abortion and other reproductive rights as some of the resources to exert influence on voters in a country that is experiencing increasingly cultural and political polarisation. Meanwhile anti-abortion organisations in the country and in the region have focused on debating the public health and epidemiological legitimation of the decriminalisation of abortion.

I conclude this paper by briefly presenting the controversy between a team of Latin American bioethics and epidemiology researchers led by the Chilean Elard Koch (Melisa Institute) and the AGI about the methodologies of estimation of legal and unsafe abortions and the impact of decriminalisation on the reduction of maternal mortality rates (MMR). This controversy has surged in the context of the debate about the decriminalisation of abortion in Chile. The Colombian case has been presented in this discussion as a model of strategic litigation. The main argument under debate is if the decriminalisation of abortion contributes to the improvement of public health.

## The double edge of numbers: Problems in the production of statistics

This controversy was triggered by a report published by the AGI in 2011 presenting statistics about induced abortions performed in Colombia. The report stated that 'an estimated 400,400 induced abortions were performed in Colombia in 2008, of which only 322 were reported as legal procedures' (AGI, 2011). Additionally it noted that the number of abortions has increased over the last decades. The institute estimated that in 1989, there were 288.400 abortions. The increase is explained in connection with a demographic expansion in the number of women of reproductive age (AGI, 2011).

This report relies on a study conducted by Prada and colleagues who have estimated the rate of abortion in Colombia in the last three decades (Prada, 2013; Prada, Singh, & Villarreal, 2012). Despite the increase in abortions the authors argue that the rate has remained relatively stable: 36 abortions per 1000 women of reproductive age in 1989, compared with 39 per 1000 in 2008. Additionally they argue that the highest rates of complications after abortion are found in the Pacific area, one of the poorest areas of the country.

In 2012 Elard Koch from the Elisa Institute and his colleagues published a paper in the journal *Ginecología y Obstetricia de México* contesting the estimations made by the AGI, specifically the estimated number of 400,400 clandestine abortions for Colombia. They specifically criticise the methodology of these studies, describing Guttmacher's methods in the following terms:

> [F]irst, (Guttmacher) authors estimated the losses from spontaneous and induced abortions from the opinion of 289 subjects who work in an equal number of Colombian health institutions through the opinion survey entitled "Health Facilities Survey". Subsequently, an expansive multiplier (×3, ×4, ×5, etc.) was applied to the numbers obtained by this survey that also emerges from a subjective opinion of another 102 respondents of the "Health Professional Survey" selected by convenience. (Koch et al., 2012, p. 360)

Koch and colleagues argue that Guttmacher methods do not work 'with objective data based on real vital events, the whole estimate is based on imaginary numbers underlying mere opinions'. Moreover, they argue that Guttmacher overestimates more than nine times the complications due to induced abortion in hospital discharges and more than 18 times the total number of induced abortions (Koch et al., 2012, p. 360). Koch's team make visible their interest behind this methodological and statistical critique. They argue that Guttmacher numbers have strong implications for the policy of the Latin American region. As they note,

> in other Latin American countries where the same methodology was applied including Argentina, Brazil, Chile, Mexico, Peru, Guatemala, and Dominican Republic, the number of induced abortions was also largely overestimated. These results call for caution with this type of report that alarms public opinion. (Koch et al., 2012, p. 370)

Koch and colleagues propose an alternative method that relies on hospitals' clinical records of postabortion events and on the use of data from Chilean healthcare to calculate missing information to be estimated in Colombia.

The AGI did not ignore such a critique and developed a detailed response. Guttmacher's researchers note that they used a method called abortion incidence complications method (AICM). 'It was developed about 20 years ago and has been widely used in studies that have appeared in reputable peer-reviewed journals. It is recognised by experts in both the academic community and international organisations, such as the World Health Organization (WHO)' (AGI, 2012, p. 2).

They argue that this method is used in countries where abortion is legally restricted and in those where, despite its legality, it is still unsafe because of social stigma or for problems with data and healthcare infrastructures. 'When abortion is illegal or stigmatised, the procedure is performed in secrecy; as a result, women are reluctant to report it, and providers are reluctant to register it' (AGI, 2012, p. 4). The social and legal complexity of abortion demands in Latin America yield estimates, rather than exact values.

The AICM relies on two types of data to estimate the number of abortions: 'the number of women who receive facility-based treatment for induced abortion complications; and the proportion of all women having abortions who receive facility-based treatment for complications'. In many cases an inflation factor is applied to the number of women treated in health facilities for induced abortion complications to yield the total number of induced abortions. In the Colombia case this is done because the quality of hospital records has 'deteriorated to an unacceptable level after decentralisation and the reform of the health system in 1993' (AGI, 2012, p. 4).

Guttmacher experts note that Koch and colleagues erroneously state that the Colombia Health Facilities Survey (HFS) is based on a convenience sample. The HFS sample is selected through use of a multistage stratified cluster sampling technique. After a detailed analysis of each element of the Koch critique, they conclude that he and his team fail in both their attempt to discredit the AICM and their attempt to present a credible alternative for estimating abortion incidence in countries where the procedure is highly restricted. 'Their approach is simplistic, highly misleading and simply wrong. Its underlying assumptions have no scientific basis and show no respect for contexts, a significant problem' (AGI, 2012, p. 9).

Koch's proposal relies on calculating abortion rates using demographic indicators based on 'real vital events' or 'standard rates from known populations'. Guttmacher notes that such methods fall into the fallacy of assuming that high-quality data from one population could be applied to other populations without any modification, and that applying such measures to a different population will generate reliable estimates for that population. 'This is not the case for any demographic measure, as such measures are influenced by many country-specific factors; it is especially erroneous with regard to abortion in settings where the procedure is illegal and stigmatised, and occurs clandestinely' (AGI, 2012, p. 9).

Koch and his colleagues have continued their critique of the Guttmacher reports. They claim epidemiological data show that abortion related complications do not significantly affect MMR in Chile. This work has been published in peer-review journals, in general interest blogs such as the AAAS (American Association of the Advancement of Science) and some of them in highly ranked journals such as the Public Library of Science's *PLOS one*. Koch's work shows a transformation in the strategies of anti-abortion groups in Latin America. They have embraced a more 'scientific' and 'technical' approach to the debate about abortion and have designed a more sophisticated strategy to influence public opinion and decision makers.

In a blog entry from the international organisation World Youth Alliance (WYA), one of the contributors notes her favourable impressions of Koch' work.

> With the use of statistics, he talked about the positive impact of the results of his studies, demonstrating that decriminalizing abortion is not related to the decrease of the MMR. The most important conclusion was that maternal mortality reduction is due to access to good infrastructure in a health care system, which includes high levels of education for women. Also, he noted that Article 119 of Chilés Health Code, which prohibits abortion, helped in the reduction of maternal mortality by 93.8%. One of the reasons why Chile has one of the lowest rates of maternal mortality in Latin America is because of this legislation, which was adopted in 1989. (WYA, 2017)

The WYA itself reflects a new type of anti-abortion organisation. It presents itself as an international collaboration of activists concerned with the reduced scope of the United Nations population policy, specifically with its focus on abortion. The organisation argues that its goal is the promotion of the dignity of the person and of alternatives to abortion. It keeps its discourse very secular, mimicking the language and style of reproductive rights organisations and other international rights movements.

On the other hand, Koch's organisation (the Melisa Institute) has set an anti-abortion research agenda in biomedicine. In addition to their work contesting the statistics that have supported the decriminalisation of the abortion in Latin America, the institute is devoted to the study of foetal malformations and the development of surgical and medical intervention to preserve its life.

This new institutional setting and the adaptation of conservative social movements represent a challenge in the promotion of sexual and reproductive rights in Latin America. These groups are adopting a more coordinated and strategic approach to intervene in public policy beyond the traditional mechanisms of the Catholic and Evangelical Christian churches. This movement has learnt about the importance of producing 'evidence' and numerical data in the legitimation of their own political agenda. Additionally, learning from the strategies of other social movements, including the experience of women's organisations in changing national policies, they are aware of the importance of thinking in terms of Latin America rather than keeping only a national specific focus. They have learnt that the constitutional order is increasingly international and that changes in regulation in other countries can affect national and local policy.

## Conclusion

This paper has shown some of the struggles of the groups that promote collective rights in Colombia, specifically of those devoted to the liberalisation of abortion and the promotion of sexual and reproductive rights. After a landmark change of regulation, decision C 355 of 2006, these groups have experienced a series of difficulties and a complex reaction from conservative sectors and social movements within Colombian society. They have faced the sabotage of high officials in the Colombian government who have used their political position to promote their personal agendas and religious beliefs. But also they have had to deal with precarious data infrastructures that make it difficult to demonstrate impacts and to monitor the impact of court decisions. Most importantly opposition to the liberalisation of abortion has adapted to a policy environment sensitive to international regulation and to technical and scientific evidence.

Opposition to abortion has triggered the engagement of citizens into politics and has empowered new advocates such as the Christian churches as influential political actors. Debates around sexual and reproductive health reveal the diversity of citizenship, the tensions within civil society and in the increasing polarisation of political cultures in Latin America. This study of abortion allows us to explore the production of values within civil society groups and the strategies of these groups to promote their own valuation strategies as normative stands.

The debate about abortion reveals a wider transformation in the definition of human life, its value and limits in Colombia and Latin America, and changes in the politics of life. The controversies around abortion show the impact that changes in reproduction technologies have had on different social groups. Some of them have embraced such transformation; others have perceived them as a threat. In recent times Colombia has experienced an increasingly cultural and political polarisation, different groups are clashing to materialise their ideas and representations of body and society.

Finally, numbers have an important role in public arenas. Statistics sometimes have been used as a mechanism to avoid political discussion in public debates, attending to the assumed 'objectivity' of numbers. However, once numbers get into the centre of discussion, they are open to debate and become a contested matter. The production of statistics in the debate about abortion in Colombia shows a transformation in the ways in which numbers are read and become entangled with wider politics. Such transformation presents a challenge to public health authorities, experts and reproductive rights activists who have to create better numbers, more accountable and more accessible to wider audiences. Citizens need to learn to distinguish between good and bad calculations, between statistics as rhetoric devices and numbers as representations of collective realities.

## Notes

1. Although there are no reported cases of unconsented embryo transplant in Colombia, the court included this condition as a legitimate cause for requesting legal abortion. This debate is relatively rare in connection with the discussion about abortion but it has been discussed in relation to the ethics of embryo transplant. This condition is understood in connection with medical practice but not regarding those cases in which women became pregnant because their sex partners did not allow them access to birth control (Andrews, 1984).
2. The debate about abortion has elicited a language deeply politically charged to call the parts in controversy. Groups in favour of abortion have called themselves 'pro-choice' while anti-abortion groups have adopted the name 'pro-life'. In this paper I have tried to avoid such politics of language by referring to 'pro-life groups as anti-abortion.
3. This policy was outrageous and clearly politically motivated. Misoprostol is widely considered a very safe and affordable drug. It was included by 17th Expert Committee on the Selection and Use of Essential Medicines in 2008 in the WHO List of Essential Medicines because of its importance for treating post-partum haemorrhage (PPH). Besides the use of misoprostol for inducing abortion, it is an important drug to stock in obstetric services around the world.

## Acknowledgements

The author would like to thank Derly Sánchez Vargas and the anonymous reviewers for their helpful and encouraging comments on earlier versions of this article.

## Disclosure statement

No potential conflict of interest was reported by the author.

## ORCID

Oscar Javier Maldonado 🔘 http://orcid.org/0000-0002-0142-3625

## References

Adams, V. (Ed.). (2016). *Metrics. What counts in global health.* Durham, NC: Duke University Press.

Akrich, M., Leaneb, M., Roberts, C., & Arriscado, J. (2014). Practising childbirth activism: A politics of evidence. *BioSocieties, 9*(2), 129–152.

Alan Guttmacher Institute (AGI). 2006. In I. K. Warriner & I. H. Shah (Eds.), *Preventing unsafe abortion and its consequences: Priorities for research and action.* New York: Guttmacher Institute.

Alan Guttmacher Institute (AGI). (2011). Unintended pregnancy and abortion in Colombia. *Causes and Consequences.* Retrieved from https://www.guttmacher.org/sites/default/files/report_pdf/unintended-pregnancy-colombia.pdf

Alan Guttmacher Institute (AGI). (2012). *Estimating induced abortion incidence: Rebuttal to a critique of a guttmacher methodology.* https://www.guttmacher.org/sites/default/files/page_files/response-to-methodology-critique.pdf

Andrews, L. (1984). Ethical considerations. In *In vitro fertilization and embryo transfer. Human in vitro fertilization and embryo transfer* (pp. 403–423). London: Springer.

Baer, J. (2002). *Historical and multicultural encyclopedia of women's reproductive rights in the United States.* Westport, CO: Greenwood Press.

Brack, C., & Rochat, R. (2016). 'Una carrera contra el reloj': A qualitative analysis of barriers to legal abortion access in Bogotá, Colombia. *Extended Abstract.* Retrieved from https://paa.confex.com/paa/2016/mediafile/ … /Brack_PAA_Extended%20Abstract_3.6.pdf

Brown, P., & Zavestoski, S. (2004). Social movements in health: An introduction. *Sociology of Health & Illness, 26*(6), 679–694.

Cotes, M. (2005). La despenalización del aborto en Colombia: una solución innecesaria. *Persona y Bioética, 25,* 88–100.

Dalén, A. (2011). *El aborto en Colombia. Cambios legales y transformaciones sociales. Tesis de maestría no publicada.* Bogotá: Universidad Nacional de Colombia, Facultad de Ciencias Humanas, Escuela de Estudios de Género.

Desrosières, A. (1998). *The politics of large numbers: A history of statistical reasoning.* Cambridge, MA: Harvard University Press.

El Tiempo. (2007, March 20). La Pastilla del Aborto Bogotano. *News Office.* Retrieved from http://www.eltiempo.com/archivo/documento/MAM-2421465

Epstein, S. (1996). *Impure science: AIDS, activism, and the politics of knowledge.* Berkeley, CA: University of California Press.

Espeland, W., & Stevens, M. (2009). A sociology of quantification. *European Journal of Sociology* [Archives Européennes de Sociologie], *49*(3), 401–436.

Faúndes, A., & Barzelatto, J. (2005). *El drama del Aborto. En busca del consenso.* Bogotá: Tercer Mundo editores.

Fourcade, M. (2011). Cents and sensibility, economic valuation and the nature of 'nature' in France and America. *American Journal of Sociology, 116*(6), 1721–1777.

Gómez, C. (2006). Visibilizar, influenciar y modificar: despenalización del aborto en Colombia. *Revista Nómadas, 24,* 92–105.

González, A. (2005). La situación del aborto en Colombia: entre la ilegalidad y la realidad. *Cadernos de Saúde Pública, 21*(2), 624–628.

Hoyos, I. (2005). *La constitución de las falacias: antecedentes de una Sentencia.* Bogotá: Temis.

Jaramillo, I., & Alonso, T. (2008). *Mujeres, cortes y medios: la reforma judicial del aborto.* Bogotá: Universidad de los Andes-Siglo del Hombre editores.

Koch, E., Bravo, M., Gatica, S., Stecher, J., Aracena, P., Valenzuela, S., & Ahlers, I. (2012). Sobrestimación del aborto inducido en Colombia y otros países latinoamericanos. *Ginecología y Obstetricia de México, 80*(5), 360–372.

La Mesa por la Vida y la Salud de las Mujeres (MVSM). (2009). *Un derecho para las mujeres: La despenalización parcial del aborto en Colombia.* Bogotá: MVSM.

Latour, B. (2004). Why has critique run out of steam? From matters of fact to matters of concern. *Critical Inquiry, 30* (2), 225–248.

Maldonado, O. (2014). Cortes, expertos y grupos de interés: Movilización y localización del conocimiento experto en la sentencia C 355 de 2006. *Universitas Humanística, 77,* 327–353.

Moreira, T. (2012). *The transformation of contemporary health care. The market, the laboratory, and the forum.* New York: Routledge.

Murphy, M. (2012). *Seizing the means of reproduction: Entanglements of feminism, health, and technoscience (experimental futures).* Durham, NC: Duke University Press.

Population Research Institute (PRI). (2005). *Amicus curiae presentado a la Corte Constitucional de la República de Colombia.* Bogotá: Corte Constitucional.

Prada, E. (2013). The cost of postabortion care and legal abortion in Colombia. *International Perspectives on Sexual and Reproductive Health, 39*(3), 114–123. doi:10.1363/3911413

Prada, E., Singh, S., & Villarreal, C. (2012). Health consequences of unsafe abortion in Colombia, 1989–2008. *International Journal of Gynecology & Obstetrics, 118*(Suppl. 2), S92–S98.

Ruibal, A. (2014). Movement and counter-movement: A history of abortion law reform and the backlash in Colombia 2006–2014. *Reproductive Health Matters, 22*(44), 42–51.

Secretaria de Salud de Bogotá. (2006). *Aborto inducido un problema de salud pública.* Bogotá: Universidad Nacional de Colombia.

Velazquez, O. (2006). Constitucional y legalmente, el nasciturus es persona y titular del derecho a la vida. *Persona y Bioética, 10*(26), 85–103.

Viveros, M. (1996). *El aborto en Colombia: debate público y dimensiones socioculturales.* Bogotá: Centro de Investigaciones sobre Dinámica Social (CIDS), Universidad Externado de Colombia, Centro de Estudios Sociales.

Viveros, M. (2003). Género y salud reproductiva en Colombia. In S. Franco (Ed.), *La salud pública hoy* (pp. 481–496). Bogotá: Universidad Nacional de Colombia.

Viveros, M., & Gil, F. (2006). De las desigualdades sociales a las diferencias culturales. Género, 'raza' y etnicidad en la salud sexual y reproductiva en Colombia. In M. Viveros (Ed.), *Saberes, culturas y derechos sexuales en Colombia* (pp. 83–109). Bogotá: CLAM, Tercer Mundo, Universidad Nacional de Colombia.

World Youth Alliance (WAY). (2017). *Dr. Elard Koch, a scientist whose work is creating a legacy.* Retrieved from https://www.wya.net/op-ed/dr-elard-koch-a-scientist-whos-work-is-creating-a-legacy/

Zamudio, L. (2000). El aborto en Colombia: dinámica sociodemográfica y tensiones socioculturales. *Revista Derecho del Estado, 8,* 45–57.

# Struggles for maintenance: Patient activism and dialysis dilemmas amidst a global diabetes epidemic

Amy Moran-Thomas ⓘ

**ABSTRACT**

Diabetes has become a leading cause of death in Belize, making this Central American country emblematic of challenges amplified by a growing global diabetes epidemic. The struggles people face as they seek care for chronic conditions like diabetes (and its complications such as kidney failure) are bringing citizens and institutions alike to revisit longstanding norms about the terms through which healthcare is accessed. Ethnographically tracing Belize's first patient-driven healthcare protests and activism – an *ad hoc* movement for public dialysis that began over a decade ago – this paper examines patients' and caregivers' struggles to probe and shape a legacy of social justice health activism, drawing on perspectives from an often-overlooked part of Central America where basic healthcare access has not historically been framed as a right of citizens. It considers these dilemmas in relation to much larger chronic struggles 'to maintain' and repair bodies, medical technologies, and health systems in the aftermath of colonial legacies – with special attention to the challenges posed for small countries now facing rising issues of diabetes injuries and chronic complications – and the role of civic media and citizen activism in this context.

## A global epidemic as seen from Belize

'We have a list of people waiting,' the nurse at the Belize City dialysis centre told me when I arrived in September 2010. 'Here, you will only meet the lucky ones.'

Most of the people I met with end-stage kidney disease during a year of chronicling diabetes experiences in Belize had been spread out, but in the dialysis centre they sat chair after chair. Many of them were restless during the hours-long treatment and full of things they wanted to say into my tape recorder: whether or not they received partial state support for this session; the ways they earned money to take the bus here; whatever they knew about the person whose death it was that opened a spot for them this room. I recognised some of their faces and names from news stories about the recent protests, including a Kriol woman who waved me over. She introduced herself as Ms. C and asked me to use a version of this name as the Belizean newspapers had; she was strategically trying to turn herself into a public figure. With changes on the horizon in partial response to their media work, the room's group of patients were learning to leverage the stories of their plights in new ways. 'Share the story when you go home. Diabetes,' Ms. C said. If it wasn't for the dialysis, she added, 'I would have died already.'

I had the sense of stepping straight into the news cycle stories that brought me to that room:

[Ms. C] ... told our newspaper that February 2009 will mark one year since she has been taking dialysis treatments. She, too, is concerned about the lack of a doctor at the dialysis unit.

'I know that it's hard, because we don't have a doctor. When our pressure goes up, God is the doctor. When my pressure goes up high I pray God please help me and I beg him because I don't have any money for any doctor,' [she] shared ....

Fighting back her tears, C. complains of having an extremely difficult time even affording the transportation expenses to get to Belize City for dialysis treatments three times a week (Ramos, 2009, p. 1; 7 News Belize, 2009, December 30).

'I didn't know how I was going to get here today,' Ms. C told me, repeating the worry she often emphasised when being interviewed by the national news stations. She wanted people to know about the dialysis situation in general, but also had a specific goal in telling her story: Ms. C was always trying to raise bus fare. The bus from Belmopan to Belize City cost $3US dollars for a ride of one hour, and required a taxi ($5US roundtrip) to reach the clinic from the bus station. The problem was that she needed to make this trip three times a week. Every Saturday, Tuesday, and Thursday, Ms. C spent most of her day telling her story to other Belizeans in hopes of raising $11 for the round trip, so that every Monday, Wednesday, and Friday she could reach the dialysis sessions the government had begun unevenly subsidising that year. Having media confirmation of the reality she was describing became a useful tool in this endless work. Ms. C felt she had been very lucky to get on the list, reciting the others with diabetes in her family: a sister and brother both already 'dead off of sugar,' but also another sister trained in nursing who had managed to get a kidney transplant in Cuba. As we spoke, a loud Spanish love ballad floated over the clinic din from the next room. 'That's my cousin,' Ms. C shook her head, smiling. 'He likes to sing on the machine.'

It felt intense to enter a space where people regarded storytelling with this sense of potential existential stakes. On a Monday morning, after visiting the week before, I heard the news alongside the room of patients that one of the country's 21 dialysis patients had died over the weekend. Someone waiting would be bumped up the list kept on a paper taped to the desk near the phone, a list which easily fit on one page. A new regular would be sitting in his chair by Wednesday. 'I was just talking with him on Friday,' reflected one man getting dialysis. 'You can be walking today and by tomorrow morning you are ... not here.' The unit's patients on once-weekly treatment were dying so quickly that it created a palpable sense that everyone was sitting in someone else's former place, and that someone new would occupy their blue chair once they were gone.

I felt myself being immediately enrolled into some much more fortunate transient rotation, one in a long line of past and future storyteller-witnesses visiting that room. At times I stopped writing in my notebook because I was listening so intently that I knew each word would be imprinted on my mind later anyway. Other times I would stop writing for the opposite reason, because bodily I just could not take in any more. Both limits left me feeling dizzy and spilling over. It was at times a physical relief to have a tape recorder rolling on those days, to think it would be possible to process later whatever could not be absorbed in real time. But later I found the tapes almost unbearable to listen to – piercing machines, background televisions, and bits of hardship coming from all sides that I found no way to pass along on a relevant interval. Many of those who were sitting in one of those chairs that day died many years ago. Others have survived against all odds.

For all the hardship assembled in one room, the stories of those waiting were also on my mind, people I'd spoken with in hospitals across the country. Some of them make the exhausting journey by school buses to Mexico for dialysis three times a week in hopes that something might change, or waited hoping for a phone call.

This was the broader backdrop when I met Jose Cruz in Belize City. By that time, he had already reached a certain level of national celebrity, after initiating the first rights-based patient activism movement in the history of Belizean national medicine. Together with his wife Mileni and a group of patients and their families from the Kidney Association of Belize, and joined by caregivers, their collective organised civic protests and eventually gathered support among the government for partnering with a U.S.-based NGO to build the country's first public dialysis centre. Since Belize does not have a constitutional right to health, Cruz's actions were not played out on judicial fronts, but rather through the national media that covered his activism. He began organising media conferences and issuing press releases about each part of his body that got amputated within a health system unable to support patients like him (Figure 1). For a time, he boycotted his own dialysis treatment until the government took steps to offer the same to other patients on the waiting list. As Cruz put it in a 2009 media interview (7 News Belize, 2009, July 1):

> I am willing to stop doing my dialysis. I am willing to die for it …

> This is nonsense. People are dying for God's sake … We have people dying, literally dying and nobody's paying attention. So I am making a stand today.

In Belize, as in much of the world, diabetes is now a leading cause of death nationwide (PAHO, 2011; IDF, 2017). Such high mortality rates are in part due to the role of diabetes as 'a prominent cause of kidney disease' (WHO, 2016, p. 73), part of the heavy toll of complications associated with globally rising rates of cardiometabolic disorders (Arredondo, Azar, & Recamán, 2017; de-Graft Aikins, Addo, Ofei, Bosu, & Agyemang, 2012; Manderson and Smith-Morris, 2010; Mendenhall and Norris, 2015; Narres et al., 2016; Sanal, 2011). Rates of kidney disease are poised to continue escalating worldwide, as diabetes is rapidly growing even among the world's poorest populations (Bukhman et al., 2015; Mendenhall & Norris, 2015; Nielson, Bahendeka, Bygbjerg, Meyrowitsch, & Whyte, 2017). According to the WHO, over half the world's countries do not currently have renal transplant available as an option, which leaves dialysis as the only possibility for survival. Yet some 54% of countries labelled 'middle-income' and 73% of countries classified 'low-income' do not currently offer access to dialysis (WHO, 2016, p. 74).

The first working dialysis machine was cobbled out of sausage casings, juice cans, and a clothes washing machine during the shortages of wartime, when Dutch physician Willem Kolff's tinkering with his vision of the world's first artificial organ in 1941 transformed the history of medicine. He never patented the invention (Figure 2), hoping that keeping the technology open-access would

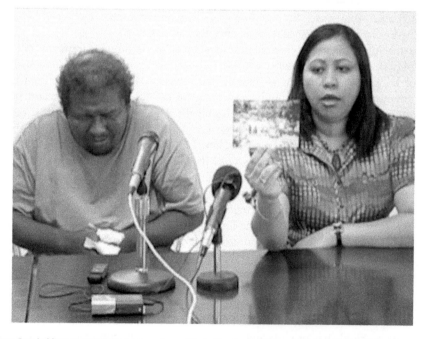

**Figure 1.** Jose Cruz holding an amputation press release (Photo Courtesy of Channel 5 Belize News. Used with permission).

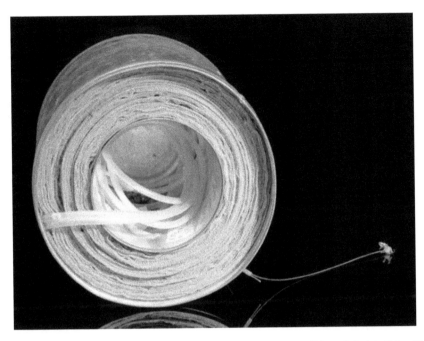

**Figure 2.** One of Kolff's kidney dialysis machine prototypes, made from an apricot can. (Science & Society Picture Library / Getty Images)

make future machines more accessible to others (Blakeslee, 2009, p. 1). In the U.S., dialysis and kidney transplants have been legally provided by the national government since 1972 (Rettig, 2011). It took more than half a century for such devices to reach Belize, when in 2003 Guatemalan kidney specialist Dr. Miguel Rosado opened the first dialysis unit at a private hospital in Belize City. After Dr. Rosado died tragically three years later in a car accident in Belize, his dialysis centre remained intact but was missing its founder's propelling vision (Belize News, 2003; 7 News Belize, 2009 July). This made for a difficult reality, because the skyrocketing diabetes rates across Central America have left an increasing number of patients in kidney failure and in need of dialysis in order to survive. But after Rosado's death, there was no nephrologist or endocrinologist working in Belize, and no public dialysis unit in the country. By the time I began this project in 2009, dialysis sessions in the private hospital were exorbitantly expensive (costing $680 a week), and any participating patients had to sign a waiver acknowledging that they wanted to accept the risks of getting dialysis even though there was usually no doctor present.

In investigating how patients and physicians alike are navigating such gaps in state infrastructures, I join scholars who return to James Scott's notion of 'infrapolitics' (1990) from a somewhat different angle and era of global politics, focusing on moments where a public's ordinary actions bear out in ways that at times unexpectedly intersect with – and may even expand or guide – directions of state development (Appel, Anand, & Gupta, 2015). This kind of ethnographic emphasis in turn 'compels us to think of people not as problems or victims, but as agents of health' (Biehl & Petryna, 2013, p. 11; see Hatch 2016; Hoover 2017; Montoya, 2013; Roberts 2017; Solomon, 2016; Yates-Doerr, 2015).

'This is the first time in [Belizean] history we have a group of actual patients suffering from an ailment come together and demanding what they want,' Cruz told one national news station. 'I hope that the Belizean people are taking notice.'

## Inventing a right to health

Belize's first patient-driven healthcare protests and activism – a movement for public dialysis – thus began unfolding in 2009, over a decade ago. This article describes patients' and caregivers' struggles to probe and shape a legacy of social justice health activism, drawing on perspectives from an often-overlooked part of Latin America where basic healthcare access has not historically been framed as a right of citizens. In a country long marked by patchwork infrastructures, Belize's diverse national population – speaking languages including Kriol, English, Spanish, Garifuna, Maya (Mopan, Yucatec, and Kekchi), and Chinese – is experimenting across registers with fragile forms of collective organising. By thinking about healthcare movements in Latin America in relation to a country frequently dismissed as marginal, this case from Belize invites comparative inquiry about the implications of particular colonial legacies for contemporary citizenship claims, as well as for reconsidering how labels like 'Caribbean' or 'Latin America' are defined and enacted in the first place (Wilk, 2006).

A few notes on regional background may be helpful as historical context for the exchanges that follow. While people often remark that Belize is 'both Latin American and Caribbean,' Michael Stone (1994) has noted that scholarship frequently tends to treat it as neither, often falling between the cracks of both regions' historiographies. But to call Belize an 'exception' in Latin America forces us to consider how we are defining the region's norms. The country has been called many things over the years: a 'colonial dead end' (Clegern, 1967); 'a meeting place for the strands of history' (Grant, 1976, pp. ix–xi); a 'strange little fragment of empire' (Huxley, 1934). In all, Belize spent over two centuries as a squatter community of uncertain status – settled by unauthorised British rogues on Spanish-owned land, yet under the consolidated control of neither England nor Spain and largely inventing their own laws – before the Settlement finally became recognised as British land in 1850. This means that Belize did not even *become* a European colony until the countries surrounding (Mexico, Guatemala and Honduras) had already won their independence from Spain and became sovereign nations. Belize thus spent much more time in this liminal phase of its existence (230 years) than it did as an officially recognised British territory (21 years), a Crown colony actually being governed by England (110 years), or as an independent nation ruled by constitutional monarchy (with an elected Belizean Prime Minister and the official head of state remaining the Queen of England) from 1981 until the present (Bolland, 1977). The former British Honduras arranged for its colonial rulers to stay two extra decades due to threat of war from Guatemala. (Even today, a very common Guatemalan saying – based on an old colonial land dispute – claims that *Belice es nuestro* (Belize is ours), while the Kriol language counter-slogan holds instead that *Da Fu Wi Belize* ('This is Our Belize') reflecting tensions finally sent to the International Court of Justice in 2019). Yet even early in its origins, the people who lived in Belize wrote of 'their country,' although the place was part of no nation's empire. When Clifford Geertz spoke of the 'central interpretative issues' raised by the 'uncenteredness of modern times,' he hit on a question that Belize has wrestled with continuously from its earliest history: 'What is a Country if It Is Not [Only] a Nation?' (Geertz, 2000, p. 228)

Belizeans have not had a constitutional right to health in the history of their nation, nor a patient activist group that had come together to leverage a particular policy demand from the state. People I spoke with seemed generally unsure what to expect from their country, in terms of health or institutional care. The public health system relies largely on rotating physicians, especially from Cuba. The expectations and norms I encountered in the national system shaped by these histories proved quite different, for example, from what Sherine Hamdy has described in her work with dialysis and transplant patients in Egypt, where people expressed an idea that both their state and their kidneys had failed (Hamdy, 2008). Yet such charges and protests in the Egyptian case that Hamdy observed also animated future demands, and spoke of a responsibility (if a largely unfulfilled and highly contested one) that the state was widely understood to have toward its citizens in the first place (see Benton, 2015).

In Belize, I struggled to understand why I never heard anything like this during my research. With so many people with diabetes dying preventable deaths and sustaining other losses all around me, patients seemed to mostly implicate themselves and to take the limits of the state system in measured stride. Some people called the opportunity to get one subsided dialysis session a week (although three were recommended to survive) a 'scholarship.' People in crisis largely focused on getting to other places they *could* receive the sessions, especially if they had some kind of mobility – some even making the three-times a week trip to Chetumal in Mexico, or more affluent citizens trying to find a route to Miami, LA, or Chicago – rather than agitating for infrastructural change within their state. Economist Albert O. Hirschman (1972) famously described the channels through which people respond to local injustices: voice, loyalty, exit. Perhaps it would be fair to say that many Belizeans facing trouble (health or otherwise) have historically been in the habit of focusing on exiting their tiny country when infrastructures become strained.

One of the key places that diabetes complications were most dramatically surfacing in Belize was around rising anxieties about injured limbs and the threat of amputations. Wear on the vascular system due to complications of high blood sugar over time can de-capacitate the body's ability to heal itself, and also contribute to the painful nerve damage of neuropathy. One U.S. study about the causes of diabetes limb amputation found at least 23 unique causal pathways in play (including 46% lost to ischemia, 59% to infection, 61% to neuropathy, 81% to faulty wound healing, 55% to gangrene, and 81% to initial minor trauma). Those numbers add up to 383% instead of 100% because most amputations are caused by several mechanisms simultaneously – which is also why remediating any one pathway will not necessarily save a limb. The biggest pattern this study found was that up to 80% of amputations were proceeded by a 'pivotal event,' usually a minor cutaneous injury (Pecoraro, Reiber, & Burgess, 1990). Tiny catastrophes such as a pebble in a shoe, an ingrown toenail, or stepping on a seashell can easily lead to a lost limb for someone with advanced diabetes, particularly once kidney complications were at play.

In 'What Wounds Enable,' anthropologist Laurence Ralph describes a phenomenon of people impacted by specific kinds of patterned injuries finding ways of 'living *through* injury,' allowing for fuller description of 'contexts in which it becomes politically strategic to inhabit the role of a 'defective body' in order to make claims' about connections between bodily injury and social injury (Ralph, 2012). I find this ethnographic concept work useful for grappling with these health struggles ongoing in Belize, and in particular the willingness of patients like Cruz to at times make their intimate injuries public in order to bring attention to wider social issues around their pending amputations.

The relaxed atmosphere in Belize often noted by tourists can easily be misrecognised for an absence of social problems in the country, rather than a hard-won effect of the way people absorbed hardship and undertook the labour of transmuting it for those around them. Yet many Belizeans also struggle with the stresses of embattled issues that adjacent countries like Guatemala and Mexico are well-known for in U.S. media – including income inequalities and persistent poverty, insecurities and traumas, murder rates that regularly rank as the leading causes of death among men and further deplete overstrained health systems (Anderson-Fye et al., 2010; Gayle et al., 2010). The normalisation of various forms of structural violence, it seemed to me, had complexly become part of 'what it means to be human in a place advertised as paradise' (Rodriguez, 2007, p. 221). There was often little opening to talk about such everyday stressors on bodies, or to probe the transnational contours of a system where healthy food and preventative care were difficult for many people to consistently access. Missing fingers, toes and limbs became a haunting endpoint of ongoing colonial legacies and at times occasioned rare discussions about the role of larger systems in shaping the choices available to people. This opened space for discussions about often-inchoate forms of 'slow violence' (Nixon, 2012; see Adams, Burke, & Whitmarsh, 2014) in the country, reflections on a system leading increasing numbers of people to need dialysis for survival in the first place (Figure 3). According to these voices, responding to compounding chronic realities would require not only maintaining but reinventing existing public infrastructures for care.

## 'Dr. Cruz'

'It is open for us to affect human history,' Jose Cruz had told me on the morning we met. By that time, in September 2010, he had already gone blind and was missing one leg and several fingers.

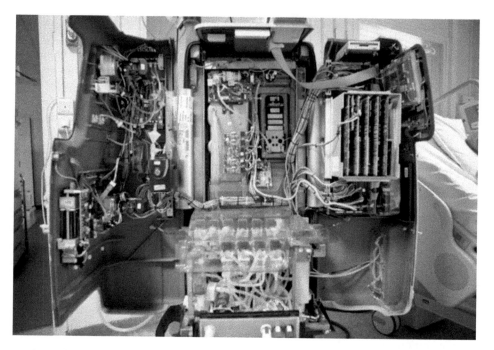

**Figure 3.** 'Hospital maintenance.' (BSIP / Getty Images).

Cruz had been holding a poster in the same injured hand the first time I had seen a picture of him in the newspaper. Cruz's unnervingly modest message scrawled on yellow posterboard – WE DON'T WANT TO DIE – could be read with different inflections against this presumed fatalism on the part of such patients. In this context of normalized deaths, what gets branded as fatalism? What are the circumstances in which someone has to announce on a poster their wish to live on? Realism about the actual proximity of death could easily blur into what could be read as a certain resignation to it. It therefore became a major feat of advocacy just to counter the assumptions about diabetes and dialysis patients that were so often repeated.

On one hand, the extreme time and travel commitment required of rural patients needing dialysis meant some people did not consider the benefits worth the costs in their particular case, a deeply personal choice that many patients uneasily faced. On the other hand, some individuals' difficult decision to forgo spottily accessible dialysis (given the numerous costs and obstacles of various kinds) certainly did not apply to everybody in Belize – an inaccurate assumption that I heard many patients worry had come to be accepted, in ways that normalised not providing dialysis to those people who *did* want and urgently need it in order to live.

'I'm a young man trapped in an old man's body,' Cruz told me with a laugh. He was first diagnosed with diabetes when he was 28 years old. 'The problem with diabetes is that it has different effects,' he said slowly. 'For example, because they did not diagnose the problem in time, I suffer retinopathy in both eyes … my vision went in a span of about two years.' It turned out that Cruz lived for many years with the diagnosis of diabetes, before finally learning that his high blood sugar was actually rooted in a deeper pathology: polycystic kidney disease. This genetic disorder causes constant little cysts on the kidneys to grow and burst, causing infection that in turn triggered Cruz's high blood sugars. 'Over 500,' he said of his glucose during times of infection. 'When that happens, it makes dialysis … complicated.' (Dialysis can also raise the sugar of the blood being returned to the body.) He preferred to arrive shirtless for his sessions and then be covered with a sheet. He was famous for making other patients laugh with his overdone singing during the awkward first part of treatment while their fistulas get connected to the machine, mostly Spanish ballads learned from his grandfathers. 'It kills the time a little faster.'

'There is going to be a lot more, because of the erasure of diabetes and hypertension,' Cruz said of kidney failure cases ahead. He described how in his western home district of Cayo, patients still had to pay for insulin and antidiabetic medications themselves, or go without them. He worried that many Belizeans accepted the fragility of healthcare system – they are 'used to it,' in his words – and often asked for nothing more. 'Because, they determine, because we're in a third-world country. That's the reason I am so much an advocate of critical dialysis,' he told me. Their advocacy had gained a powerful immediate goal when the group learned about a letter from a U.S.-based organisation, which had offered to supply dialysis machines and train personnel if the Belizean government agreed to refurbish two unit locations and commit to certain care criteria over time. Cruz called the U.S. organisation himself when he learned that the letter had gone unanswered. He recalled their office hung up the first time he telephoned, suspecting a prank because they were unfamiliar with his accent.

Cruz called back. 'I was told it couldn't be done,' he said, flashing a mischievous grin. 'We deserve to have good healthcare in this country … .For the individual … in the population, no? As part of the population.' At some point, fellow kidney patients and their families began calling him 'Dr. Cruz,' a striking nickname to emerge from a context where patients were getting dialysis without a physician. Cruz became both patient in and doctor of the system. 'But you can see the doctors are circling up already. That is what I'm doing. Despite the fact that I'm always fighting with them. That is part of it, fighting all the time or it is never going to happen.'

One young woman a few years older than me, who I'll call Katherine, said the chances this opened had changed her life. She wore her long dark hair straight down her shoulders, and travelled 250 miles each week for the sessions. Her son loved Spiderman, she smiled. In her late twenties, Katherine said, the diabetes and kidney troubles developed during pregnancy. Her son was five by the time we met, and lived far south with her parents in Toledo; Katherine didn't want him to move to Belize City because so many children had been caught in the violence, and she worried about putting him in danger. Her strategy, instead, was to arrive with her suitcase packed at every Friday session, ready to undergo the trip to her parents' village to see him for the day on Saturday before making the return trip on Sunday to be back in Belize City for Monday dialysis.

As Katherine told me this, intricate feats of fluid mechanics were occurring in tubes inside the machines around us. Blood flowed in one direction, and clear dialysate fluid (technically, 'a buffered electrolyte solution') in the other. The liquids were being brought together inside an encased plastic cylinder about a foot long, which is the dialyzer cartridge that actually serves as 'artificial kidney,' dwarfed and fed by the larger mechanical apparatus. The cartridge simulates the work of a glomerulus (Latin meaning 'little ball of yarn') – the knotted balls of vessels and fibres that make up the kidney's semi-permeable membrane for filtering toxins. Today most semi-permeable membrane simulations use a new mechanism, a far cry from the original sausage casings model: Blood is channelled inside tiny hollow fibres, each only about the width of three human hairs, capillaries submerged in a bath of dialysis solution inside the cartridge's inner chamber. Very small pores in the fibres' walls keep larger molecules, such as blood cells and proteins that need to be returned to the body inside the filtering membrane. But smaller molecules of accumulating toxins, including chemicals like potassium, sodium, and bicarbonate that can rise to dangerous levels in the blood without a kidney, spin out through the tiny pores and dissolve into the chamber's fluid. Invisibly laden with waste, salt, and extra water from the blood, the used dialysis solution drains into the wall behind the machine.

When I left the dialysis centre the last time we spoke, Cruz was belting out *I'm Singing in the Rain* in a comedic operatic voice, the patients around him laughing with a shake of their heads. The image of him waving goodbye with a three-fingered hand while singing so theatrically stuck with me. His routine performances' feeling of a serious joke remained larger than life in my memory. And so did the first picture I had seen of him on the news in 2009. Cruz had both legs then, marching in the midst of a protest in Belize City. One of his hands still had all the fingers. But he held the sign in the other side, and the missing few read as part of his message: A PROMISE IS A CONSOLATION TO A FOOL.

## Pressure and the press

João Biehl (2016) describes two ways that patient-citizens in Brazil are learning, in their words, 'to enter justice' around their state's constitutional right to health: one can either enter through the court' (by filing a lawsuit for access to medications), or 'enter through the press' (by getting media coverage about missing rights that puts public pressure on the state for upholding them). In some ways, the press side of this work reminds me of Jose Cruz's press releases. But in a country like Belize without any right to health written into a constitution or otherwise legible in a court of law, what do such tactics become when they rely on media outlets alone? What bodies are they meant to put pressure on?

People in Belize spoke constantly of rising 'pressure,' which commonly went hand in hand with high sugar (especially when diabetes complications such as kidney failure begin to show their signs). Indeed, in the common phrasing ('I have *pressure*') it was often literally impossible to tell if someone meant high blood pressure or escalating social pressure, or simply both at the place where they could not be separated (Banerjee, 2013). The work of transforming it from lethal blood pressure straining individual biologies, to creating 'fields of pressure in public consciousness' (Fischer, 2003, p. 265) that might drive state institutions toward building a healthcare or regulatory system that could potentially redress these risks, required a bold experiment in collective solidarity.

Cruz's strategy of leveraging media publicity began as something improvised, rather than planned in advance. When Cruz's foot became infected, the dialysis nurse 'complained to management that she needed a doctor but could not get one' (Ramos, 2009, p. 1). As a consequence, Cruz lost part of his foot. National papers covered the story. One article quoted the patient: '"I'm gonna be having a toeless Christmas. It's sad," said Cruz, laughing to lighten the mood.' Shortly afterwards, the only dialysis nurse in Belize quit, saying she would come back only if a doctor was also on staff. 'Only in Belize can you get dialysis without a nephrologist present, only in Belize. That is not right,' Cruz said; the patients had joined together refused to sign the permanent waiver that a doctor need not be present for patients on the dialysis machine. 'When our pressure goes up, God is the doctor,' added Jose's cousin [Ms. C] (Ramos, 2009). Cruz campaigned the Belizean media, calling into radio and TV stations: 'From a patient standpoint we want a doctor, if it's even a General Practitioner … along with our nurse. We want our nurse back'.

In the wake of public protest, the hospital accepted the dialysis collective's terms. Their momentum grew. Shortly afterward, another story about Cruz appeared in the paper. 'I need $150,000 by Monday because I could lose my whole hand,' Cruz told the media; his left foot had been amputated only the month before (7 News Belize, 2010, January 15). The papers ran his bank account number and cell, for Belizeans to contact him directly. Support poured in from around the country. Amazingly, he got the large sum (though it took costly time), and departed for Guatemala on 10 February 2010. With this medical intervention, Cruz lost two fingers but kept the rest of his hand. Even after his leg was later amputated, he continued leading protests in his wheelchair. In another photo, the stump of his leg still wrapped in a fresh bandage, Cruz holds another handprinted sign painted with a skull and crossbones.

In trying to puzzle out what such media images might ask of us, I remembered Ariella Azoulay's notion that some photographs might act as 'civil contracts' (2012) that at times capture specific injustices that cannot be addressed in their own context or political moment. Maybe it is possible, she writes, that they will make a claim on people in another place or time. Perhaps it was in a similar spirit to Azoulay's hope for images that Cruz organised these impromptu press conferences for his amputations, or that so many patients I met wanted people in other countries to see their pictures. Photographs of these street protests, strategic press releases, and personal stories became the vital materials through which patients like Cruz were attempting to cobble an alternative possibility of politics or reassemble future visions of rights, at times choosing to publicly share and reconceive of their hardships – even seeking out public platforms to actively perform and display them – as they tried to press for a different future.

The doctors, nurses, family members and policy makers who eventually came to join in this struggle recognised that this particular struggle contained larger questions: How does a body extend into structures around it? Where does an injury begin or end? Organs, limbs, and senses will wear down without care. A common answer to *How are you doing?* in Belizean Kriol is 'trying to maintain.' Treating the complications of diabetes has long entailed what E. Brown calls 'halfway technologies' (1996; see also Feudtner, 2003) – devices that help address 'symptoms or manifestations of disease, rather than the underlying pathogenesis.' Such *halfway technology* 'does not treat the underlying disease itself, but reflects the absolute failure of all efforts at medical and conservative therapy and is a last ditch, gerry-rigged lifesaving solution.' And yet, Brown adds, 'when a 'halfway' technology is also lifesaving, its value cannot be underestimated by the individual patient.' Preventative and prosthetic devices might allow health to be extended, but requires that bodies and infrastructures be maintained together (Russel & Vinsel, 2018).

## Holding measures

Annemarie Mol describes 'tinkering' around chronic conditions as 'an open-ended process: Try, adjust, try again. In dealing with a disease that is chronic, the care process is chronic, too. It only ends the day you die' (2008, p. 20). Because Cruz's work to create an idea of rights took place largely through the news stories written about him, I am trying to take seriously the different work of narrating them myself. As anthropologists have shown in thinking with Stanley Cavell's 'active awaiting' to reexamine care relations, time is a key horizon, and the centre of gravity shifts depending on where you stop or start the story (Han, 2012). I could choose to end here, for example, by telling you about people I knew who died over the years tinkering and waiting for the dream of dialysis to become a reality – like Sulma, whose daughter once called me at midnight to come over, but there was nothing either of us could really do as we stood together while her fifty-year-old mother ran frenetically around the house. She was flailing but unable to breathe as her lung condition was exacerbated by the sequelae of kidney damage, appearing to choke on the air as if underwater. Or Jordan, whose organs failed for the last time at the age of twenty one, after a brief lifetime as a Type 1 patient unable to consistently access insulin. There was nothing really to say when he showed me his bloated feet and said that he was not even on the dialysis waiting list; apparently his kidneys were so badly damaged that he was considered a poor candidate for the costly treatment.

But I could also tell a more heartening story about what I saw when I returned to Belize and saw the same location where, almost five years before, Ethan had shown me around the hospital's garage of abandoned machines and the old watchman's quarters being converted to make space for the newly arriving dialyzers they hoped to install. He was gone by the time I returned, moved on to mission work elsewhere. Jose Cruz died on a December morning, three months after I interviewed him in 2010. But there it was on the hill, landscaped with dirt rumoured to come from recently dug oil wells: a low building and a small sign directing patients into a Memorial Dialysis Unit.

It took me a minute to compose myself enough to take a picture of the open clinic, thinking of the past lives its sign marked and ongoing ones it might now extend. But I suppose you can't freeze-frame a happy ending any more than a tragic one. Inside the unit, two visiting dialysis nurses bustled around, reflecting the transnational circuits of dialysis nursing expertise. Later that week, a government official worried aloud that the U.S. donor who had originally funded the centre had now withdrawn after three years of training and support (as had been planned), leaving the machines to the state for maintenance. A significant percentage of Ministry's entire operating budget was being spent to keep the dialysis centres running, leaving nationwide limitations in more basic technologies – such as glucometers and strips for home testing (which were too expensive to be provided by the state) and insulin (now provided in 3 of its 6 districts) – which will mean more Belizeans needing dialysis in years ahead. Government officials are now looking for investors to help them maintain the units, and hoping to find a partner state abroad. Some in the Ministry of Health have become key dialysis advocates themselves, while balancing tough resource issues of scaling up (7 News Belize, 2011, February 4). By 2018, the programme's coverage expanded to reach 25% of patients on the waiting list.

Among this number, getting dialysis in the room that morning I checked back in, was my old friend Guillerma. We had first met many years ago when her mother, a renowned midwife and herbalist, had hosted an ancestral ritual for health and protection during a time when she worried Guillerma might be dying from diabetes complications and could not get dialysis at all. The last time I had seen Guillerma was in a Belize City hospital in fall of 2010, when she had just started getting one of the three dialysis sessions that she needed each week, due in large part to Jose Cruz's advocacy. It was a fraction of the care she needed, but had still opened some precarious margin of survival.

Sitting there years later in the new dialysis unit, where Guillerma was now getting between two and three weekly sessions, these histories meant something different already. But they were also part of the repair work (Schubert, 2019) that had sustained her until now. I showed Guillerma the picture I had taken during my last visit, when she had been sitting in the same chair in Belize City where Jose Cruz once received treatment; though the two had never met, she told me. 'Tell them, I am still right here fighting it,' she said, many years later then. Three days every week, she woke up at 4am and took a taxi and then a public school bus three hours in each direction in order to receive her hard-won session.

The dialysis machine whirred and beeped next to us the entire time we spoke, like a shrill but persistent third voice in our conversation, as it removed accreted toxins from Guillerma's blood. In many parts of the world, dialysis is considered a 'holding measure' (Mitaishvili, 2010) until renal transplant becomes possible. But in Belize, where no renal transplant has yet been performed in the country's history, dialysis instead became a 'holding measure' against death. It is waiting in this holding measure with Guillerma that I want to end here, trying to co-envision how to remain with these long-term maintenance projects – including ethnographic ones – now unspooling further contingencies ahead.

I remember how mechanical those exact machines had looked back in 2010, still stiffly wrapped in factory plastic, when I had photographed them in their storage room with the AC blasting to preserve their delicate parts. Seeing them surrounded by people and care, it was somehow comforting

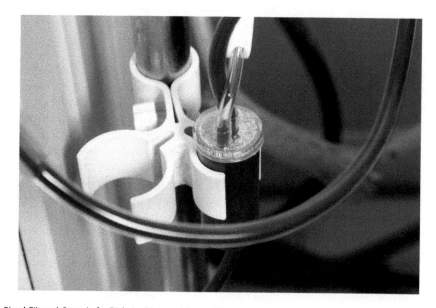

**Figure 4.** Blood Filtered Cannula for Dialysis. (Universal Group / Getty Images)

that the medical tubes carrying her blood into the machine for cleansing looked more pliable than I expected: less the electrical circuitry of a cyborg, more like an umbilical cord (Figure 4). Guillerma followed my eyes. 'Still alive,' she smiled. The electrodes and wires thread the air between us, awkward and alive, into its tenuous machinery. Together we watched the centrifuge wheel her blood backwards like a wildly broken clock, trying to turn back enough time for the week ahead.

## Acknowledgements

I am deeply grateful to all of those who spoke with me in Belize, and hope this is a gesture of recognition both for those 'still fighting it' and those 'not here.' Special thanks are also due to the Belize Institute for Social and Culture Research (ISCR) and the Belize Ministry of Health for their collaborative input and research approvals that launched this project, and the guidance of patients, families, and physicians in Belize. The complexities described offered here are offered here in the spirit of mutual care and critical inquiry, with much respect for all of these actors' difficult work. Thanks to the institutional funders below that generously supported this project; to my great teachers in the Department of Anthropology at Princeton and to my wonderful colleagues in MIT Anthropology; and to Emily Vasquez for her exceptionally caring editorial work on this special issue.

## Disclosure statement

No potential conflict of interest was reported by the author.

## Funding

This work was supported by Mellon-American Council of Learned Societies; Princeton Program in Latin American Studies; Wenner-Gren Foundation for Anthropological Research; Princeton Center for Health and Wellbeing and the MIT School of Humanities, Arts and Social Sciences (SHASS) Dean's Fund.

## ORCID

*Amy Moran-Thomas*  http://orcid.org/0000-0001-5411-1046

## References

7 News Belize. (2009, December 30). Dialysis patients protest. Retrieved from http://7newsbelize.com/sstory.php?nid=15872

7 News Belize. (2009, July 1). Jose Cruz refuses dialysis in protest. Retrieved from http://www.7newsbelize.com/sstory.php?nid=14397

7 News Belize. (2010, January 15). Jose Cruz needs $15,000 to save his fingers. Retrieved from http://www.7newsbelize.com/sstory.php?nid=15995

7 News Belize. (2011, February 4). Dialysis, finally a public health reality. Retrieved from http://7newsbelize.com/sstory.php?nid=18867

Adams, V., Burke, N. J., & Whitmarsh, I. (2014). Slow research: Thoughts for a movement in global health. *Medical Anthropology*, 33(3), 179–197.

Anderson-Fye, E., et al. (2010). Cultural change and posttraumatic stress in the life of a Belizean adolescent girl. In C. Worthman (Ed.), *Formative experiences: The Interaction of caregiving, culture, and developmental psychobiology* (pp. 331–343). Cambridge, MA: Cambridge University Press.

Appel, H., Anand, N., & Gupta, A. (2015). Introduction: The infrastructure toolbox. *Cultural Anthropology* online series, "Theorizing the Contemporary". Retrieved from https://culanth.org/fieldsights/714-introduction-the-infrastructure-toolbox

Arredondo, A., Azar, A., & Recamán, A. L. (2017). Diabetes, a global public health challenge with a high epidemiological and economic burden on health systems in Latin America. *Global Public Health*. Retrieved from http://www.tandfonline.com/doi/full/10.1080/17441692.2017.1316414

Azoulay, A. (2012). *The civil contract of photography*. Cambridge: MIT Press.

Banerjee, D. (2013). Writing the disaster: Substance activism after Bhopal. *Contemporary South Asia*, 21(3), 230–242.

Belize News 5. (2003). First dialysis centre opens in Belize. Retrieved from http://edition.channel5belize.com/archives/15509

Benton, A. (2015). *HIV exceptionalism: Development through disease in Sierra Leone*. Minneapolis, MN: University of Minnesota Press.

Biehl, J. (2016). *Patient-citizen-consumers: Claiming the right to health in Brazilian courts*. Cambridge, MA: MIT Global Health and Medical Humanities Colloquia. April 14, 2016.

Biehl, J., & Petryna, A. (Eds.). (2013). *When people come first: Critical studies in global health*. Princeton, NJ: Princeton University Press.

Blakeslee, S. (2009, February 12). Williem Kolff, doctor who invented kidney and heart machines, dies at 97. *New York Times*, online edition. Retrieved from www.nytimes.com.

Bolland, N. O. (1977). *The formation of colonial society: Belize, from conquest to crown colony*. Johns Hopkins Studies in Atlantic History and Culture. Baltimore, MD: The Johns Hopkins University Press.

Brown, E. 1996. Halfway technologies. *Physician Executive, 22*(12), 44–45.

Bukhman, G., Bavuma, C., Gishoma, C., Gupta, N., Kwan, G. F., Laing, R., & Beran, D. (2015). Endemic diabetes in the world's poorest people. *The Lancet. Diabetes & Endocrinology, 3*, 402–403.

Clegern, W. (1967). *British Honduras: Colonial dead end, 1859–1900*. Baton Rouge, LA: Louisiana University Press.

de-Graft Aikins, A., Addo, J., Ofei, F., Bosu, W., & Agyemang, C. (2012). Ghana's burden of chronic non-communicable diseases: Future directions in research, practice, and policy. *Ghana Medical Journal, 46*(2S), 1–3.

Feudtner, C. (2003). *Bittersweet: Diabetes, insulin, and the transformation of illness*. Chapel Hill, NC: University of North Carolina Press.

Fischer, M. M. J. (2003). *Emergent forms of life and the anthropological voice*. Durham, NC: Duke University Press.

Gayle, H., Mortis, N., Vasquez, J., Mossiah, R. J., Hewlett, M., & Amaya, A. (2010). *Report: Male social participation and violence in urban Belize*. Belize City: Belize Ministry of Education.

Grant, C. H. (1976). *The making of modern Belize: Politics, society and British colonialism in Central America*. New York, NY: Cambridge University Press.

Geertz, C. (2000). *Available light: Anthropological reflections on philosophical topics*. Princeton, NJ: Princeton University Press.

Gough, E., Emmanuel, E., Jenkins, V., Thompson, L., et al. (2011). *Survey of diabetes, hypertension, and chronic disease risk factors: CAMDI survey of Central America*. Washington, DC: PAHO/WHO. Retrieved from http://www.paho.org/hq/index.php?option = com_content&view = article&id = 6345%3A2012-camdi-survey-diabetes-hypertension-chronic-disease-risk-factors-centro-america-2012&catid = 4045%3Achronic-diseases-news&Itemid = 40276&lang = en

Hamdy, S. (2008). When the state and your kidneys fail: Political etiologies in an Egyptian dialysis ward. *American Ethnologist, 35*(4), 553–569.

Han, C. (2012). *Life in debt: Times of care and violence in neoliberal Chile*. Berkeley, CA: University of California Press.

Hatch, A. R. (2016). *Blood sugar: Racial pharmacology and food justice in Black America*. Minneapolis: University of Minnesota Press.

Hirschman, A. O. (1972). *Exit, voice, and loyalty*. Cambridge: Harvard University Press.

Hoover, E. (2017). *The river is in us: Fighting toxics in a Mohawk community*. Minnesota: University of Minnesota Press.

Huxley, A. (1934). *Beyond the Mexique Bay*. London: Chatto & Windus.

International Diabetes Federation (IDF). (2017). *Diabetes atlas* (8th ed.). Retrieved from https://diabetesatlas.org/resources/2017-atlas.html

Manderson, L., & Smith-Morris, C. (Eds.). (2010). *Chronic conditions, fluid states: Chronicity and the Anthropology of Illness*. New Brunswick, NJ: Rutgers University Press.

Mendenhall, E., & Norris, S. (2015). When HIV is ordinary and diabetes new: Remaking suffering in a South African Township. *Global Public Health, 10*(4), 449–462.

Mitaishvili, R. (2010). *Dialysis: Complete textbook of dialysis*. Los Angeles, CA: RM Global Health.

Mol, A. (2008). *The logic of care: Health and the problem of patient choice*. New York, NY: Routledge.

Montoya, M. (2013). Potential futures for a healthy city: Community, knowledge, and hope for the sciences of life. *Current Anthropology, 54*(S7), S45–S55.

Narres, M., Claessen, H., Droste, S., Kvitkina, T., Koch, M., Kuss, O, & Icks, A. (2016). The incidence of end-stage renal disease in the diabetic (compared to the non-diabetic) population: A systemic review. *PLoS One, 11*, e0147329. Retrieved from http://journals.plos.org/plosone/article?id = 10.1371/journal.pone.0147329

Nielson, J., Bahendeka, S. K., Bygbjerg, I. C., Meyrowitsch, D. W., & Whyte, S. R. (2017). Accessing diabetes care in rural Uganda: Economic and social resources. *Global Public Health, 12*(7), 892–908.

Nixon, R. (2012). *Slow violence and the environmentalism of the poor*. Cambridge, MA: Harvard University Press.

Pecoraro, R., Reiber, G., & Burgess, E. (1990). Pathways to diabetic limb amputation: Basis for prevention. *Diabetes Care, 13*(5), 513–521.

Ralph, L. (2012). What wounds enable: The politics of disability and violence in Chicago. *Disability Studies Quarterly, 32*(3). Retrieved from https://scholar.harvard.edu/lauralph/publications/what-wounds-enable-politics-disability-and-violence-chicago

Ramos, A. (2009). Dialysis patients, kidney association cry for help. *Amandala*, December 15.

Rettig, R. A. (2011). Special treatment—The story of Medicare's ESRD entitlement. *New England Journal of Medicine*, *364*, 596–598.

Roberts, E. (2017). What gets inside: Violent entanglements and toxic boundaries in Mexico City. *Cultural Anthropology*, 32(4), 592–619.

Rodriguez, R. (2007). Disappointment. In D. F. Wallace (Ed.), *Best American essays* (pp. 221–233). New York, NY: Mariner Books.

Russell, A., & Vinsel, L. (2018). After innovation, turn to naintenance. *Technology and Culture, 59*(1), 1–25.

Sanal, A. (2011). *New organs within us: Transplants and the moral economy.* Durham, NC: Duke University Press.

Scott, J. (1990). *Domination and arts of resistance: Hidden transcripts.* New Haven, CT: Yale University Press.

Schubert, C. (2019). Repair work as inquiry and improvisation. In I. Strebel, A. Bovet, & P. Sormani (Eds.), *Repair work ethnographies: Revisiting breakdown, relocating materiality.* London: Palgrave Macmillan.

Solomon, H. (2016). *Metabolic living: Food, fat, and the absorption of illness in India.* Durham, NC: Duke University Press.

Stone, M. (1994). *Caribbean nation, central American state: Ethnicity, race, and national formation in Belize, 1798–1990* (PhD diss.). University of Texas, Austin.

Wilk, R. (2006). *Home cooking in the global village.* Oxford and New York: Berg.

World Health Organization (WHO). (2016). *Global report on diabetes.* Geneva, Switzerland. Retrieved from http://apps.who.int/iris/bitstream/10665/204871/1/9789241565257_eng.pdf

Yates-Doerr, E. (2015). *The weight of obesity: Hunger and global health in postwar Guatemala.* Berkley, CA: University of California Press.

# Index

Milton Keynes UK
Ingram Content Group UK Ltd.
UKHW051853071024
449327UK00025B/1936

9 780367 498726